MENTAL HEALTH AND AGING WOMEN

MENTAL HEALTH AND AGING WOMEN

Important Correlates

Editors
Prof. Parul Dave
Prof. Pallavi Mehta

PUBLICATIONS
KALPAZ PUBLICATIONS
DELHI-110052

Mental Health and Aging Women : Important Correlates

Rs. 1190

ISBN: 81-7835-673-2

Published in 2008 in India by
Kalpaz Publications
C-30, Satyawati Nagar,
Delhi-110052
E-mail: kalpaz@hotmail.com
Phone : 9212729499

Printed at : Excel Prints, Naraina, New Delhi.

Contents

SECTION-III
SOCIAL REALITIES AND MENTAL HEALTH OF WOMEN

SECTION-IV
SOME ASPECTS OF PHYSICAL AND MENTAL HEALTH IN AGING WOMEN

Foreword

About thirty years ago, I met a distinguished British psychiatrist at a conference on mental health amongst immigrant women. He was working in a hospital in one of the multicultural cities of Britain, and treated male and female patients all nationalities, ages, and occupations. In his address he remarked that he found South Asian patients most difficult to deal with. His professional training did not include them or even a passing mention of them, and there was no reliable literature that he could read up to familiarise himself with them. He went on to say that South Asian patients invariably equated mental ill health with madness, felt deeply ashamed of it, and did not want to talk about it. They came to him most reluctantly, and only because their doctors had referred them to him. When he met them, they refused to talk about their problems. And when they did, they had no technical vocabulary to express themselves, and talked in vague and general terms. I asked him if I could sit in on one of his sessions involving Indian women. He agreed.

The session a few weeks later involved an Indian woman in her late forties. She talked about loss of appetite, fatigue, sleeplessness, and a general sense of unease and anomie. He diagnosed her as suffering from depression, and asked me for its equivalent in Hindi. I could not think of one, just as I could not think of Hindi or Gujarati equivalents of other terms such as schizophrenia and anxiety disorder. The only course of action open to me was to describe at some length the state of mind depression referred to, and to ask her if she suffered from it. This helped us up to a point, but not very much. My psychiatrist friend did not know what to do, and prescribed her some drugs and asked her to talk about her problems more freely with her family members and to go and see him whenever she wanted.

This experience and a few others like it raised a number of questions in my mind. Mental ill health is a real problem, among Indian men and women, as it is amongst other groups of people, but it is not taken seriously because it is stigmatised, associated with madness, and invites rejection, infantalisation and all kinds of social sanctions. It is difficult to deal with because patients have no vocabulary in which to articulate and express it. The paucity of literature on mental health in India adds to the difficulty. Unlike physical illness up to a point, Inental ill health is distinctly socio-cultural in its nature and origin, and hence not an1enable to the conceptual and diagnostic tools developed in the West. If we are to deal with it effectively, we need to understand the structures of social relations in which individual Indians live their lives as well as their deepest hopes, fears and forms of self-understanding. The limited research that has been done in India in the past is conceptually somewhat untidy, methodologically rather weak, and disconcertingly patchy. Things are no doubt beginning to improve, but we still have a long way to go.

In one of our discussions, I raised this matter with Professor Parul Dave. By serendipitous coincidence, she was already moving in that direction, and was thinking of undertaking a systematic study of the incidence and forms of mental ill health in Gujarat. She needed funds, and these were made available by Nirman Foundation of which my brother Dr. Chandrakant Shroff and I are president and vice-president respectively. Together with her colleagues and after consulting experts in the field, Professor Dave designed an interdisciplinary project. It was carried out in two phases. In the first phase it covered six cities in which over 17,000 records were assiduously collected from general hospitals and private practitioners. It showed that depression and schizophrenia were the most common mental health disorders, follow by anxiety and bipolar disorders. They were found to be particularly common among those between twenty and forty years of age, and varied with age. The research also showed that the quality of treatment remains poor, and largely consists in prescribing drugs or ECT. In the second phase Parol Dave's research involved in-depth intervieyvs with a small group of carefully selected women in the city of Baroda, with particular focus on their psycho-social characteristics and nutritional practices (investigated by Prof. Pallavi Mehta). As one would expect, these interviews show that while the traditional Indian family with its supportive but also claustrophobic and rigid structure guards its rmembers against certain forms of mental ill-health, it also generates and intensifies others. The increasing transformation of Indian society, brought about by industrialisation and social atornisation, complicates the situation and gives rise to new forms of mental ill health. It generates familial and intergenerational tensions, emotional disorientation, loneliness, isolation, and feelings of abandonment and insecurity. The fact that many women lack wider interest, have a limited circle of friends, and do not consume proper diet aggravates the situation and generates a vicious cycle.

This book includes the research findings of Professor Parul Dave and her colleagues as well as the scholarly papers they commissioned to discuss the issues raised by these findings. It rightly concentrates on mental health as it relates to aging women, a largely neglected area that is nevertheless of considerable growing importance. The book has both theoretical and practical dimensions, and should be a valuable reference for future researchers and practitioners At the practical level it shows what needs to be done and offers many valuable suggestions. At the theoretical level it opens up new areas of inquiry and represents a considerable intellectual achievenlent. It shows that if Indian scholars are to understand and address mental ill health, they cannot continue to mechanically reproduce Westen1 researches and practices. They need to ask new questions, develop an indigenous vocabulary, and explore new ways of defining, diagnosing and dealing with mental ill health. I congratulate the editors and the authors, and very much hope that their trail blazing book will inspire others of its kind, and over time lead to distinctly Indian theories of mental health.

Bhikhu Parekh FBA

University of Westminster and House of Lords.

Preface

It gives us immense pleasure to publish this book titled "Mental Health and Aging: Psychosocial and Physical Health Issues of Women".

The book is a result of the ideas generated from our earlier research project on "Mental Health and Aging: Focus on Women with Depression". A major part of this research was funded by Nirman Foundation, through the Women's Studies Research Centre (WSRC) of the Maharaja Sayajirao University of Baroda.

Our interest was initially on menopausal depression and the factors contributing to it, because depression, if left undiagnosed and untreated, could have a negative impact on women's health, both physical and mental, in the later years of their lives. Hence the need for a life-cycle approach to women's health.

However, the causes of depression in women are not just due to hormonal fluctuations, but are often a mix of biological (hormonal fluctuations throughout life span, malnutrition, and greater burden of reproductive health related problems) and psychosocial and cultural factors (among others: poverty, powerlessness, alienation, unequal work distribution and work overload, low self-esteem, stress of multiple social roles, low status in the family, experience of violence and abuse, experience of stressful life events). Hence the need also for a social-ecological approach to women's mental health.

Although depression is said to affect anyone regardless of their age, gender, race, or class, there is sufficient research evidence from around the world to show that women and older people have higher rates of depression. Our research on mental health of aging women in Gujarat, focusing on women with depression showed high prevalence of mental illnesses like depression and schizophrenia and an increasing prevalence of depression in women and in older persons. However, more men than women had availed of mental health services, indicating underutilization of health services as well as underreporting of illness by women. Besides lack of awareness about mental illnesses, it is the stigma attached to mental illness that keeps women from seeking psychiatric treatment even for common mental disorders.

The process of aging and all the biological and social outcomes related to this process - poor health, undernutrition, decreasing ability to function, loss of spouse and other significant relations, feelings of isolation, insecurity, economic dependency, declining status in the family, etc. - impact on the mental health of older persons. The process of aging also makes diagnosis of psychiatric disorders in older people difficult. For instance, depression, a common mental disorder in older people, is difficult to diagnose because it may be confused with the symptoms of other ailments commonly occurring in older people such as Parkinson's or Alzheimer's disease, dementia, thyroid disease, arthritis, etc.

Therefore we strongly felt the need for a cross-disciplinary understanding of mental health of women, that of aging women in particular.

As part of the research on "Mental Health and Aging: Focus on Women with Depression", a two-day National Seminar was organized in April 2005, on the theme Mental Health and Aging: A Gender Perspective. The aim was to share findings of research on the theme and discuss issues related to mental health and aging from various disciplinary perspectives. Experts from the fields of medicine, psychology, psychiatry, social work, human development and family studies, education, nutrition, geriatrics, etc., presented review and research papers on the theme, many of which have been compiled in this book.

This book is unique in that it presents cross cutting issues in the areas of aging, mental health and women's health. It is aimed at a broad audience, at both experts and lay persons, who may be students, psychologists, psychiatrists, social scientists, nutritionists, gerontologists, and professionals from allied fields. It is hoped that this book would not only serve as a reference but also help build a perspective to the problems of the elderly in India, their mental health and the problems of aging women in particular.

We hope that the reader will find the contents comprehensive, crisp and illustrative covering many areas affecting women's health. If this be so, our efforts are amply rewarded.

Parul Dave **Pallavi Mehta**

Acknowledgements

We gratefully acknowledge and thank the trustees of Nirman Foundation for the constant support and inspiration provided during the entire course of the Project, 'Mental Health and Aging: Focus on Women with Depression'.

We specially convey our profound thanks to Lord Bhikhu Parekh for his personal interest and interactions in funding pertinent issues and encouragement in publishing this book.

Many thanks to all the contributors for their informative material.

All our team members, Purnima Khanna, Bhavika Thakkar, Anna Marie Nainan, Tejal Vasavada, Bhavisha Doshi, Neha Shah, Priyanka Bishnoi, Yamini Venkatachalam and Rita Bhatt for their hard work and sincere involvement in completing the work.

We owe a special thanks to Yamini Venkatachalam and Purnima Khanna who have assisted in carefully editing and putting together this publication.

We are grateful to Dr. Prakash Desai for readily accepting our request to write the epilogue for this work and enriching it by giving future directions.

We also thank Kalpaz Publications for publishing our book.

Finally, we acknowledge with great respect the contribution of all the subjects of our project, who extended their unconditional cooperation and provided valuable information for our project.

Parul Dave
Pallavi Mehta

Introduction

The book is divided into eight sections on broad topics. The first section is a status paper on the elderly in India. Drawing heavily from Census data, the recent National Family Health Surveys and the National Sample Surveys, the paper discusses the socio-economic and health conditions of the current aged population of India. The paper highlights the greying of India, caused by the sharp fall in fertility during the last two to three decades, which has resulted in changes in the age structure of the population, with a sharp decline at the younger ages (0-14 years) and a corresponding increase in the proportion of population in the older ages. Given the current trends, the proportion of elderly persons is expected to increase by about two percent between 2001 and 2016, in absolute numbers, from about 71 million in 2001 to 113 million in 2016. Not only has the elderly population in the country): grown at a relatively faster rate than the general population, among the elderly population increase is greater for females than for males. The trends in sex-ratio and the projected age-sex structure show an increase in the number of elderly females. Like other developed countries, in India, elderly women are likely to outnumber men. The paper also highlights the economic-dependency of the elderly population, with as high as 70 per cent of the aged population being partially or fully dependent on others for the fulfillment of their livelihood and little over half having some financial assets and property. Widowhood is more among elderly women than men, increasing their dependency on others and their vulnerability.

Failing physical health adds further to their dependency. There is a high rate of chronic diseases among the elderly. Problem of the joints is one of the most severe health conditions. Prevalence of tuberculosis and asthma is high. Among disabilities reported are visual, auditory, locomotor and speech. Partial or complete loss of vision heads the list of disabilities among the elderly. Habits such as consumption of tobacco and *paan masala* as well as alcohol by both elderly men and women is likely to further compromise their health.

In the second chapter *Glimpses of the WSRC Project,* the WSRC project team describes the findings of their project on Mental Health and Aging. The project had a research as well as an intervention component. The study supports the WHO finding that depression is indeed very common, with as many as 42 per cent of women over 40 years of age who were surveyed having moderate depression. Analysis of hospital records of cases of mental disorders from six major cities of Gujarat show that depression and schizophrenia are the most prevalent mental disorders, followed by anxiety and bipolar disorders. Not only are there gender differences in the prevalence of these disorders but also in the utilization of mental health services, with more men than women availing of these services. The review of medical records also highlighted the problem of lack of detailed documentation of cases, particularly recording of precipitating factors for mental disorders, and the poor doctor-patient ratio, which in turn affects the quality of care. Utilization of mental health services in-depth interviews of women with moderate depression have identified psychosocial factors such as low status within the family, increased burden of responsibility, conflict in relationships, experience of loneliness, isolation, neglect and abuse as causes of stress and depression in women. The study has also found an association between factors such as satisfaction with the existing power structure within the family, feeling of isolation, experience of stressful life events and self-esteem, and the nutrient intake of women with depression. Also, nutrient intake of women was greatly reduced by depression. The intervention of providing Folic Acid supplementation to women with depression had beneficial effects on the severity of depression, nutritional status, dietary intake, and minor health complaints.

The third section of the book, *Aging Women and Mental Health: Issues and Concerns,* contains two papers. In the first paper, Archana Sinha, lays the ground for a gender perspective in aging and mental health.

The second paper by Dipti Oza is based on a study of 500 elderly women, who were administered a Standardized Adjustment Inventory and a semi-structured interview guide. The study identified the adjustment problems of elderly women, which were related to their health, financial condition, role at home and family. In addition to various health problems, financial dependency, and loss of decision making power and importance in the family, elderly women experienced loneliness, isolation, rejection, misery, loss of self-esteem and feeling of self-worth.

In section four, *Gender and Depression,* Tushar Agravat presents findings from a hospital based study of gender differences in depression. The study examined the gender differences in major depression in 50 men and 50 women with respect to their demographic characteristics, clinical manifestations of major depression, experience of stressful life events, and risk factors. The study did not find any difference in the severity of depression between male and female patients, but has found that factors such as lack of a confiding relationship, substance abuse and unemployment of the spouse (husband), parental separation during childhood, housing problems, problems with in-laws, are associated with depression in women more than in men.

Aruna Khasgiwala's community-based study of *Depression in Middle aged Women,* covering 50 Muslim women, aged 45-50 years, found over half of the women to have moderate depression on the 21-point Beck's Depression Inventory. The study has found stressful life events such as financial crisis, economic and social insecurity of children and continued dependence of children, adjustment problems with children, childlessness, death and loss of important family members causing depression in women.

The papers presented in the section, *Social Realities and Mental Health of Women,* have explored the factors that are said to negatively impact mental health of women such as loss of spouse or widowhood, experience of domestic violence, out migration of children (the 'empty nest' syndrome). Geeta Challa and K. Mayuri describe the findings of their study of *Determinants of Stress in Older Women.* The study found most of the elderly women participants to be experiencing medium to low level of stress. In these women, stress was exhibited mostly by physiological and psychological symptoms and very rarely by behavioral symptoms. The study also found that that age, religion, income, health status, family type, type of house, self esteem and resources availability affect the symptomatic stress among elderly women.

The papers *Traumatic Widowhood and Major Depression: A study of Widows affected by Communal Violence* and *Mental Illness: A Risk Factor for Domestic Violence in Women?* are both hospital-based studies conducted among women patients seeking psychiatric treatment. Both studies are unique and pioneering works, as very few studies in India have explored or established traumatic bereavement and experience of violence as causes of major depressive disorders.

Indira Mallya and Parul Dave's paper *Is there a Light at the End of the Tunnel?* is a review of life events through oral histories of six widows whose children have out-migrated to other countries. The widowed women give an account of major events during their life course that included births, marriages, deaths, major trauma and life satisfactions. They also express feelings about life events and the future, and, their concept of old age.

The papers presented in the sixth section, *Some Aspects of Physical and Mental Health in Aging Women,* cover a range of problems related to physical and mental health of elderly persons, and women in particular. The papers on Oral Care for Elderly People and Common Medical Problems of the Elderly, have been contributed by medical practitioners, giving an overview of various problems specific to elderly women, treatment options, and tips for prevention. The paper by Gayatree Jadeja and S. Rema, *Osteoporosis in Aging Women* is a study of the prevalence of osteoporosis among adult and elderly women in a community of Gujarat. Using anthropometric measurement and radiographic techniques, the authors found decrease in bone mineral density beyond the age of 45 years and a high prevalence of low bone mass in the aging women of the community under study.

The paper *Physical and Mental Status of Geriatric Women of a District of Gujarat,* is a community-based, house-to-house survey of rural and urban women age 60 years and above. The study found that elderly women had more chronic morbidity and disability than other age groups. The level of depression was also higher among these women. Given the difference in the pattern of morbidity and depression in urban and rural areas, the authors recommend that the problems of elderly women be addressed through a multi-pronged approach - through medical, economic, social and mental health interventions.

Jayashree Mehta, surgeon, in her paper, discusses the psychological and social aspects of breast cancer and dealing with breast cancer.

Anand Khorana, psychiatrist, in his paper *Depression and Comorbid Anxiety in Older People: Diagnosis and Treatment Options,* highlights the difficulty in recognizing depression in older people, as overt sadness is often absent and many of the symptoms characteristic of depression overlap with those associated with the ageing process and with the range of physical illnesses often found in elderly persons. It is necessary, though sometimes difficult, to make a distinction between depression and dementia to decide on appropriate management. Cognitive behavior therapy is recommended as a psychological treatment option.

Two papers in this section discuss the role of nutrition in mental health. One by N. Somashekara, C. N. Ramchand and Sandeep Shah, review existing evidence on the role of nutrition mental disorders, and using nutrigenomics, a whole new area of research to address depressive disorders through nutrition intervention. The study by Pallavi Mehta, Komal Chauhan and Swati Khurana, assess the effect of Iron and Folic Acid Supplementation on the physical and mental performance of elderly, anemic women. The supplementation for a period of six weeks was found to be effective in improving their hemoglobin levels, which in turn reflected on their physical performance and mental functioning.

The seventh section, *Intervention Strategies,* contains five papers. Three papers discuss alternative therapies in mental health. These papers mark an attempt to go beyond allopathy and psychiatry to explore alternative healing techniques and therapies. In his paper, *Panch-Kosha Purification in Mental Health Management,* the author, B. M. Palan, describes the relation between stress and aging and cellular aging, and the application of the concept of "Panch-Kosha" or five sheaths and their purification, in stress management. The purification of each of these five sheaths by the use of several techniques suggested in the system of eight fold Yoga (Ashtang Yoga) and remaining aware about certain spiritual concepts can help one break the cycle of stress and aging and reduce the rate of aging.

In their paper, *Brahmi: An alternative therapy for Depression in Elderly Women,* Pallavi Mehta, Tejal Vasavda, Arpita Shah, and Komal Chauhan discuss the use of the Ayurvedic herb Brahmi (bacopa monniera), as an alternative therapy in the treatment of depression. The paper is based on a study of the impact of Brahmi supplementation on elderly women with depression. After being provided a supplementation of Brahmi for a period of six weeks, these women showed an improvement in the severity of depression, cognitive function, food and nutrient intake, blood pressure and number of health complaints.

Monali Desai, a medical practitioner, gives useful pointers to dealing with depression during menopause. Her paper, *Dealing with Depression During Menopause: Recommendations from Praxis,* advocates life style modification as the most important option to treat depression during menopause. A positive attitude may be cultivated by channelizing one's energies and attention to being creative, sharing one's experience and wisdom with the younger generation developing a positive attitude towards one's sexuality, learning to deal with children leaving home. High fiber, low fat, high calcium and food rich in soya isoflavones can help counter menopausal depression. Yoga, cardiovascular exercises can help keep one physically and mentally fit. Medical practitioners and physicians treating women must emphasize positive attitude, diet alterations and physical fitness to help them deal with menopause and depression.

The last part of the book, is an annotated bibliography of over 50 relevant literature on Aging, Gender and Mental Health available at the Women's Studies Research Centre, M. S. University Baroda. The literature has been collected from various sources like journals, edited books, essays, internet publications, newspapers, covering a wide range of topics such as gender differentials in the prevalence of mental disorders, psycho-social, economic and adjustment problems of the elderly, geriatric depression, geriatric psychiatry, health concerm of elderly women, diet pattern and diseases of elderly, postmenopausal women, reviews of the mental health practices, policies and programs, alternative treatment options to psychotherapy.

List of Contributors

1. ***Dr. Agravat Tushar***, Consultant Psychiatrist, E-1, Psychiatry Ward New Civil Hospital and B.J. Medical College, Asawara, Ahmedabad 380016,

2. ***Dr. Challa Geeta***, Dept. of Human Development and Family Studies, College of Home Science, Hyderabad.

3. ***Dr. Chauhan, Biren Roy***, MD Medicine, Consultant, Sarveshwar Hospital, Opp. Navjivan Post Office, Ajwa Road, V adodara- 390019.

4. ***Ms. Chauhan Koma*l**, Sr. Lecturer, Dept. of Foods and Nutrition, Faculty of Family and Community Sciences. The M.S. University of Baroda, Vadodara- 390002.

5. ***Prof. Das N.P.***, Director, Population Research Centre, Faculty of Science, The M.S. University of Baroda, Vadodara- 390002.

6. ***Prof. Dave Parul***, Former Director, WSRC 2, Vrundavan Society, Elora Park, Vadodara-390007.

7. ***Dr. Desai Monali***, Consultant Gynaecologist, Bhailal Amin General Hospital, Vadodara.

8. ***Dr. Jadeja Gayatree***, Post Graduate Dept. of Home Science, S.P. University, Vallabh Vidyanagar.

9. ***Ms. Khanna Punima*** Program Officer, Women's Studies Research Centre (WSRC), The M.S. University of Baroda, Vadodara- 390002.

10. ***Prof. Aruna***, Khasgiwala Dean Faculty of Social Work, The M.S. University of Baroda, Vadodara- 390002.

11. ***Dr. Khurana Anand***, Consultant Psychiatrist, 103, Race Cource Medical Centre, Race Cource Towers, Vadodara-390007.

12. ***Ms. Khurana Swati***, Dept. of Foods and Nutrition, Faculty of Family and Community Sciences, The M.S. University of Baroda, Vadodara- 390002.

13. ***Dr. Mallya Indira***, Reader, Dept. of Human Development and Family Studies, Faculty of Family and Community Sciences, The M.S. University of Baroda Vadodara- 390002.

14. ***Dr. Mehta Jayshree***, Vice Chancellor, Sumandeep Vidyapeeth University, Waghodia, Baroda, Avsar 404, (Residence) 2 Pratapgunj Vadodara.

15. ***Dr. Mehta Khyatia*** Dept. of Psychiatry B.J. Medical College and Civil Hospital, Ahmedabad-380016.

16. ***Prof. Pallavi Mehta***, Head, Dept. of Foods and Nutrition, Faculty of Family and Community Sciences, M.S. University of Baroda Vadodara-390002.

17. ***Dr. Oza Dipti***, Reader, Dept. of Education, Faculty of Education and Psychology, The M.S. University of Baroda, Vadodara-390002,

18. ***Dr. Palan B.M.*** M.D. Dip. Clin. Hypno. B.M. (USA) 12, Gulmohar Park, Opp. Akota Garden, Vadodara- 390020.

19. ***Dr. Pandit Niraj,*** Asstt. Professor, Dept. of Community Medicine, P.S. Medical College, Karamsad, Gujarat.

20. ***Dr. Parekh Amit***, Consulting Dentist, Ramway Plaza, Dandia Bazaar, Vadodara.

21.. ***Dr.Ramchand C.N.*** K -104, 16th street. Annanagar east, Chennai C.N. - 600102.

22. ***Dr. Saiyad M.S.*** Dept. of Psychiatry B.J. Medical College and Civil Hospital, Ahmedabad-380016.

23. ***Ms. Shah Arpita*** Dept. of Foods and Nutrition, Faculty of family and Community Sciences, The M.S. University of Vadaodara-390002.

24. ***Dr Shah Sandeep*** Consultant Psychiatrist, Brij Clinic, Opp. Nimbalkar Chambers, Jambubet, Dandia Bazaar, Vadodara.

25. ***Dr. Shah Urvi***, Population Research Centre, Faculty of Science, The M.S. University of Baroda Vadodara- 390002.

26. ***Dr. Sinha Archana***, Senior Programme Officer, Rural Development Unit, Dept. of Research, Indian Social Institute, New Delhi.

27. ***Dr. S. Rema Hon***. Director, WSRC, Post Graduate Dept. of Home Science, S.P. University, Vallabh Vidyanagar.

28. ***Dr. Vankar O.K*** Head, Dept. of Psychiatry New Civil Hospital, Asarwa, Ahmedab-380016

29. ***Ms.Vasavada T ej al*** Clini Research Asdate min Pharma, 01-Blue Bell Complex,Opp PNB bank,Atmajyoti Asram Road, Ellora Park, V adodara-l

1

The Socio-Demographic and Health Status of the Elderly in India: Evidence from Recent National Level Data

Narayan P. Das and Urvi Shah

The study of ageing in developing countries like India has its roots in the growing concern over the perceived increase in dependency on the state of large numbers of elderly persons who are likely to impose a rising burden in terms of social security, pension, health and other services, on a relatively diminishing working population. The United Nations World Assembly on Ageing. held at Vienna in 1982, formulated a package of recommendations which gives high priority to research related to developmental and humanitarian aspects of ageing (United Nations, 1987). The plan of action specifically recommended, "International exchange and research cooperation as well as data collection should be promoted in all the fields having a bearing on ageing, in order to provide a rational basis for future social policies and action. Special emphasis should be placed on comparative and cross-cultural studies in ageing". Very few studies, however, exist that focus on the social, economic and health aspects about ageing in India, as it has not yet become an issue for serious consideration in India. This might be due to a preoccupation with the severe problems of a huge child and youth population or perhaps because social security for the elderly is still maintained under the traditional family system. But with the spread of education, industrialization and social mobility, population ageing is likely to pose problems for elderly care in India in the near future.

It is therefore in the recent years that the policy makers and administrators at central and state governments, and voluntary organizations have begun to plan for these anticipated changes and consider alternatives for the care of the elderly population. In fact, this concern is reflected in the adoption of a National Policy on Older persons by the Ministry of Social Justice and Empowerment in 1999 and is also echoed in the National Population Policy 2000, which articulates the need for providing for the country's elderly population through sensitization and training of health staff and equipping rural and urban health centers and hospitals to provide appropriate health care services, such as screening for cancer, osteoporosis and cardio-vascular conditions. It is therefore important to have these concerns translated into viable programmes and services by developing a complete health and welfare package for the elderly at the grassroots level. To develop such a complete welfare package for the elderly population, there is a need for a study of elderly persons on various aspects and initiate social, economic and health policy debate about ageing in India. To this end, a serious effort, based on census data was made by the Office of the Registrar General and Census Commissioner, India to study the socio-economic and demographic characteristics of the aged in India (Sharma and Xenos, 1992). The census data however have very limited scope to examine the various aspects of the elderly population in detail and do not provide data on standard of living, housing condition, social status, family support and most importantly of their health condition. Apart from small surveys and studies, the recently concluded two rounds of the National Family Health Surveys (I and II) conducted during 1992-93 and 1998-99 provide an opportunity to review the socio-economic and health condition of the elderly persons at the national and state level in India. Yet another major source of information is data from the two rounds of the National Sample Survey (NSS). The National Sample Survey Organisation (NSSO) for the first time, conducted a survey on the elderly (persons of age 60 years and above), along with the survey on social consumption in it's 42nd round (July 1986 – June 1987), to assess the nature and dimensions of the socio-economic problems of the aged. After a time lag of 9 years, the NSSO repeated the survey on social consumption in its 52nd round (July 1995 – June 1996). Among the information on the socio-economic condition of the aged, data on some chronic diseases and physical disabilities were also collected during these two rounds of the NSS. The details of the methodology, procedure and results can be obtained from the respective reports (Government of India, 1991; 1998). The main objective of this study is therefore to focus on the socio-economic and health conditions of the current aged population, and the emerging policy issues for elderly care in India in the coming years. Before addressing such issues it is imperative to look at the demography of ageing, that is, the changing age structure of the population and the emerging demographic characteristics of the aged population in India.

Demography of Ageing

This section is therefore basically concerned with the change in absolute number and proportionate size, growth and composition of the elderly population in India since 1901, to understand the economic implications of emerging population structure and change and to look at the gender differences in longevity and other demographic parameters which have resulted due to a changing age structure of the population.

Before going any further in the discussion of the dynamic process of population ageing and the demographic characteristics of the aged population, it is necessary to understand the concept and measures used to define population ageing. Population can become older or younger depending on the changes in the proportion of people in different age groups. The age of a population is normally measured in one of three ways: by the proportion of elderly persons in the population, generally taken in India as those of ages 60 and over for both men and women (considering the socio-economic situation and pension ages in India); by the proportion of children in the population, usually taken as those under age 15; and by the median age of the population. Throughout the present study unless stated otherwise, references to the 'aged' or 'elderly' relate to persons aged 60 years and over.

By any of the measures discussed above, India can now be said to have an aged population. Throughout the twentieth century the proportion of population aged 60 or over has increased in all the countries of the world. This trend started earlier in the industrialized countries but developing countries are also experiencing the same changes in population structure. It was estimated that about two-thirds of the world's estimated 600 million people aged 60 or over were living in Third World countries during the year 2000 and in the first twenty years of the twenty-first century the number of people aged 60 and over throughout the world is expected to increase from some 600 million to over 1000 million (Bond and Coleman, 1993). The increase in the elderly population will be most marked in Asia, particularly China and India, which could essentially be attributed to the large base of the population in these countries.

The changes in the age structure which occurred in the developed countries, leading to the ageing of the population, are primarily because of the long term downward trend in the birth rates in these economically advanced countries. Secondly, there is substantial improvement in life expectancy throughout the world. This is particularly due to a reduction in child mortality which reflects improvement in public health and medical advances in the prevention of many fatal infectious diseases in childhood. Since the mortality level of the developed countries was already low and the expectation of life at birth was very high, further improvement in mortality condition in these countries affected the older age groups and led to a further ageing of the population. On the other hand, the age structure of the developing countries has remained virtually unchanged because their birth rates have remained more or less at high levels, though their death rates have been declining since the 1950s. These developing countries have also started experiencing the fall in their birth rates since the last two to three decades. The relatively faster decline in birth rates than in the death rates in the developing countries like India is however a recent phenomenon. The review of trend in fertility and mortality, based on census estimates for the early period (1901 – 1971) and SRS and NFHS estimates for the latter period reveals that in India the crude death rate (CDR) had started declining as early as the 1920s but a sharp fall was seen after 1951 when a CDR of 22.8 was recorded during

Table 1: Percent Distribution of Population by Broad Age Groups, India, 1951-2021

Year	*Age Groups*			
	0-14	*15-59*	*60+*	*Total*
1951	38.4	56.1	5.5	100.0
1961	41.1	53.3	5.6	100.0
1971	42.0	52.0	6.0	100.0
1981	39.7	53.9	6.4	100.0
1991	37.6	55.7	6.7	100.0
2001	35.4	57.1	7.5	100.0
2011*	28.8	63.1	8.1	100.0
2021*	25.8	64.0	10.2	100.0

* Projected figures

Sources: (1) Census data for the period 1951-81 are taken from Occasional Paper No.2 of 1992 – Ageing in India: Demographic Background and Analysis Based on Census Materials, Office of the Registrar General and Census Commissioner, India, New Delhi.

(2) Census data for the year 1991 and 2001 are taken from the data file of Census of India, 1991 and 2001 respectively, Office of the Registrar General and Census Commissioner, India, New Delhi.

(3) Projected population for the period 2001-2016 have been taken from Dyson, 2002.

1951-61. Since then it has fallen further and reached a level of 15.0 during 1971-81, which again dropped to 11.4 during 1981-91. The downward trend in the CDR continued during 1991-2001 and although a bit slow, it was noted to be below 10 during 1996-2001. As a result of the decline in mortality at all ages, the expectation of life at birth (e^{o}) had increased substantially during the last century. As a result of the decline in fertility, the ageing of the population has been evident in these countries during the latter part of the twentieth century.

The crude birth rate (CBR) for India was about 49.2 during 1901-11, which came down to 41.2 during 1961-71. Thereafter, there has been a continuous fall in the crude birth rate. A CBR of 37.2 recorded during 1971-81, fell to 32.5 during 1981-91, which further dropped to 29.1 during 1991-96 and it was about 25-27 during 1996-2001. It is expected to fall further in the future as per the estimates of the Expert Committee on Population Projections (Government of India, 1996), and is likely to be about 22.8 during 2001-2006 and 21.4 during 2011-2016.

The sharp fall in fertility during the last two to three decades has been reflected in the changing age structure of the population in India. It can be seen from Table 1 that the proportion of the population in the younger age groups (0-14 years) has dropped sharply after 1971, and accordingly the proportion of population in the 15-59 and 60+ age groups has shown a tendency to increase. The proportion of population in the 0-14 age group, which was 42 percent in 1971, dropped to about 35 percent in 2001 and is expected to reduce further to 26 percent by 2021, while the proportion of elderly population (60+) which was about 6 percent during 1971 and 7.5 percent during 2001, is expected to increase to about 10 percent by 2021. In other words, the process of ageing of population has already begun in India. The size and growth of the elderly population is discussed in the next section.

Size and growth of elderly population

In India, as a result of the change in the age composition of the population over time, there has been a progressive increase in both the number and proportion of aged people. As can be seen from Table 2, the proportion of the population that is aged 60 or

Table 2: Number and Proportion of Older People in India, 1901-2021

Census year	*Population age 60 or over*					
	Number (millions)			*Proportion to total population (percent)*		
	Men	*Women*	*Total*	*Men*	*Women*	*Total*
1901	5.50	6.56	12.06	4.55	5.59	5.06
1911	6.18	6.99	13.17	4.81	5.65	5.22
1921	6.48	7.00	13.48	5.04	5.70	5.37
1931	6.94	7.27	14.21	4.86	5.35	5.09
1941	8.89	9.15	18.04	5.43	5.91	5.66
1951	9.67	9.94	19.61	5.21	5.66	5.43
1961	12.36	12.35	24.71	5.46	5.80	5.63
1971	16.87	15.83	32.70	5.94	5.99	5.97
1981	22.49	21.49	43.98	6.35	6.50	6.42
1991	29.28	27.17	56.45	6.67	6.67	6.67
2001	37.77	38.85	76.62	7.12	7.85	7.47
2011*	-	-	97.52	-	-	8.10
2021*	-	-	138.93	-	-	10.20

* Projected figures

Sources:

(1) Population figures from 1901 to 1981 have been taken from Occasional Paper No.2 of 1992 – Ageing in India: Demographic Background and Analysis Based on Census Materials, Office of the Registrar General and Census Commissioner, India, 1992, pp.94-97.

(2) Population figures for 1991 have been taken from Census of India, 1991 data file as well as from Paper 2 of 1992 – Final Population Totals, Office of the Registrar General and Census Commissioner, India, New Delhi, 1992.

(3) Projected population figures for the period 2006-2016 have been taken from Dyson 2002.

Table 3: Percent increase in the general population and the population aged 60 years and over by sex, India 1901

Period	*% Decadal variation of general population*			*% Decadal variation of population aged 60 & over*		
	Males	*Females*	*Total*	*Males*	*Females*	*Total*
1901-11	+6.29	+5.41	+5.75	+12.4	+6.6	+9.2
1911-21	+0.13	-0.75	-0.31	+4.9	+0.2	+2.4
1921-31	+11.19	+10.60	+11.00	+7.1	+3.7	+5.4
1931-41	+14.52	+13.92	+14.22	+28.0	+25.9	+27.0
1941-51	+13.34	+13.49	+13.31	+8.8	+8.7	+8.7
1951-61	+21.97	+21.29	+21.64	+27.8	+24.3	+26.0
1961-71	+25.52	+24.03	+24.80	+36.6	+28.0	+32.2
1971-81	+24.77	+25.25	+25.00	+33.3	+35.8	+34.5
1981-91	+24.31	23.35	23.85	+30.2	+26.4	+28.4
1991-01	21.23	21.87	21.54	+22.5	+30.1	+26.3
2001-11*	-	-	17.28	-	-	27.23
2011–21*	-	-	13.10	-	-	42.46

* Projected figures

Source: (1) Govt. of India, 1998. Family Welfare Programme in India, Year Book, 1996-97, Ministry of Health and Family Welfare, Dept. of Family Welfare, Govt. of India, New Delhi.

(2) Computed from data file of Census of India 1991 & 2001, Office of the Registrar General, India, New Delhi.

(3) Projected population figures for the period 2006-2016 have been taken from Dyson, 2002.

over has been increasing consistently over the last century, particularly after 1951. In 1901 the proportion of the population aged 60 or over in India was about 5 percent, which marginally increased to 5.4 percent in 1951, and by 2001 this share was found to have risen to about 7.5 percent. Table 2 also shows the absolute growth in elderly population over time. The size of the elderly population has risen in absolute terms by more than five times during the last century; from 12.1 million in 1901 to approximately 76.6 million in 2001. According to recent population projections, the number of elderly persons will rise to about 97.5 million in 2011, and further to approximately 138.9 million in 2021 (Table 2). In other words, the proportion of elderly persons (i.e. aged 60 or over) in the population of India is expected to rise from less than 8 percent in 2011 to approximately 10 percent by 2021.

The decadal growth rate of India's elderly population and of the general population, for the period 1901 to 2021, shown in Table 3, reveals once again that the aged population in India has grown very steadily since 1951 and is likely to grow relatively faster from 2001. A decadal growth rate of 26 percent, recorded for the elderly population during 1951-61, increased to 35 percent during the 1971-81 decade, though there was a decline in the decadal growth rate during 1981-2001. According to population projections, this rate is likely to increase further to approximately 42 percent during 2011-2021. When the changes in the decadal growth rate in the general population are compared with those for the elderly population, it is found that the elderly population has grown at a relatively much faster rate than the general population, particularly since 1951. It is further observed that the decadal percent increase in the elderly population for the period 2001-2011 is likely to be more than three times the rate of increase of the general population. The decadal growth rate of the elderly population by sex, also shown in Table 3, reveals that the increase is greater for elderly females since 1991 and such an increase is also expected to be greater after 2001.

The trend in the sex ratio of elderly population

The progressive increase in the proportion of females to males in the elderly population is also evident in the trend in the sex ratio of elderly population aged 60 years or over. Table 4 shows the sex ratios (females per 1000 males) of elderly population and of general population from 1901 to 2021. It is evident from this table that the proportion of females in the elderly population is increasing,

Table 4: Sex ratio (females per 1000 Males) of elderly population and general population, India, 1901-2021

Year	*Sex ratio (Females per 1000 males)*	
	Elderly population (Age 60+)	*General population (All ages)*
1901	1193	972
1911	1131	964
1921	1080	955
1931	1048	950
1941	1029	945
1951	1028	946
1961	999	941
1971	938	930
1981	956	934
1991	928	927
2001	1029	933
2011*	-	939
2021*	-	947

Source:

(1) The data for the period 1901 to 1951 have been taken from Occasional Paper No.2 of 1992 – Ageing in India: Demographic Background and Analysis Based on Census Materials. Office of the Registrar General & Census Commissioner, India, New Delhi, 1992.

(2) The data for the period 1961-81 have been taken from the Social and Cultural Tables of respective census reports (a) Census of India, 1961, Series 1, Part II-C, 1964, (b) Census of India, 1971, Series 1, Part II-C(ii), 1977, (c) Census of India, 1981, Series 1, Part IVA, 1987; Controller of Publications, Govt. of India, New Delhi.

(3) The data for 1991 have been obtained from data file of Census of India, 1991.

(4) Projected population for the period 2006-2016 have been taken from Dyson, 2002.

particularly since 1991. The sex ratio among elderly people was about 928 in 1991 which increased to about 1029 in 2001 and is expected to increase further. The projected age-sex structure of the population indicates that gender differentials among those aged over 60 are expected to decline with time and like the pattern in the developed countries, women may outnumber men especially at the older ages. The excess of females over males is not a new phenomenon. From Table 4, it can be seen that in 1901 there were 1193 women aged 60 or over for every 1000 men of the same age.

Like the pattern in the general population, this ratio of females to males in the elderly population declined consistently until 1991, although the outnumbering of women to men in the elderly population continued until 1951. Table 4 further reveals a relatively higher ratio of females to males in the elderly population than in the general population which is evident for all the years since 1901, indicating once again the preponderance of women in the elderly population.

Sex differentials in mortality

This progressive advantage in favour of women in the elderly population is primarily due to the increasingly lower mortality rates of women at middle to late ages compared with men, as evident from the recent two rounds of NFHS data (IIPS, 1995; IIPS and ORC-Macro 2000). The fall in overall mortality has been accompanied by differential changes in sex-specific mortality rates. As can be seen from Table 5, between 1946 and 1991 the life expectancy of a man aged 60 increased by 4.8 years from 10.1 years to 14.9 years, whereas for a woman of the same age the increase was nearly 5 years, from 11.3 years to 16.2 years. As regards the fall in overall mortality, the expectation of life at birth during the same period increased by about 28 years from 31.7 years to 59.7 years for females, while the corresponding increase was 26.5 years from 32.5 years to 59.0 years for males.

An important feature of population ageing is therefore the greater longevity of women than men, a differential that has increased during the latter half of the twentieth century. The female/ male discrepancy in life expectancy increased during 1996-2001 and is expected to continue (Table 5). The reason for this differential

Table 5: Expectation of life at different ages by sex, India, 1941-2021

Period	*Mid-year*	*Expectation of life at*			
		Birth		*Age 60*	
		Males	*Females*	*Males*	*Females*
1941-50	1946	32.5	31.7	10.1	11.3
1951-60	1956	41.8	40.6	11.8	13.0
1970-75	1973	50.5	49.0	13.4	14.3
1976-80	1978	52.5	52.1	14.1	15.9
1981-85	1983	55.4	55.7	14.6	16.4
1987-91	1989	58.1	58.6	14.8	16.2
1989-93	1991	59.0	59.7	14.9	16.2
1996-2001	1998	61.5	63.1	-	-
2001-2006*	2003	63.2	64.8	-	-
2006-2011*	2008	64.6	66.8	-	-
2011-2016*	2013	66.1	68.7	-	-
2016-2021*	2018	66.9	69.7	-	-

* Projected figures - Not available

Source: (1) Census Life Tables

(2) SRS Based Life Tables, Occasional Paper 1 of 1 of 1989. Office of the Registrar General, India, New Delhi, 1990.

(3) SRS Based Life Tables, Occasional Paper

(4) Projected population for the period 2006-2016 have been taken from Dyson, 2002.

decline is not yet very clear, particularly in view of the fact that status of women is very low which is reflected in the neglect of their health and well-being at all ages in the developing countries like India. However, the improvement in life expectancy is particularly due to a reduction in child mortality, which reflects improvements in public health and medical advances in the prevention of many fatal infectious diseases in childhood. Increases in the life expectancy of older people reflect improvement in the quality of life in the latter part of the twentieth century and to a limited extent some of the achievements of medical science, although we are not yet successful in combating some of the illnesses that are major causes of death among the elderly such as heart attacks, lung cancer, stroke and circulatory diseases. These are major causes of death for both men and women at older ages, but they do not become as important for women until later in the age curve. Thus these factors differentially affect the sexes within the same age cohort and contribute to the increasing longevity of women to men. The morbidity condition, life style and health status of elderly men and women are discussed later in a separate section.

Dependency ratios

The total dependency ratio is often used as an indicator of the economic potential, the principal argument being that a low dependency implies more workers and the need to divert fewer resources to dependent populations. It has also been argued that the shift in the age composition of the population (in favour of ageing of population) is likely to damage the economy. As older people consume a higher proportion of the national budget for health, social services and social security, these become somewhat self-evident aspects, particularly in the developed countries. For example, for the USA it is estimated that per capita costs for elderly persons are approximately three times those incurred by youth. Comparable figures for the developing world indicate that the costs of elderly people are 1.5 times higher than for young people (Johnson, 1993).

To understand the economic implications of the changing population structure, we will look briefly at the trend in the dependency ratio over time. However, it may be noted that dependency ratio is not a completely accurate measure for assessing

Table 6: Dependency Ratios and Index of Ageing, India, 1951-2021

Year	Dependency ratio			Index of Ageing[4]
	Young (child)[1]	*Gerontic (old age)*[2]	*Total*[3]	
1951	68.5	9.8	78.3	14.3
1961	77.0	10.6	87.6	13.7
1971	80.8	11.5	92.3	14.2
1981	73.6	11.9	85.5	16.2
1991	68.0	12.0	80.0	17.7
2001	62.1	13.1	75.2	21.1
2011*	45.6	12.8	58.4	28.1
2021*	40.1	15.9	56.0	39.7

[1] Number of persons age 0-14 per 100 persons age 15-59 (a)

[2] Number of persons age 60 and above per 100 persons age 15-59 (b)

[3] Number of persons age 0-14 and 60 and above per 100 persons age 15-59 (a+b)

[4] Number of persons age 60 and above per 100 persons age 0-14

* Projected figures

Sources: (1) The data for 1951 have been taken from Occasional Paper No.2 of 1992 – Ageing in India: Demographic Background and Analysis Based on Census Materials, Office of the Registrar General and Census Commissioner, India, 1992, pp.94-97.

(2) Population figures for 1991 have been taken from Census of India, 1991 data file as well as from Paper 2 of 1992 – Final Population Totals, Office of the Registrar General and Census Commissioner, India, New Delhi, 1992.

(3) Projected population for the period 2006-2016 have been taken from Dyson, 2002.

the dependency burden, as not all persons in the working age group are employed; or all those in the dependent age economically dependent. This measure, nevertheless, gives us a broad idea of the economic dependency in any population. As can be seen from Table 6, the geriatric (old age) ratio (number of people aged 60 and over, divided by the population of working age, aged 15-59) had increased during the latter half of the last century from almost 10 old people per 100 in the working ages in 1951 to 13 in 2001 and this figure is expected to increase to about 16 by 2021. During the same period the young (child) dependency ratio (number of young people aged 0-14, divided by the population of working age, aged 15-59) had initially increased from about 69 in 1951 to 81 in 1971, mainly as a result of the decline in mortality and subsequently fallen to 62 in 2001. Projections indicate that it is expected to fall further to 40 by 2021. Thus, the total dependency burden is likely to fall as a result of the decline in young dependency, although there is a need to divert more resources to old dependent populations in view of the rising geriatric ratio and relatively higher costs of supporting elderly people.

The study of the dependency ratios over time helps not only to examine the nature and extent of dependency but also the changing age structure including ageing of population. The geriatric ratio will inevitably rise as the population ages. In fact, these data are sometimes used to compute a composite index, viz. the index of ageing. It is defined as the number of elderly persons to the number of children in a population and is a useful measure of the ageing process, as it is very sensitive to changes in the age structure of the population. The computed ratios for the period 1951-2021 are also shown in Table 6. The ageing of the Indian population is succinctly illustrated by the fact that there were nearly 14 elderly persons for every 100 children in 1951, and this ratio has been rising continuously and is expected to reach 40 by 2021.

Socio-Economic Status of Elderly Population

This section examines the current scenario of the elderly population with respect to their age-sex composition, marital status, household composition, rural-urban residential patterns, religious and caste composition, other social and economic conditions including occupational pattern and standard of living and lifestyle pattern.

Table 7: Percent distribution of elderly population (aged 60+) by their age and sex, India, 1961-2001

Year	*Age Groups*						*Total (Aged 60+)*	
	60-64		*65-69*		*70+*			
	Male	*Female*	*Male*	*Female*	*Male*	*Female*	*Male*	*Female*
1961	46.2	44.8	20.0	19.2	33.8	36.0	100.0	100.0
1971	44.3	43.6	21.6	21.2	34.1	35.3	100.0	100.0
1981	42.6	41.5	21.9	22.4	35.5	36.1	100.0	100.0
1991	39.7	39.7	22.1	23.5	38.2	36.8	100.0	100.0
1998-99 (NFHS-2)	35.8	38.5	24.7	25.6	39.5	35.9	100.0	100.0
2001	36.0	35.9	25.1	26.6	38.9	37.5	100.0	100.0

* In the absence of age-sex data for 2001 census, official projected figures are used.

Sources: (1) Census data for the period 1951-81 are taken from Occasional Paper No.2 of 1992 – Ageing in India: Demographic Background and Analysis Based on Census Materials, Office of the Registrar General and Census Commissioner, India, New Delhi.

(2) Census data for the year 1991 & 2001are taken from the online data file of Census of India, 1991 & 2001 respectively, Office of the Registrar General and Census Commissioner, India, New Delhi.

(3) The data for the period 1992-93 and 1998-99 are obtained from NFHS-2 (All India) published report (IIPS & ORC-Macro 2000).

The age and sex pattern

To understand the changing age-sex structure of the elderly population, the percentage distribution of the elderly (aged 60+) by sex for the age groups 60-64, 65-69 and 70+ for the period 1961-2001 is presented in Table 7.

It is evident from Table 7, that the proportion of the elderly population aged 60-64 to the total elderly population aged 60 and above declined consistently for both males and females during the last four decades, particularly after 1991, and is expected to decline further in the future. Accordingly, the proportion of elderly population in the higher age groups (65-69 and 70 years and above) increased over time for both the sexes, indicating that India's population has grown continuously older. The process of ageing is however noted to be slow, but is relatively faster for females than males, particularly during the recent period.

Ageing at the state level

To understand whether the pattern observed at the all-India level also holds for the state level, the 2001 Census data are examined here briefly, before proceeding to examine the other characteristics of elderly population in India. Table 8 shows the proportion of elderly population at ages 60+ and 65+ by place of residence, according to state. It is evident from this table that the proportion of elderly population aged 60 and above was noted to be 7.5 percent and those aged 65 and above was about 4.8 percent in India during 2001, while the corresponding figures for the rural areas was slightly higher.

At the state level, the corresponding figures are relatively much higher than the national average for a number of states, indicating that the ageing process is relatively faster in these states. Such states in the first place, include Kerala, Tamil Nadu, Maharashtra, Punjab, Himachal Pradesh and Orissa. For example, the proportion of population at ages 60+ and 65+ years was as high as 9 percent or more and 6 percent or more, respectively, for the states like Kerala, Punjab, Tamil Nadu and Himachal Pradesh. This steady increase in the proportion of elderly population is a reflection of the long-term decline in fertility and mortality and a higher expectation of life at birth and at ages 60 and above in these states.

Table 8: Proportion of elderly persons to total population by residence, according to major states, India, 2001

State	Percentage of elderly persons to total population					
	Rural		Urban		Total	
	Age 60+	Age 65+	Age 60+	Age 65+	Age 60+	Age 65+
India	7.8	5.0	6.7	4.3	7.5	4.8
North						
Delhi	4.5	2.9	5.3	3.4	5.2	3.3
Haryana	8.0	5.5	6.4	4.3	7.5	5.2
Himachal Pradesh	9.3	6.4	6.3	4.1	9.0	6.2
Jammu & Kashmir	6.8	4.4	6.4	4.0	6.7	4.3
Punjab	9.9	6.9	7.4	5.0	9.0	6.3
Rajasthan	7.0	4.5	6.0	3.9	6.8	4.4
Central						
Chattisgadh	7.6	4.8	5.6	3.4	7.2	4.5
Madhya Pradesh	7.4	4.8	5.3	4.1	7.1	4.5
Uttar Pradesh	7.3	4.6	5.9	3.7	7.0	4.4
Uttranchal	8.3	5.4	6.0	3.9	7.7	5.0

(Contd.)

(Contd. Table 8)

State	*Percentage of elderly persons to total population*					
	Rural		*Urban*		*Total*	
	Age 60+	*Age 65+*	*Age 60+*	*Age 65+*	*Age 60+*	*Age 65+*
East						
Bihar	6.7	4.1	6.2	3.9	6.6	4.1
Jharkhand	6.1	3.7	5.1	3.1	5.9	3.5
Orissa	8.6	5.5	6.4	4.1	8.3	5.3
West Bengal	6.6	4.3	8.4	5.6	7.1	4.7
Northeast						
Assam	5.9	3.7	5.8	3.7	5.9	3.7
West						
Gujarat	7.3	4.6	6.2	3.9	6.9	4.3
Maharashtra	10.3	7.0	6.7	4.4	8.7	5.9
South						
Andhra Pradesh	8.1	4.9	6.2	3.7	7.6	4.5
Karnataka	8.3	5.2	6.5	4.1	7.7	4.9
Kerala	10.5	7.3	10.4	7.1	10.5	7.2
Tamil nadu	9.3	5.8	8.4	5.3	8.9	5.6

Source: Computed from the data file of Census of India, 2001, Office of the Registrar General and Census of Commissioner, India, New Delhi.

Some of the states like Andhra Pradesh, Karnataka, Haryana and Uttranchal are found to have values closer to the national average, while other states, including developed states like Gujarat and West Bengal, have a relatively low proportion of elderly population. It is further evident from Table 8 that like the pattern obtained at the all-India level, the proportion of elderly population is relatively greater in rural areas than in the urban areas in most of the states, indicating once again that the rural population is older than the urban population in most parts of India. Having discussed the state level ageing pattern, we turn back to examine the basic characteristics of the elderly population in India.

Age and marital status

As mentioned earlier, the second round of NFHS (1998-99) data for all the states were mainly analysed to study the characteristics of the elderly population. The age-sex composition of the elderly population by rural-urban residence has already been discussed in the earlier section. Nevertheless it is important to note once again, to understand the age pattern of the surveyed elderly population, that less than two-fifths of the elderly male and female population aged 60 and above (36 to 39 percent) belong to ages 60-64 years, while less than one-fifth of the elderly population are aged 75 years or above (Table 9). The remaining proportion of elderly population falls in the age group of 65-74 years.

As regards the marital status of the elderly population, about three-fifths (62 percent) were found married at the point of survey and less than two-fifths (37 percent) was widowed, while 1 percent each was either single or separated/divorced. The sex wise marital status of the elderly population differs significantly. As can be seen from Table 9, more than four-fifths of the elderly men are married and 17 percent are widowed, while the proportion of married among elderly women reduces to two-fifths (40 percent) and the proportion of widows among them increases to almost three-fifths (58 percent). A similar pattern is noted in the rural and urban areas. Given the large number of widows in India and their special vulnerability to ill-health and related deprivations, they deserve an important place in the formulation of health policy and economic development in India. Very few attempts have been made at studying the special needs of this disadvantaged group in the state as well as in the country as a whole. There is much less public concern for the deprivations experienced by these elderly widows in their day-to-day lives. Widowhood and the helplessness that is often associated with it might have an influence on the health and well being of these women.

The vulnerability due to widowhood in old age may be an important motive for high fertility and strong son preference among Indian women, presuming that surviving sons are the only source of social support for the elderly widows, with resultant adverse consequences on the health of women and children. In fact, some studies indicate that the economic deprivation and social neglect in turn are the factors behind high morbidity and mortality rates among widows, compared to married women in the same age cohorts.

Elderly as heads of household

In the traditional Indian value system, the authority of the elderly in the family was always supported, often in opposition to rationality and the right of the individual conscience. The joint family system, which is the core of the traditional Indian way of living, was like a patriarchal organization where the eldest male controlled all economic and social affairs. The senior female member also gained in power and wielded considerable influence in household and other general matters. In this context the elderly as heads of households is a key indicator of the prevailing traditional value system as it is likely to reflect the elder persons' control and decision making power in familial matters. As can be seen from Table 9, 49 percent of the elderly are reported to be the heads of the household in both rural and urban areas. This proportion differs essentially by sex, as 79-80 percent of the elderly men are found as heads of households as against only 15-19 percent of elderly female in both the rural and urban areas. This however does not reflect the economic or other control of the elderly. We now examine the other socio-cultural aspects of the elderly viz. their religious and caste affiliations and educational background.

Religion and caste composition

As is known, the caste system forms one of the basic structural features of the Indian society. Caste and religion together constitute

Table 9: Percent distribution of elderly persons age 60 years and above by selected background characteristics, according to sex and residence, India, 1998-99

Characteristics	*Percentage of Elderly Persons Age 60+*								
	Urban			*Rural*			*Combined*		
	Male	*Female*	*Total*	*Male*	*Female*	*Total*	*Male*	*Female*	*Total*
Age									
60-64	35.9	35.2	35.5	35.5	40.0	37.6	35.6	38.8	37.1
65-69	25.4	26.4	25.9	24.2	25.3	24.7	24.5	25.6	25.0
70-74	20.1	18.6	19.4	21.3	17.7	19.6	21.0	17.9	19.5
75+	18.6	19.8	19.2	19.0	17.0	18.1	19.0	17.7	18.4
Marital status									
Single	1.5	1.2	1.3	1.2	.6	.9	1.3	.7	1.0
Married	83.9	36.4	60.2	80.4	41.6	62.1	81.2	40.3	61.6
Widowed	14.3	61.7	37.9	18.0	57.1	36.5	17.1	58.3	36.8
Divorced	.1	.4	.2	.1	.2	.1	.1	.2	.2
Not living together	.2	.3	.3	.3	.6	.4	.3	.5	.4
Head of household									
Self	79.5	19.0	49.4	78.7	15.1	48.7	78.9	16.1	48.8
Others	20.5	81.0	50.6	21.3	84.9	51.3	21.1	83.9	51.2

(Contd.)

(Contd. Table 9)

Characteristics	Percentage of Elderly Persons Age 60+								
	Urban			Rural			Combined		
	Male	Female	Total	Male	Female	Total	Male	Female	Total
Religion									
Hindu	77.6	77.7	77.7	84.0	84.3	84.2	82.5	82.6	82.6
Muslim	14.3	14.5	14.4	9.5	9.2	9.4	10.6	10.6	10.6
Christians	3.4	3.4	3.4	2.5	2.6	2.5	2.7	2.8	2.7
Sikh	2.3	1.7	2.0	2.8	2.5	2.7	2.7	2.3	2.5
Buddhist	1.1	1.3	1.2	.6	.7	.7	.7	.9	.8
Jain	1.1	1.1	1.1	.3	.3	.3	.5	.5	.5
Others	.2	.3	.2	.4	.4	.4	.3	.3	.3
Caste									
Scheduled caste	13.1	12.2	12.7	19.8	19.3	19.6	18.2	17.5	17.9
Scheduled tribe	2.9	2.9	2.9	10.1	9.6	9.8	8.4	7.9	8.2
OBC	30.7	30.8	30.7	35.3	35.1	35.2	34.2	34.0	34.1
Others	53.3	54.1	53.7	34.9	36.0	35.4	39.2	40.6	39.8
Education									
Illiterate	23.1	60.3	41.6	55.5	87.7	70.7	47.9	80.7	63.6
Primary	25.9	21.0	23.4	27.0	9.8	18.8	26.7	12.6	19.9
Secondary	31.9	15.1	23.5	15.2	2.4	9.1	19.1	5.6	12.6
Higher	19.2	3.7	11.5	2.3	.2	1.3	6.3	1.1	3.8

(Contd. Table 9)

Characteristics	Percentage of Elderly Persons Age 60+								
	Urban			Rural			Combined		
	Male	Female	Total	Male	Female	Total	Male	Female	Total
Occupation									
Professional	4.7	.6	2.7	1.3	.2	.8	2.1	.3	1.2
Clerks and related workers	1.7	.1	.9	.4	.1	.2	.7	.1	.4
Service workers	1.5	.2	.9	1.1	.1	.6	1.2	.1	.7
Sales workers	11.8	1.8	6.8	3.3	.7	2.0	5.3	1.0	3.2
Maids & Labourer	4.5	2.5	3.5	4.8	2.3	3.6	4.7	2.4	3.6
Agricultural and related workers	5.3	1.4	3.4	43.6	11.3	28.4	34.6	8.8	22.3
Skill workers	10.7	1.8	6.3	4.4	.8	2.7	5.9	1.0	3.6
None +	59.7	91.6	75.6	41.2	84.6	61.7	45.5	86.4	65.1
Total percent	**100.0**	**100.0**	**100.0**	**100.0**	**100.0**	**100.0**	**100.0**	**100.0**	**100.0**
Number of usual residents age 60 & above	**5977**	**5842**	**11819**	**14988**	**13159**	**28147**	**20965**	**19001**	**39966**

Source: Computed from NFHS-2 (1998-99), India data file (IIPS, 1999).

+ Includes housewives, unemployed and retired.

the social, economic and cultural background as well as reflect the values and belief system that guide the daily living of individuals and communities. An examination of the recent NFHS data reveals that the religion and caste composition of the elderly population is similar to the pattern generally observed in the general population (Table 9). A large majority of the elderly persons are Hindus (83 percent) and 11 percent of them are Muslims, while more than 2 percent each are Christians or Sikhs and the rest are either Jains, Buddhists or belong to other religious groups. By sex and residence, the religious composition follows almost the same pattern, except the fact that the proportion of Muslims, Christians and Jains to the total elderly population are relatively more in urban areas than in the rural areas. A broad classification of elder persons by their caste reveals that about 18 percent of them belong to the scheduled castes, 8 percent belong to the scheduled tribes and 34 percent belong to other backward castes (OBCs), while the remaining 40 percent belong to other caste groups (Table 9). However, the proportion of other caste groups increases to almost 54 percent in the urban areas, as only a very small proportion of scheduled tribes (less than 3 percent) reside in the urban areas. Similarly, the proportion of scheduled castes among the elderly population reduces to less than 13 percent in urban areas. In other words, a higher proportion (29 percent) of the scheduled caste and scheduled tribe elderly population reside in the rural areas.

Educational status

Education, in its broadest sense is a means of transference of knowledge and information among the members of a society, which in turn helps develop secular and individualistic ideas. The formal education system not only helps the individual acquire skills in reading, writing and calculating to be able to meet the requirements of the employment sector in later life, but equally importantly enables the development of rationality. Despite the spread of education over time, however, its benefits have not reached the elderly population.

A large majority of the elderly population (64 percent) is non-literate (Table 9). This proportion increases to almost 71 percent in the rural areas. Among those who are literate, only less than 4 percent of the total elderly population has higher secondary or above education, less than 13 percent have completed high school education while the remaining 20 percent have primary or less education. In rural areas, more than 1 percent have completed higher secondary or above, and 9 percent have reported a high school education while 19 percent have primary or less education. The corresponding proportions are however relatively higher in the urban areas. Similarly, the educational attainment of the elderly men is higher than that of the elderly women in both rural and urban areas in India. However, it is important to note that only 12 percent of the elderly women and 44 percent of the elderly men in rural India are literate, indicating the need to design socio-economic development and health programmes in light of the low level of literacy for their effective utilization by the elderly, particularly in the rural areas.

Work participation and economic status

The financial and economic well being of the elderly is closely linked to their level of education and past work status. Under usual circumstances, most of the elderly in the formal sector would have retired from the labour force. However, given the Indian situation where the unorganized sector accounts for a larger share of the work force and where rural labour is predominantly in agriculture or allied activities, there is no question of formal retirement for the elderly. In fact, being economically active is probably a positive feature of the aged population in India since it helps to keep at bay many of the age related health problems that arise from a feeling of being unwanted, isolated and useless.

The occupational pattern of the elderly population, based on the recent NFHS data reveals that the majority of them were not engaged in any occupation for one reason or the other (Table 9). This proportion increases to 26 percent for females, while it is only 46 percent for males, which includes mainly those who are retired, unemployed or disabled due to old age and are unable to work (Table 9). Furthermore, it may be noted that a large proportion of the elderly, particularly females, are essentially carrying out household activities. Thus, two thirds of the elderly are not engaged in any economic activity. This proportion is higher in the urban areas (76 percent) than in the rural areas (62 percent) in view of the fact that the rural elderly continued to work in the agriculture sector which has no formal age of retirement. In other words, about one-third of the elderly persons in India are engaged in some occupation, although this proportion varies by sex and residence. In the rural areas, more than two fifths (44 percent) of the elderly men are engaged in agriculture and related work, 5 percent are in labour work, 4 percent in caste occupation, another 3 percent in petty business and only 2 percent in white collar jobs while more than four-fifths of the elderly women are engaged in household activities, 11 percent are in agriculture and related work, 2 percent are engaged as labourers / domestic help, less than 1 percent in sales jobs and the rest in other jobs. In the urban areas, 13 percent of the men are engaged as sales and service workers, 11 percent are engaged as skill workers, 5 percent are in agriculture and related work, less than 5 percent in labour work and only 6 percent are in white collar jobs, while as high as 92 percent of the elderly urban women are engaged in household activity, less than 3 percent as labourers / domestic help, less than 1 percent in white collar jobs and the rest in other petty jobs.

Data from the Ageing Survey (Rajan et al., 1999) also confirm a similar work participation pattern among the elderly. The authors noted that about 44 percent of the elderly were engaged in some economic activity. Sex differentials were also noted with 56 percent of males reporting that they were currently working, the corresponding figure being 28 percent for females. Such a differential may however be due to the invisibility of women's work within the domestic domain. Turning to the other major source of information on work participation and economic status, the recent NSS data reveals a much lower work participation rate among the elderly compared to that obtained from other surveys. The NSS data (Table 10) reveals that about 21 percent of the elderly in the urban areas (35 percent males and 8 percent females) was currently working while the corresponding figure for the rural areas was 39 percent (60 percent among males and 17 percent among females). The higher work participation rate in the rural areas obtained from the various surveys can largely be attributed to the fact that such occupations are generally in agrarian activities wherein there is no formal retirement and therefore the elderly also continue working beyond the age of 60 years.

Table 10: Economic independence, financial status and living arrangements of elderly persons (age 60 & above) by their sex and place of residence, India, 1995-96

	Percentage distribution of elderly persons					
	Urban			*Rural*		
	Male	*Female*	*Total*	*Male*	*Female*	*Total*
State of economic dependence on others⁺						
Not dependent	51.5	11.5	31.1	48.5	12.1	30.1
	(45.7)	(4.8)	(28.9)	(51.1)	(8.8)	(34.0)
Partially dependent	16.9	11.0	13.9	18.0	14.6	16.3
	(16.9)	(9.1)	(13.7)	(16.2)	(13.7)	(15.2)
Fully dependent	29.7	75.7	53.2	31.3	70.6	51.1
	(37.4)	(86.0)	(57.4)	(32.7)	(77.5)	(50.8)
Total	100.0	100.0	100.0	100.0	100.0	100.0
Work participation rate⁺⁺						
Proportion working to earn their livelihood	35.3	7.9	21.4	60.3	17.3	38.6
	(42.9)	(9.2)	(25.5)	(68.3)	(17.3)	(43.3)
Possession of financial assets and property⁺						
Proportion having financial assets[1]	70.2	37.6	53.5	69.5	39.1	54.2
	(52.5)	(37.1)	(46.2)	(58.1)	(48.2)	(54.1)
Proportion having property[2]	74.2	42.0	57.8	80.4	45.6	62.9
	(70.0)	(48.1)	(61.1)	(82.0)	(63.3)	(74.5)

(Contd.)

(Contd. Table 10)

	Percentage distribution of elderly persons					
	Urban			Rural		
	Male	Female	Total	Male	Female	Total
Living arrangements of the elderly+						
Living alone as an inmate of home for the aged	0.5 (0.5)	1.1 (0.2)	0.8 (0.4)	0.8 (0.7)	1.0 (0.7)	0.9 (0.7)
Living alone but not as an inmate of home for the aged	2.5 (9.0)	4.9 (0.6)	3.7 (5.5)	1.7 (11.8)	5.1 (0.7)	3.4 (7.3)
Living with family members or others	97.0 (91.5)	94.0 (99.2)	95.5 (94.1)	97.5 (87.5)	93.9 (98.6)	95.7 (92.0)
Total	**100.0**	**100.0**	**100.0**	**100.0**	**100.0**	**100.0**

Note: NSS 42nd round (1986-87) covered 49,693 households (32,237 from rural and 17,456 from urban areas), while NSS 52nd round (1995-96) covered 72,883 households (43,076 from rural and 29,807 from urban) areas across the country to assess the nature and dimensions of the socio-economic and health problems of the aged, i.e. persons of age 60 years and above.

*Source:*1 Government of India. 1991. Socio-Economic Profile of the Aged Persons: NSS 42nd Round (July 1986 – June 1987). Sarvekshana, Vol.15, No.2, Issue No.49, October-December 1991, National Sample Survey Organization (NSSO), Department of Statistics, Ministry of Planning, New Delhi.

2 Government of India. 1998. The Aged in India: A Socio-Economic Profile. NSS 52nd Round, July 1995 – June 1996, NSSO, Department of Statistics, Ministry of Planning and Programme Implementation, New Delhi.

1 Includes company shares, government securities, Unit Trusts, National Saving Certificates etc.

2 Includes land and buildings

\+ Figures in parenthesis give the corresponding estimates obtained from NSS 42nd Round (1986-87)

++ Figures in parenthesis give the corresponding estimates obtained from NSS 47th Round (1991)

The economic status and living arrangements of the elderly can also be assessed from the data of the NSS. As high as 70 percent of the elderly are partially or fully dependent on others for the fulfillment of their livelihood. This situation is worse for elderly females in the rural and urban areas since 88 percent of them are economically dependent on others in India. The corresponding dependence among males is much lower as about 48-51 percent of the elderly males in the rural and urban areas are partially or completely dependent on others for their livelihood. The economic condition of the elderly, especially the gender differentials, are further reiterated from an examination of the data on possession of financial assets and property. About 54 percent of the elderly reported about having some financial assets in both rural and urban areas. However, the ownership of such assets varies by sex.

The definite edge that males have over females is evident here as 70 percent of the elderly males in both the rural and urban areas had financial assets such as company shares, government securities, investment in unit trust, while 38-39 percent of the females reported having such financial assets (Table 10). On the other hand, the proportion of elderly who reported having some property (land, building) was much higher (58-63 percent) in the rural and urban areas in the country. Sex differentials are noted here also as 74-80 percent of the elderly men reported having some property as against 42-46 percent of the females. Finally, Table 10 provides information on the living arrangements of the elderly. The strong familial ties prevalent in the Indian society are clearly evident as the majority of the elderly (94-98 percent) reported that they were living either with family members or others. The table further reveals that about 2 to 5 percent of the elderly were living alone and only about 1 percent of them were found to be living as inmates of homes for the aged.

Thus, it is evident from various sources of data that the majority of the elderly in India do not have sufficient financial assets and property nor are currently earning their livelihood and are therefore dependent on others, usually family members, for their care and day to day physical maintenance.

Table 11: Percent distribution of elderly population by their standard of living and by their access to mass media in the household, according to sex and residence, India, 1998-99

Standard of living / access to mass media	*Percentage of Elderly Persons Age 60 and above*								
	Urban			*Rural*			*Combined*		
	Male	*Female*	*Total*	*Male*	*Female*	*Total*	*Male*	*Female*	*Total*
Standard of living index+									
Low	11.6	13.4	12.5	35.6	38.4	36.9	29.9	32.0	31.0
Medium	39.2	39.5	39.3	49.2	46.4	47.9	46.8	44.6	45.8
High	49.2	47.1	48.2	15.3	15.2	15.2	23.2	23.3	23.3
Total percent	100.0	100.0	100.0	100.0	100.0	100.0	100.0	100.0	100.0
Access to mass media: Household ownership of									
A radio/ transistor	59.4	57.2	58.3	36.1	34.1	35.2	41.6	40.0	40.8
A television	73.8	72.1	73.0	23.6	23.8	23.7	35.4	36.1	35.7
Number of elderly persons age 60 & above	**5977**	**5842**	**11819**	**14988**	**13159**	**28147**	**20965**	**19001**	**39966**

Source: Computed from NFHS-1 (1992-93), India data file (IIPS, 1995).

\+ It is a summary household measure which is calculated by adding scores received by the household to which respondent(s) belong, on the following items: house type, toilet facility, source of lighting, main fuel for cooking, source of drinking water, availability of separate room for cooking, ownership of agricultural land, ownership of irrigated land, ownership of live-stock and ownership of various durable goods. On the basis of total scores, the elderly population are divided into three standard of living index (SLI) categories viz. (i) a low SLI (0-12), (ii) a medium SLI (13-22) and (iii) a high SLI (23-48)

Standard of living

Having discussed the socio-economic condition of elderly persons which depicts a rather unsatisfactory scenario it is important to understand their overall standard of living based on the household characteristics and amenities as well as based on the availability of consumer durable goods in the household. In this context, a summary household measure called the standard of living index (SLI) developed and applied to the data of NFHS-2 is used here for assessing the socio-economic status of the elderly population surveyed during NFHS-2.

Each household was judged on a number of indicators, and given a score accordingly, to understand the overall standard of living of the household. On the basis of the total score received by a household on the SLI, the elderly persons are broadly classified into three categories viz., low, medium and high. Index scores range from 0-12 for a low SLI, 13-22 for a medium SLI and 23-48 for a high SLI. The classification of elderly persons by this measure, according to sex and residence is shown in Table 11.

It is evident that as high as 46 percent of the elderly have a medium standard of living, followed by 31 percent who fall in the low standard of living category, while only 23 percent enjoy a high standard of living. In other words, not even one-fourth of the elderly have access to basic amenities, some degree of comfort in their daily living and exposure to some means of mass communication.

Sharp rural-urban differences in standard of living are also clearly evident. While only 15 percent of the rural elderly fall in the high index category, almost half of them (48 percent) in the urban areas belong to this category. The pattern virtually reverses, when one looks at the proportions in the low index category, with only 13 percent of the urban elderly in this group which rises to 37 percent in the rural areas.

Access to mass media in the household

The possession of durable goods is an important indicator of a household's socio-economic level and various consumer durable goods, as mentioned earlier, were considered in the computation of, the Standard of Living Index. Some of these may also have other benefits. For example, availability of a refrigerator in the household prolongs the wholesomeness of food, while the availability of some means of transportation (such as scooter, motorcycle or a car) in the household allows greater access to many services outside the local area. Similarly, having access to a radio/transistor or television may expose household members to innovative ideas or important information about health and welfare programmes and various services under them in addition to providing entertainment. Therefore, the latter two indicators are separately examined here to understand the access to such mass media among the elderly persons in the household. As can be seen from Table 11, only two-fifths of the elderly persons (41 percent) might have access to a radio/transistor and 36 percent reported to have access to a television in India. These proportions among elderly however differ significantly by their place of residence. In the urban areas, 58 percent of the elderly have access to a radio or transistor, as against 35 percent in the rural areas, while about 73 percent have access to a television in the urban areas as against only 24 percent in the rural areas. In other words, as expected, urban households are much more likely than rural households to own such durable goods and are likely to be exposed to mass media.

Lifestyle of the elderly

The second round of the National Family Health Survey (1998-99) provides certain aspects of the lifestyle of household members for the first time. The NFHS-2 Household Questionnaire sought information about all men and women aged 15 and above who chewed *paan masala* or tobacco, consumed alcohol, or smoked. These lifestyle indicators are of considerable interest because the use of *paan masala*, tobacco, and alcohol all has detrimental effects on health, particularly among the elderly population.

In the absence of the relevant data file of NFHS-2, the limited published data in the all-India report (IIPS and ORC-Macro, 2000, pp. 41-43) are used here to examine these lifestyle indicators of elderly persons in the household. This information is summarized in Table 12. It may however be noted that information on these lifestyle indicators for all persons in the household are obtained from the person who responded to the Household Question and not from each person above 15 years of age. Although the household

Table 12: Percentage of usual household members age 60 years and above who chew paan masala or tobacco, drink alcohol, currently smoke or have ever smoked by sex, India, 1998-99

Lifestyle indicator	*Percentage of usual household membersage 60 and above*	
	Male	*Female*
Chew paan masala or tobacco	37.6	25.0
Drink alcohol	18.6	3.1
Currently smoke	38.2	5.3
Ever smoked[1]	46.6	6.0
Number of household members age 60 and above	**20571**	**18588**

[1] Includes household members who currently smoke

Source: National Family Health Survey (NFHS-2), 1998-99, India. IIPS, Mumbai, India and ORG Macro, Calverton, Maryland, USA, October 2000. p. 42.

respondent was usually a responsible adult he/she may not be aware of the habits of all members especially related to tobacco and alcohol consumption outside the household. In addition, under-reporting is likely, to the extent that social stigma may be attached to the use of some of substances (IIPS and ORC-Macro, 2000, p.43). Therefore the results should be interpreted with caution. The results, summarized in Table 12, reveal that about 38 percent of the elderly men and 25 percent of the elderly women in the country are reported to chew *paan masala* or tobacco. On the other hand, about 19 percent of the elderly men and 3 percent of the elderly women are reported to drink alcohol. Similarly, only 6 percent of the elderly women are reported to have ever smoked and 5 percent currently smoke, while as high as 47 percent of the elderly men are reported to have ever smoked and about 38 percent currently smoke. Eighty-two percent of the elderly men and 88 percent of the elderly women who ever smoked were still smokers at the point of survey. Thus, chewing of *paan masala* or tobacco, drinking alcohol and smoking are more frequent among elderly men than among women. While we do not have detailed data of such practices among the elderly by rural-urban residence, it is noted from the published all-India NFHS-2 report that such practices by household members (age 15 and above) are relatively much higher in the rural areas than in the urban areas. The proportion of men who chewed *paan masala* or tobacco, consumed alcohol or smoked, is one and one-half times as high in rural areas as in urban areas. Similarly, such practices are two-three times as high among non-literate men and among men with a low standard of living, as among men who have completed at least high school and men with a high standard of living. The pattern of differentials for elderly population is expected to resemble that observed for general population, indicating that such practices are expected to be more common among those who are non-literates, with a low standard of living and reside in the rural areas, than others.

Health and Morbidity

The process of biological ageing brings with it several accompanying health problems or diseases. The decline in the efficient functioning of the various organ systems of the body including the immune system renders the elderly particularly vulnerable to several diseases. The sight of the elderly fail as a result of the development of cataract or glaucoma, their sense of hearing is also not as sharp and poor salivation and loss of taste buds causes a decrease in the taste of food and dryness of the mouth. They are also prone to suffer from diseases of the cardio-vascular system (hypertension, artherosclerosis, heart trouble), respiratory system (decreased breathing capacity), central nervous system (dizziness, slow movements, loss of memory, altered sleep pattern) and the muscular-skeletal system (decreased strength, susceptibility to loss of teeth and fracture of bones). Endocrinal deficiency diseases like diabetes are also a result of poor functioning of the organ system.

Evidence from a study in the rural areas near Madurai on various aspects of life of 1910 elderly men and women age 60+ years (including their health status) revealed that visual handicap, reported by 89 percent was ranked first amongst all illnesses, followed by degenerative joint diseases (50 percent), sleeplessness (40), body ache (38), backache and giddiness (34 percent each) and numbness (26 percent). Each elderly respondent reported an average of 5 or 6 symptoms (Rao, et al., 1982). Clinical diagnosis revealed visual disability to be the primary illness condition (88 percent) followed by locomotor disabilities (40). Diseases of the central nervous system were identified in 19 percent of the cases, respiratory disorders were diagnosed among 16 percent and hearing impairment was diagnosed among 8 percent of the elderly men and women.

The combined effects of deteriorating physical health and psycho-social factors (retirement from active professional life, bereavement, disintegration of their personal lives) leads to poor mental health and mental disorders among the elderly. Data from general epidemiological studies and community based surveys among the elderly have revealed a varied rate of mental illness or psychiatric morbidity which was found to be as high as 34 percent in some studies. Depression contributed to 67 percent of psychiatric morbidity among a sample of 686 men and women aged sixty years and above (Sharma, 1999). It is thus of utmost importance to establish the morbidity pattern among the elderly to meet their health care needs. The available national level data from the two major sources viz. NSS and NFHS are examined to have a complete picture, to some extent, of the likely illnesses that we know generally prevail among the elderly persons.

I - Evidence from NSS Data

As mentioned earlier, the two rounds of NSS viz. 42nd and 52nd, sought information on chronic diseases and physical disabilities prevailing among the elderly persons (aged 60 years and above). The data of these surveys are examined in the following sections.

Chronic ailments

The prevalence rate of some specified ailments for elderly males and elderly females for the rural and urban areas, were obtained and these rates (per 100,000) are given in Table 13. In the survey schedule, information on morbidity was collected in detail for each household member irrespective of age. In the module for the aged, information on some specific chronic diseases was also collected separately. However, it may be noted that strict definitions and procedures were not followed to identify the chronic diseases. If one had suffered from any of the specified chronic diseases at any time in the past, he/she had also been considered to be suffering from that chronic disease irrespective of whether or not he/she was suffering from the chronic disease on the date of the survey. This was done with the assumption that some of the chronic diseases could be controlled but might not be cured.

It is evident from Table 13 that the prevalence of chronic diseases among the aged is very high, as more than half of the elderly persons surveyed during 1995-96, reported to be suffering from one or the other type of chronic ailment and it is relatively higher in the urban areas (54,459 per 100,000) than in the rural areas (52,034 per 100,000). A comparison of this estimate with that obtained during the NSS 42nd round (1986-87) indicates that the prevalence of these chronic ailments has increased significantly during this gap of 9 years (Table 16). 'Problems of joints', 'cough' and 'blood pressure (high/low)' appear to be the most severe diseases for the aged. As high as 38,395 persons from rural areas and 34,000 persons from urban areas out of 100,000 elderly population reported to be suffering from problem of joints and 22,241 per 100,000 in the rural areas and 15,982 per 100,000 in the urban areas indicated to be suffering from cough, while 10,635 per 100,000 in the rural areas and 22,557 per 100,000 reported to have high or low blood pressure. These data also indicate that problem of joints and cough are more prevalent in the rural areas than in the urban areas while the problem of high or low blood pressure is more common in the urban than in the rural areas. A study of these diseases among the elderly by sex reveals that problem of joints and blood pressure are more severe among elderly females than among elderly males, while cough is more common among elderly males than elderly females.

Diabetes and heart diseases are the other health problems among the elderly that were reported next in order of severity (Table 13). These diseases are more prevalent in the urban than in the

Table 13: Number of aged persons (60 and above) suffering from a chronic disease and having physical disability per 100,000 aged persons by type of disease/disability for each sex in rural and urban areas, India, 1995-96

Type of chronic disease / physical disability	*Urban*			*Rural*		
	Male	*Female*	*Total*	*Male*	*Female*	*Total*
Chronic ailments						
Cough	17855	14187	15982	24995	19533	22241
Piles	3218	1831	2510	3289	1605	2440
Problem of joints	28540	39254	34010	36306	40448	38395
Blood pressure (high/low)	20022	25086	22557	10791	10474	10635
Heart disease	6828	5309	6062	3385	2658	3025
Urinary problem	4917	2407	3649	3846	2273	3063
Diabetes	8525	6582	7544	3617	2815	3223
Cancer	183	392	290	197	312	254
Any of the above ailments	52822	56029	54459	52670	51409	52034
	44344)+	(45493)	(44816)	(45097)	(44849)	(44997)

(Contd.)

(Contd. Table 13)

Type of chronic disease / physical disability	Urban			Rural		
	Male	Female	Total	Male	Female	Total
Physical disabilities						
Visual	22547	26016	24318	24886	29133	27028
Hearing	11083	13182	12155	13944	15607	14783
Speech	2930	3439	3190	3203	3763	3485
Locomotor	7957	9374	8681	10671	11535	11107
Amnesia/Senility	6076	7977	7047	9551	11344	10455
Any of the above disabilities++	33285	36696	35027	38002	42455	40247
Number of sample aged persons (NSS 52nd round)	6434	6601	13035	10739	10216	20955

Note: NSS 42nd round (1986-87) covered 49,693 household (32,237 from rural and 17,456 from urban areas), while NSS 52nd round (1995-96) covered 72,883 households (43,076 from rural and 29,807 from urban areas) across the country to assess the nature and dimensions of the socio-economic and health problems of the aged, i.e. persons of age 60 years and above.

Source: 1 Government of India. 1991. Socio-Economic Profile of the Aged Persons: NSS 42nd Round (July 1986 – June 1987). Sarvekshana, Vol.15, No.2, Issue No.49, October-December 1991, National Sample Survey Organization (NSSO), Department of Statistics, Ministry of Planning, New Delhi.

2 Government of India 1998. The Aged in India: A Socio-Economic Profile. NSS 52nd Round, July 1995– June 1996, NSSO, Department of Statistics, Ministry of Planning & Programme Implementation, New Delhi.

\+ Figures in parenthesis give the corresponding estimates obtained from NSS 42nd Round (1986-87)

++ Figures in parenthesis give the corresponding estimates obtained from NSS 47th Round (1991) rural areas. The prevalence rate of heart disease and diabetes for the urban areas (6062 to 7544 per 100,000) is just twice that in the rural areas (3,025 to 3,223 per 100,000). Elderly men were more prone to suffer from these diseases than elderly women in both rural and urban areas.

Urinary problem and piles are the other chronic diseases that are reported by more than 2 to 4 percent of the elderly population. Another disease, viz. cancer that is considered to be fatal, is also reported by a number of elderly persons in India. The prevalence rate of this disease is relatively higher in the urban areas (290 per 100,000) than in the rural areas (254 per 100,000). Further, it is very important to note that the prevalence of this dreaded disease is much higher among elderly females than elderly males in both rural and urban areas.

Physical disability

Physical disability of the elderly persons is also a cause of concern. Disability increases with age even among the aged. It prevents them from carrying out work or occupation for their livelihood, maintaining economic independence and at the same time prevents their participation in some social and religious activities and household chores. In other words, such physical disabilities denies them the right to lead an active life or pursue the activities of their interest. As can be seen from Table 13, the prevalence of various disabilities such as visual, hearing, amnesia/ senility, speech and locomotor, among the aged are very high. The prevalence rate per 100,000 elderly for each sex in the rural and urban areas of India based on estimates obtained from NSS 52nd round (1995-96) have been presented in Table 13. It was seen in general that more than two-fifths of the elderly persons in rural areas (40,247 per 100,000) and more than one-thirds of elderly in urban areas (35,027 per 100,000) had one or the other type of physical disability. Such problems are relatively higher among elderly females than elderly males in both rural and urban areas.

The problem of **visual disability** happened to be the most severe physical disability condition for the aged. Loss or lack of ability to execute tasks requiring adequate visual acuity is considered as visual disability. The visually disabled, for the purpose of the survey (NSS), include those who do not have any light perception, both eyes taken together and those who have light perception but cannot correctly count fingers of a hand (with spectacles/contact lenses in the case of those who are normally using these) from a distance of 3 meters (or 10 feet) in good daylight with both eyes open (Government of India, 1998, p.3). The prevalence rate of this disease condition varies from 24,318 per 100,000 in urban areas to 27,028 per 100,000 in the rural areas (Table 13). The sex differential in visual disability is also very large in both rural and urban areas, with relatively more proportion of elderly females than elderly males having the problem of visual disability. The NFHS estimate on complete or partial blindness is quite low (Table 17), compared to this NSS estimate, which could be due to differences in concepts, definitions and procedures used in the two surveys.

The problem of **hearing disability** (persons' ability to hear properly) came next in order of severity. Hearing disability was judged taking into consideration the disability of the better ear but without taking into consideration the use of hearing aids (Government of India, 1998, p.3). The prevalence rate of this disease condition varies from 12,155 per 100,000 in urban areas to 14,783 per 100,000 in rural areas (Table 13). Here again, elderly females are more prone to this problem than elderly males.

Locomotor disability and **amnesia/senility** (loss of memory) are also quite common among the aged. Persons having locomotor disability (i.e. an individual's loss or lack of ability to execute distinctive activities associated with the movement of himself/herself and objects from place to place and physical deformities) are those with loss or absence or inactivity of whole or part of hand or leg or both due to amputation, paralysis, deformity and dysfunction of joints and those with physical deformities in the body (other than limbs) which do not affect normal movement, such as hunchback, deformed spine etc. (Government of India, 1998, p.4). The prevalence of locomotor disability among the aged is as high as 11,107 per 100,000 in rural areas while it is 8,781 per 100,000 in urban areas. The elderly females are more likely to have suffered from this problem than elderly males. Similarly, the prevalence of amnesia/senility was also seen to be equally high and it was higher in rural areas (10,455 per 100,000) than in the urban areas (7,047 per 100,000) and it is much higher for elderly females than for elderly males.

Finally, Table 13 also provides the prevalence of **speech disability** among the aged. It refers to a person's inability to speak properly. Here, persons with speech disability include those who cannot speak, those who speak only a limited number of words and those with loss of voice. It also includes those having speech but with defects in speech such as stammering, nasal voice, hoarse voice, discordant voice and articulation defects, etc. (Government of India, 1998, pp.3-4). The prevalence of this disability condition appears to be the least among the aged, compared to other physical disabilities probed under the survey. As can be seen from Table 13, the prevalence rate of speech disability is of the order of 3,485 per 100,000 in the rural areas and 3,190 per 100,000 in the urban areas, with relatively higher proportion of elderly females than elderly males affected by this disease condition in both rural and urban areas.

II – Evidence from NFHS Data

The two rounds of NFHS which collected data on diseases such as asthma, tuberculosis and blindness for all household members are examined here to understand the health profile of the elderly with respect to these three diseases. The data were collected from the head of the household or other responsible adult member of the household and not from the individual having the illness. Furthermore, no clinical or medical examinations were made for the reported conditions. Therefore the results need to be interpreted with caution. Nevertheless, each of the disease conditions probed under both the surveys is discussed in the following section. Table 14 shows the prevalence of asthma, tuberculosis and partial and complete blindness, among the elderly population by sex and place of residence in India. We examine each of these disease conditions by their prevalence among elderly men and women in the rural and urban areas.

Asthma

Asthma is one of the common health problems among the elderly population in India. It is a chronic respiratory disease characterized by sudden attacks of laboured breathing, chest constriction and coughing. There has been a substantial increase in asthma cases in recent years. Moreover, the prevalence of asthma increases rapidly with age, from say, 950 per 100,000 at age 0-14 to 10,271 per 100,000 at age 60 and over (IIPS & ORC-Macro, 2000, pp.197-198). The prevalence of asthma is much higher among males (11,943) than among females (8454). As can further be seen from Table 14, the prevalence of asthma among the elderly population is considerably higher in the rural areas (10,944 per 100,000 population) than in the urban areas (8,194 per 100,000 population).

Tuberculosis

The prevalence of tuberculosis is also likely to be high among the elderly population. The NFHS-2 data reveal that the prevalence of tuberculosis is substantially higher among persons age 60 and above (1,374 per 100,000) than among those age 15-59 (675 per 100,000) or age 0-14 (153 per 100,000) (IIPS, 2000, p.197). It is an infectious disease that affects the lungs and other body tissues. Tuberculosis of the lungs, the most commonly known form, is characterized by coughing up mucus and sputum, fever, weight loss and chest pain (IIPS, 2000, p.198). The estimate of the prevalence of this disease among the elderly differs between the two rounds of NFHS (Table 14). According to NFHS-1 (1992-93), the overall prevalence of tuberculosis among elderly in India was 1,600 per 100,000 population while the corresponding estimate as per NFHS-2 (1998-99) was much lower at 1,363 per 100,000 population. Such a difference is particularly noted in the rural areas. It is difficult to presume that the prevalence of tuberculosis among the elderly population might have reduced between the two surveys (six years), while the overall prevalence of tuberculosis among all ages is on the rise in India, the rate being 467 per 100,000 population during NFHS-1 (1992-93) and 544 per 100,000 population during NFHS-2 (1998-99). Nevertheless, the prevalence of tuberculosis appears to be very high among the elderly population and is expected to be in the range of 1,363-1,600 per 100,000 population. Further, as can be seen from Table 14, the prevalence rate is much higher in the rural areas (1446-1774 per 100,000 population) than in the urban areas (1028-1108 per 100,000 population). Similarly, the prevalence of tuberculosis is quite high for elderly males (1746-2096 per 100,000 population than for elderly females (946-1035 per 100,000 population) as per estimates from NFHS-1 and NFHS – 2. A similar pattern by

Table 14: Number of elderly persons (age 60 and above) per 100,000 usual household residents suffering from asthma, tuberculosis and blindness and by sex and place of residence, India, 1992-99

Illness/ Disease condition/ Year of study	*Number of elderly persons per 100,000 suffering from a particular illness*								
	Urban			*Rural*			*Combined*		
	Male	*Female*	*Total*	*Male*	*Female*	*Total*	*Male*	*Female*	*Total*
Asthma:									
1992-93	-	-	-	-	-	-	-	-	-
1998-99	9481	6899	8194	12700	8985	10944	11943	8454	10271
Tuberculosis:									
1992-93	1486	560	1028	2276	1190	1774	2096	1035	1600
1998-99	1505	709	1108	1821	1028	1446	1746	946	1363
Blindness(1992- 93)+									
Partial	13109	16118	14597	15901	19055	17350	15284	18334	16709
Complete	1158	1455	1305	1619	2424	1992	1517	2186	1829
Number of usual residents age 60 and above									
1992-93	4577	4467	9043	16125	13697	29822	20702	18163	38865
1998-99	-	-	9488	-	-	29737	-	-	39224

Source: 1992-93: Computed from NFHS-1, (1992-92) India data file (IIPS, 1995)
1998-99: Computed from NFHS-2, (1998-99), India data file (IIPS and ORC-Macro, 2000)
+ Data not collected under NFHS – 2

sex is noted in the rural and urban areas, although the sex differential is more marked in the urban areas than in the rural areas. The possible reasons for the much higher prevalence of tuberculosis among males than females are that men are more exposed to the outside world and likely to come in contact with people who suffer from active tuberculosis and that men smoke more than women in India, while the higher prevalence rate in the rural areas than in the urban areas could be attributed to the fact that poor nutrition makes rural population more susceptible to the tuberculosis virus.

Partial and complete blindness

As mentioned earlier, among the various disease conditions probed under the NFHS, blindness (partial or complete) has the highest incidence among elderly population in India. The results of NFHS-1 (data on this aspect were not collected under NFHS-2) clearly reveal that the prevalence rate increases sharply with age. The much higher prevalence of blindness among elderly persons is quite striking and this tendency for blindness to increase with age is evident at all periods in history. In the country as a whole, the prevalence of partial blindness is as high as 16,709 per 100,000 for elderly persons (Table 14). This overall prevalence of partial blindness is much higher in rural areas (19,055 per 100,000) than in the urban areas (14,597 per 100,000. In both rural and urban areas, elderly females are more prone to partial blindness than elderly males. The overall prevalence of partial blindness is 18,334 per 100,000 for elderly females and 15,284 per 100,000 for elderly males.

The overall prevalence of complete blindness is 1,829 per 100,000 population for the elderly persons (Table 14). Here again, the prevalence of complete blindness is much higher in the rural areas (1,992 per 100,000) than in the urban areas (1,305 per 100,000). Similarly, in both rural and urban areas elderly females are more prone to complete blindness than elderly males. The overall prevalence of complete blindness is 2,186 per 100,000 for elderly females and 1,517 per 100,000 for elderly males in India. The NSS data as noted earlier, reveals a similar pattern but a very high incidence of this. The prevalence of any visual disabilities was as high as 24,000 to 27,000 per 100,000 in the rural and urban areas of India.

Summary and Conclusions

The twentieth century has witnessed an increase in the proportion of elderly population aged 60 years and over in all countries of the world. While the ageing of population began earlier in the industrialized countries, the developing countries too are experiencing similar changes in their population structure. In fact, the increase in the elderly population is expected to be markedly more in China and India due to the large base of the population in these countries. The growing numbers of the elderly, in the country merit a special study to understand their current social, economic and health status, and the familial and other supports available to them so as to address the special needs of this vulnerable population. This study of the elderly has mainly utilised data of the recently conducted National Family Health Surveys and the National Sample Surveys.

Demography of ageing

The proportion of the elderly population (age 60+) has been increasing consistently over the last century, particularly after 1951. In 1901 the proportion of this population was about 5.1 percent, which increased to about 5.4 percent in 1951, and to about 6.7 percent in 1991. As per official population projections, this proportion is expected to be about 7.0 percent by 2001.

The sharp fall in fertility during the last two to three decades has resulted in changes in the age structure of the population in the country with a sharp decline at the younger ages (0-14 years) and a corresponding increase in the proportion of population in the older ages. This trend is likely to continue in the future and the proportion of elderly persons is expected to register an increase of about two percent between 2001 and 2016. In terms of absolute growth, the population of the elderly, which had grown from about 12.1 million in 1901 to approximately 56.5 million in 1991 (increase of about 37 percent), is expected to be about 71 million in 2001 and reach a phenomenal 113 million in 2016. Furthermore, it has been noted that the elderly population has grown at a relatively faster rate than the general population and among the elderly the increase is greater for females than for males. The sex ratios over time also reveal an increase in the number of elderly females while the projected age-sex structure of the population indicates that with time, India too will have a pattern similar to the developed countries where women are likely to outnumber men. The excess of females over males is not a new phenomenon and had been evident since the 1901 when there were 1193 women aged 60 years or more for every 1000 men in that age group. This trend continued until 1951, despite a decline in the sex ratio among the elderly. Thereafter, the pattern reversed once again in favour of women.

The progressive advantage of females over time among the elderly is essentially due to lower mortality rates of women at middle and late ages compared to men. Between 1946 and 1991 the expectation of life at birth for males increased by about 26 years as against 28 years for females. In view of the relatively low status of women in India, which is also reflected in the neglect of their health at all ages, the greater life span of the women is indeed a paradox. However, what it indicates is the need to plan for various services particularly health and welfare services, for the elderly in general and for elderly women in particular.

The study of dependency ratios is yet another parameter to estimate the needs of various dependent population and in turn helps assess the economic potential of a populations since a low dependency reflects more workers who produce services as against a high dependency which has more "consumers" of services. An increase in the elderly population, therefore, is likely to damage the economy since they consume a higher proportion of various services. In this context, it has been noted that the geriatric ratio had increased during the latter half of the last century from almost 9 older persons per 100 in the working ages in 1951 to 12 in 1991 and is likely to increase to about 14 by 2016. The ageing of the Indian population is also illustrated by the fact that there were nearly 14 elderly persons for every 100 children in 1951 and is expected to more than double and reach 32 by 2016. Furthermore, the changing age-sex structure of the elderly during the last three to four decades also indicates that there has been a proportionate decline in those aged 60-64, which is offset by an increase in the proportion of elderly population at higher ages (65-69 and 70 years and above) over time for both the sexes. In other words, India's population has grown continuously older, although this process of ageing is noted to be slow, but is relatively faster for females than males particular during the recent period.

Ageing at the state level

The analysis of NFHS-1 data has revealed that the proportion of the elderly aged 60 and above was about 8 percent and that age 65 and above was about 5 percent in India during 1992-93 while the corresponding figures for the rural areas were slightly higher. The corresponding figures are much higher than the national average for a number of states (particularly in the rural areas) such as Kerala, Tamil Nadu, Andhra Pradesh, Haryana, Punjab, Himachal Pradesh, Jammu and Orissa, indicating that the ageing process is relatively faster in these states. These states therefore need to be well prepared to provide for their growing numbers of elderly.

Socio-economic status

The socio-economic status of the elderly has indicated that on some of these parameters, their characteristics are like those found in the general population in the country. For example, about 74 of the total population and 78 percent of the elderly population was found residing in the rural areas. The proportion of elderly females is also more in the rural areas than the urban areas, a pattern that has been noted since the 1960s.

An examination of the availability of basic amenities and access to mass media at the household level, which in turn reflects the standard of living enjoyed by the elderly, has revealed that less than one fifth of the elderly reside in households which have access to basic amenities like safe drinking water, electricity, ownership of land and ownership of consumer durable goods (radio, television, sofa, bed etc.), which provide some degree of comfort in daily living and increase the exposure of household members to some means of mass communication. Sharp rural-urban differentials in living standard were noted with only ten percent of the rural elderly falling in relatively high standard of living category as against 49 percent in the urban areas.

As regards the marital status of the elderly population, about 61 percent were found married, more than one third (37 percent) was widowed, while 1 percent each was either single or separated/

divorced. A significant feature of marital status among the elderly is the greater percent of widows (58 percent) as against only 17 percent of widowers. This indicates the greater social and economic vulnerability of elderly women in the context of the traditional patriarchal familial structure in the country.

The religion and caste composition of the elderly population is also similar to the pattern observed in the general population with the majority being Hindus, followed by Muslims with negligible proportions of Christians, Sikhs, Jains and Buddhists. The proportion of Muslims, Christians and Jains are relatively more in the urban areas than in the rural areas. The caste composition also reflects the pattern of the general population with four fifths belonging to castes other than scheduled castes or tribes. The proportion of the elderly belonging to the scheduled castes and tribes was higher in the rural areas than in the urban areas.

The educational background of the elderly reveals that the benefits of schooling have not reached this group since 70 percent was found to be non-literate. Among the literate, the majority reported having only primary or less education. Rural-urban and gender differentials were noted with a greater proportion of rural population and women reporting less education than the urban and male population. The occupational pattern of the elderly reveals that about two-fifths of them were engaged in some occupation which increases to almost fifty percent for elderly males in the rural areas. The higher work participation rate in the rural areas is attributed to the fact that such occupations are generally in agrarian activities wherein there is no formal retirement unlike in the organized sector.

Yet another dimension of the economic well being of the elderly is noted from their possession of financial assets and property and their degree of economic dependence on others. As high as seventy percent of the elderly were partially or fully dependent on others for the fulfillment of their livelihood and little over half reported having some financial assets and property. Gender differentials are particularly striking and the situation of elderly females is worse on both counts with a higher proportion of females reporting economic dependence on others and a much lower proportion reporting possession of financial assets and property. Since financial security is closely linked to the ability of the elderly to care for them independently, this aspect has implications on the living arrangements they make for themselves.

It is indeed fortunate therefore that the strong familial ties still prevail in the Indian society and the majority of the elderly (almost cent percent) reported to be living either with family members or others. With the gradual break down of the traditional patterns of joint familial living as a result of urbanization and modernization, the picture is likely to change in the future and today's younger generation is quite likely to need the help of the state to make suitable institutional arrangements for this young population as it reaches the stage of senescence.

Health and morbidity

The socio-economic status of the elderly thus reveals their dependency on others for fulfilling their basic needs. Yet another facet of the elderly that would further add to their dependency is their failing physical health as a result of ageing. In this regard the data examined in the present study has revealed a high rate of various chronic diseases among the elderly. Degenerative changes are reflected by the fact that the problem of the joints is one of the most severe health conditions mentioned while visual, auditory, locomotor and speech disabilities were the other health problems reported with visual disability heading the list of ailments. In fact partial or complete loss of vision among the elderly has been evident at all periods in history.

Among the other disease conditions reported from various surveys are asthma and tuberculosis. The prevalence of asthma increases with the increase in age of an individual as a result of the decreasing efficiency of the lungs. Similarly, the prevalence of tuberculosis was also found to be high among the elderly, which again may be attributed to their overall lowered resistance to diseases coupled with their poor nutritional intake. Data on these diseases further highlight the urban-rural differentials with the rural population being more susceptible to these diseases.

In addition to the vulnerability of the elderly as a result of the biological process of ageing, certain individual habits further compromise their health. Data on this aspect has revealed the consumption of tobacco and *paan masala* as well as alcohol by both elderly men and women. Smoking was another habit reported by both men and women. Such practices were found more common among those who had no education, had a low standard of living and resided in the rural areas. The need to therefore educate this group on the harmful effects of such practices is clearly evident to safeguard the already deteriorating health of the elderly.

In view of the various chronic ailments and physical disabilities that prevail among the elderly, as a result of their failing immune system, the need to design a special health care package is critical to minimize their suffering and enable them to lead an active and productive life.

Programmes and policies

It is therefore encouraging to note that the National Policy for Older Persons announced in 1999 has identified principal areas of intervention and action strategies. These include financial security for the elderly in both the formal as well as those working in the informal sector, health care and nutrition, shelter and housing, development of trained manpower in medical colleges and schools of social work, attention to the needs of vulnerable groups among the elderly such as the destitute, widows and those who are disabled (GOI, 2000).

In addition, the policy suggests the formulation of a National Council and a National Association of Older Persons, the establishment of a separate bureau for older persons in the Ministry, preparation of Sectoral Annual and Five Year Plans for the Elderly and a detailed review of the implementation of the National Policy every three years (GOI, 2000). The translation of the suggested strategies is envisaged through the Social Justice Committees of the Village Panchayat and by involving experts of public administration to co-ordinate and monitor the implementation of the policy. The government also has a scheme of assistance tc Panchayati Raj Institutions/Voluntary Organizations or other self help groups for the construction of old age homes or multi-service centers for older persons. Under the scheme, a one time grant of Rs.30 lakhs per Home/Centre is provided to eligible organizations for the construction of old age homes or a multi service centre comprising day care centre for those elderly who are mobile and outreach units for the home bound as well as Old Age Homes for the destitute.

While the thrust of the various programmes is on the elderly persons of age 60 years and above, particularly the infirm, destitute and widows among them, the need to implement broad based interventions targeting the family and community with the aim of improving the quality of life of the elderly, is also articulated in the policy. In light of the findings of the present study, any welfare package for the elderly has to be developed considering the low levels of literacy among them, their concentration in the rural areas and their primary occupation in the unorganized agricultural sector, poor financial security in terms of possession of assets, property and income, their dependence on others, their overall low standard of living which denies them basic amenities of daily living and poor access to means of mass communication to inform them about various programmes and services designed especially for them.

Furthermore those states that already have a larger share of the elderly population need to prioritise the development of a suitable package for their elderly. In addition, in view of the varied diseases and disabilities affecting the elderly as well as their life style patterns which further threatens their health, the government health services need to be equipped in terms of infrastructure and manpower training to address these special health needs of the elderly.

Finally, in view of the break up of the traditional familial way of life and industrialization and urbanization, the social and economic security of the elderly is also threatened. The state therefore needs to provide suitable institutional and other economic support to address the socio-economic needs of the elderly.

References

Dandekar, K. (1993). The aged, their problems and social intervention in Maharashtra, *Economic and Political Weekly, 27*(23), 1188 – 94.

Das, N. P., and Shah, U. (2001). *The social and health status of the elderly in India: Evidence from recent national level data*. A special report prepared as a part of the research initiative at the Population Research Centre, Baroda for the Ministry of Health and Family Welfare, New Delhi.

Dyson, T. (2002). *India's Population –The Future.* Paper presented at the workshop on India's Future: Population, Environment and Human Development, India International Centre, New Delhi, January 14 – 15, 2002.

Government of India (GOI). (2000). *Elderly in India: Profile and Programmes 2000*. New Delhi: Central Statistical Organization, Ministry of Statistics and Programme Implementation.

Government of India (GOI). (1998). The aged in India: A socio-economic profile: NSS 52nd Round, (July 1995 – June 1996). New Delhi: National Sample Survey Organization (NSSO), Department of Statistics, Ministry of Planning and Programme Implementation.

Government of India (GOI). (1991, October - December). Socio-economic profile of the aged persons: NSS 42nd Round (July, 1986 – June 1987). *Sarvekshana, Vol. 15, No. 2, Issue no.49.* New Delhi: National Sample Survey Organization (NSSO), Department of Statistics, Ministry of Planning.

Rajan I.S., Mishra, U. S., and Sankara Sarma, P. (1999). *India's Elderly: Burden or Challenge*. New Delhi: Sage Publications.

Rao, V.A., Vasudevan, P.M. and Madhavan, T. (1982). Psychosocial aspects of geriatric population: A community study in rural area near Madurai. In A. Kiev and A. Venkoba Rao (Eds.), *Readings in Transcultural Psychiatry*. Madras: Higginbothams.

Sharma, S. (1999). Elderly in India: Their Mental Health Poblems. In A. P. Bali (Ed.), *Understanding Greying People of India*. New Delhi: Inter-India Publications.

Sharma, S.P. and Xenos, P. (1992). *Ageing in India. Demographic Background and Analysis Based on Census Materials*. Occasional Paper No. 2, Office of the Registrar General and Census Commissioner, Government of India. New Delhi.

United Nations. (1987). *Population Ageing: Review of emerging issues*. Asian Population Studies, Series No.80. Bangkok, Thailand: United Nations Economic and Social Commission for Asia and the Pacific (UNESCAP).

2

Mental Health and Aging: Glimpses of the WSRC Project

Parul Dave, Pallavi Mehta, Purnima Khanna

Introduction

According to the definition in the World Health Organization (WHO) constitution, Health is a state of complete physical, mental and social well-being and not merely the absence of disease or infirmity. The WHO definition of health has been a landmark in two ways: one, its focus on positive health, and second, its holistic approach which includes the aspects of mental health and social well-being. This concept of health implies that a healthy person must actualize all the potentials of growth and development without being unduly tense or unhappy (Dutta Ray, 1993). Thus, mental health refers to emotional and psychological well-being along with others aspects of health that enable a person to lead a productive and fulfilling life.

The development of the field of mental health has been gradual and multidimensional. The journey of the shift from treatment of mental illness to promotion of mental health can be traced back to the seventeenth century. Until the seventeenth century, abnormal behavior was looked upon as an act of the 'Devil' or as possession by an evil spirit. In the later period, abnormal behavior was considered as 'criminal' (Murthy, 1993). Between the seventeenth and nineteenth centuries, the concept of 'insanity' as a medically treatable problem began to gain currency (Murthy and Burns, 1992). The impact of these shifts in understanding of and attitudes towards mental illness was seen on the treatment and services provided to mentally ill persons. From witchcraft, social isolation, confinement, and punishment the measures changed to medical treatment and institutionalization. With greater understanding of the role of psycho-social factors in mental health besides bio-medical factors, the scope for interventions also became broader. From asylums and institutions to psychiatric units in hospitals, and now the emergence of community mental health, the changes in the field of mental health albeit slow, have been remarkable and positive. The broadening of understanding about mental health has increased the scope for various kinds of interventions ranging from care and treatment of the ill to promotion of mental health.

Depression: The 'Common Cold' among Mental illnesses

At the global level, mental health problems currently are said to constitute about 8 percent of the global burden of diseases and more than 15 percent of adults in the developing societies are estimated to suffer from mental illness (Desjarlais et al., 1995). Mental disorders are projected to increase to 15 percent of the global disease burden by the year 2020 (Lewis and Araya, 2001). It is also estimated that at least 15 million people at some time in their lives will suffer from a truly severe, long-term disability (Vishwanathan and Wetzel, 1993).

In India, according to a north Indian Survey, the rate of psychiatric morbidity is 82 per 1000 population. This survey estimated that about 15 million people suffer from one or the other serious psychiatric illness and about 30 million people suffer from depressing and socially incapacitating emotional disorders (Bhatia, 1990 as cited in Ray, 1993). Prabhu and Raghuram (1987) have estimated that more than 30 million individuals suffer from mental illness every year and that 0 .175 million new cases are added every year.

In Gujarat, as per the Mission Report 2003 commissioned by the Government of Gujarat, there are an estimated 2.8 million adults with common and severe mental disorders at any given point in

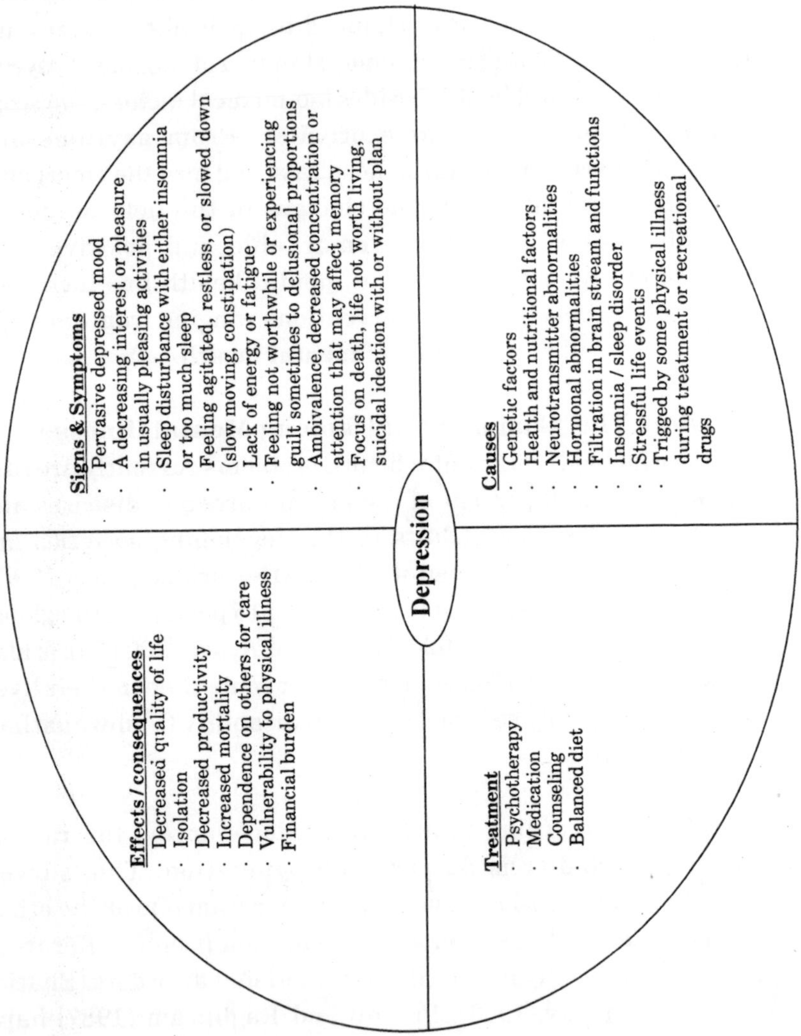
Depression
Signs & Symptoms
· Pervasive depressed mood
· A decreasing interest or pleasure in usually pleasing activities
· Sleep disturbance with either insomnia or too much sleep
· Feeling agitated, restless, or slowed down (slow moving, constipation)
· Lack of energy or fatigue
· Feeling not worthwhile or experiencing guilt sometimes to delusional proportions
· Ambivalence, decreased concentration or attention that may affect memory
· Focus on death, life not worth living, suicidal ideation with or without plan
Causes
· Genetic factors
· Health and nutritional factors
· Neurotransmitter abnormalities
· Hormonal abnormalities
· Filtration in brain stream and functions
· Insomnia / sleep disorder
· Stressful life events
· Trigged by some physical illness during treatment or recreational drugs
Effects / consequences
· Decreased quality of life
· Isolation
· Decreased productivity
· Increased mortality
· Dependence on others for care
· Vulnerability to physical illness
· Financial burden
Treatment
· Psychotherapy
· Medication
· Counseling
· Balanced diet

time in Gujarat. The occurrences of natural disaster and communal violence in the recent past are understood as significant contributors to the number of reported cases of depression, trauma and anxiety.

Depression is one of the most common psychiatric disorders that can affect anyone regardless of age, race, class or gender and hence referred to as the 'common cold' among mental illnesses. There is evidence to suggest that depression has increased over recent decades (A.D.A.M. Inc. Well-Connected reports).

The WHO estimates that within 20 years, recurrent depressive disorder will be the second most serious cause of morbidity in the world. According to the US Department of Health and Human Services, in Western industrialized nations, the lifetime risk for depression is 7-12 percent for men and 20-25 percent for women. Affective disorders like depression and mania are estimated to account for 50 percent of psychiatric inpatients. There are more than 400 million men and women in the world suffering from depression, out of which 40 million are from India (Vaishnav, 2002). In India, depression constitutes between 17 percent and 20 percent of all diagnosed psychiatric disorders in patients (Sharma, 1987).

Depression as often understood commonly by people is feeling sad or feeling low. Depression as a psychiatric disorder is different from feelings of sadness or lowness that we may experience in day to day life following setbacks or losses that we may face. Depressive disorder is identified on the basis of its persistence, severity, duration and the presence of other symptoms, which can be distinguished from the feelings of sadness that a person normally feels. The American Psychiatric Association (1994) has listed signs and symptoms of depression as shown in the following diagram. The presence of five or more of these symptoms over a period of two weeks is indicative of depression.

Causes of Depression

The causes of depression are however not fully known. Most likely a combination of genetic, biological (i.e. health and nutrition related) and environmental factors are at work. Available researches suggest a genetic or familial link to some of the psychiatric disorders, including depression (A.D.A.M. Inc. Well-Connected Report Series, 1999).

Nutritional deficiencies have been found to be widely prevalent among depressed people. Alterations in the manufacture and release of neurotransmitters in the human brain which are made of nutrients from food can also affect the way one feels and behaves. Thus besides genetic factors, intake of certain foods and medicines can also affect the chemical reactions of the brain, making one vulnerable to depression. Besides these there are several environmental factors which are found to be linked with depression. Changing social structures and value systems, break down of the family, lack of confiding relationships, family support, increased responsibilities, widowhood and divorce have been found to be associated with depression (Sethi and Manchanda, 1978; Amin, Shah and Vankar, 1998) Socio-economic factors like low income, low educational attainment, cramped living conditions, and stressful live experiences like loss of employment, end of a relationship or lack of positive relationships, may trigger depression (Net Doctor.co.uk, 2003; Brown and Harris, 1978; Blacker and Clare, 1987; Blue, et al., 1995).

Consequences of depression

The effects and consequences of depression are felt at various levels. Depression places excessive burden on individuals, families and the society. The burden refers to not only the economic burden in terms of direct cost of treatment, mortality and lost productivity but also the negative impact on the quality of life of the individual and the family. Although depression is a disorder that affects mental well being, it also proves harmful to the physical and social well-being of an individual. A study by Broadhead, Blazer and Tse (1990) found that people with symptoms of depression have 4.8 times higher risk than people without symptoms. Depression is often an exceptionally disabling condition, leading to difficulties in working and carrying out household tasks. Nearly 15 percent of people with depression commit suicide (Rider, 2000). Unlike many physical conditions, depression can also lead to a profound deterioration of relationships with friends, family and work colleagues that can give rise to particular difficulties (Lewis and Araya, 2001).

Depression in Adult and Older Women: Prevalence and Causes

The prevalence and diagnosis of mental health conditions are found to vary with gender. Women are more likely to be diagnosed with depression, anxiety disorders and eating disorders, whereas men are more likely to be diagnosed with substance abuse and certain types of personality disorders such as antisocial personality (Eichier and Parrot, 1987). According to the United Nations, women have higher rates of mental illness throughout the world (Women's International Network, 1993) in which depression and anxiety top the list (Vishwanathan and Wetzel, 1993). Women, regardless of their nationality or socio-economic status, have significantly higher rates of depression than do men. The chances that a woman will experience major depression at sometime during her life time range anywhere between 10 percent and 25 percent (APA, 1994).

Evidence for the higher depression rates among women is provided by community based studies of depression. These studies have reported sex ratio of depressed patients (female: male) as 2:1; in general practice this ratio rises to 3:1 or even to 4:1 (Blacker and Clare, 1987; Dunn and Skuse, 1981). Several other studies have indicated that both major depressive disorder and dysthymic disorders are two to four times more common in women than men (Kersler, McGonagle and Zhao 1994; McGrath, Keita, Strickland and Russo, 1990; Nolen-Hocksema, 1990; Sporck and Yoder, 1997). According to Davar (1995) where mental illness has biological bases, frequency of illness is same for both genders but where mental illness has a psycho-social basis, more women are mentally ill. Depression being one of the disorders that has a psycho-social basis explains higher prevalence of depression in women. Diane and Susan (2003) point out that the 2:1 ratio for prevalence of depression in women and men has been documented across different countries and ethnic groups. Besides prevalence, differences have also been reported between men and women in the nature of depressive symptoms, course of illness and response to treatment (Diane and Susan, 2003).

The prevalence of mental disorders is likely to rise as life expectancy increases (Vishwanathan and Wetzel, 1993). Depression is one of the most common psychiatric disorders in older persons.

In old age, depression is generally accompanied by other morbidities making the diagnosis more complex. Because of the complex relationship between depression, serious physical illnesses and drug interaction in older persons, an accurate diagnosis in this group is important, but not always easy (Well-Connected Reports, 1999). Many symptoms of depression, e.g. weight loss, fatigue, insomnia, are common to a number of physical ailments in old age, often resulting in mistaken diagnosis (Scanion). Some of the symptoms may be misunderstood to be normal symptoms of aging. The symptoms of depression in older persons are also often ignored or confused with other ailments common in the older persons including Parkinson's or Alzheimer's disease, dementia, thyroid disease, arthritis, stroke, cancer, heart disease and other chronic conditions (Well-Connected Reports, 1999).

Depression is also a side effect of many drugs that are commonly prescribed for the older persons. It thus becomes difficult to determine whether depression is a psychological reaction to the illness, caused by disease itself or is completely independent of the medical condition. Combination of these factors makes the diagnosis of depression in older persons a difficult task.

Malnutrition and Depression

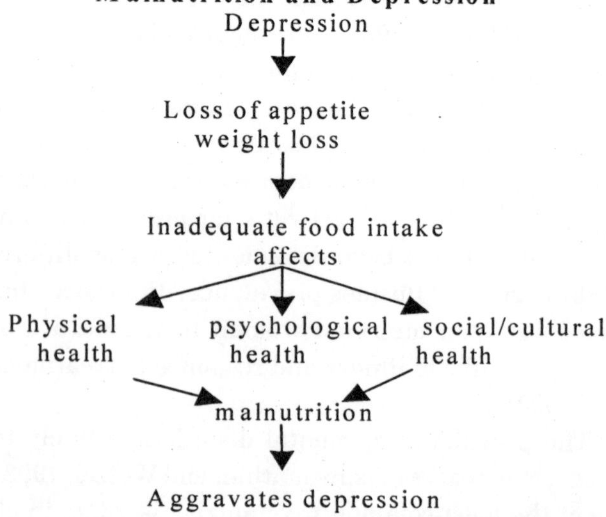

Despite the difficulties in diagnosing the psychiatric disorders in the older population, available data suggest high rates of depression in the older persons. Studies show that, in general, a third of the older population is depressed (Well Connected Reports, 1999). In India around 4 million people aged 60 and above are said to be suffering from mental illness (Lewis, 1988 as cited in Jaiprakash, 1997) and two-thirds of these are diagnosed as depressed (Jaiprakash, 1997). Rao and Madhavan (1997) estimated the prevalence of mental morbidity in those aged 60 or above at 89/1000 population in semi-urban area. The prevalence of depression in the community varies from 60/1000 (Rao and Madhavan, 1982 as cited in Rao, 1992) to 241/1000 (Kurup as cited in Rao, 1992).

Factors leading to Depression in Adult and Older Women

The causes for higher rate of depression amongst women are numerous and are often a mix of biological and cultural factors.

Nutritional factors

Nutrition is "the combination of process by which the during organism recess and utilizes the materials necessary for the maintenance of its functions and for the growth and renewal of its component" (Turner, 1959)

Malnutrition is an impairment of health resulting from a deficiency (under- nutrition), excess or imbalance of nutrients (over nutrition).

Depression leading to Malnutrition or vice versa is a vicious cycle that cannot be broken unless proper nutrient care and intervention strategies are developed to reduce the frequency and aggravation.

Available research suggests that nutrition does play a role in the development or maintenance of depression. Tanskanen and colleagues (2001) in Finland found 31 percent likelihood of having mild to severe of depression in 3204 males and females of age 25-64 years who consumed fish less than once a week which are all rich in omega – 3 PUFA (Poly Unsaturated Fatty Acid).

Tolmunen and associates (2003) investigated the association between dietary folate, cobalamine, pyridoxine and riboflavin. It was found that lower folate intake was significantly associated with depression.

In 1993, Christensen and colleagues studied the relation between carbohydrate craving and depression and found that carbohydrate helped in improving the symptoms of depression.

Specific Role of Nutrients in Depression

Nutrients	*Role in Depression*
Amino Acids Tryptophan, phenylalamines, Tyrosine Methnonine	Play a role in serotonin synthesis, conversation in the body act as endogenous stimulant and anti depressive substance.
Vitamins Folic acid and vitamin B12	Stimulate the synthesized form which is an essential co-engine in the formation of several neurotransmitters.
Vitamin B6	Vital for blood formation and healthy nervous system. It is believed to help in the break down of the estrogen hormone in the liver and may have an indirect effect over mood. Involved in the synthesis of monoamine neurotransmitters which is frequently deficient on people with depression.
Vitamin B1, D and C	Nerve vitamins, aids the absorption of calcium which is needed for relaxing nerves inducing sound sleep, antioxidant activity and facilitate synthesis of neurotransmitters.
Choline	It is considered as one of the major chemical messengers of the brain. It is precursor of the neurotransmitter acetylcholine essential for optimal memory functions.
Minerals Iron	Haemoglobin the carrier of oxygen to brain affects the attention and concentration resulting in low productivity.

Contd.

(Contd. Table)

Nutrients	*Role in Depression*
Copper	Brain has the second highest amount of Copper (370 mg/g) next to liver which itself reflects its role in the central nervous system.
Magnesium	Acts as a natural tranquilizer
Selenium	is a "good mood" seafood mineral because seafood is a rich source of this trace mental. Also has antioxidant properly.
Omega - 3 fatty acids	Mainly involved in oxidative mechanism acids majority Dihydroxy Acid and Eicasapentanoic Acid are needed for normal nervous system function.

Recent evidence indicates that naturally occurring low cholesterol concentration is associated with depression. Suarez (1999) conducted a study on 121 adult women, aged 18-27 years, and found significant association between low lipid and lipoprotein concentration with higher rates of depression anxiety.

Role of Nutrients in Aging

No.	*Nutrient*	*Physiological Role*	*Specific Role in Aging*
1.	Iron	Immune-competence	Preventing vulnerability of infectious disease
2.	Iron/Folate	Prevention of anemia	Maintaining appropriate level of activity in old age
3.	Calcium	Bone calcification	Preventing free radical damage in biological process
4.	Selenium	Antioxidant	Preventing free radical damage in biological process
5.	Vita-A Beta carotene, vita-C, E, lycopene	Antioxidant	Preventing free radical damage in old age e.g. arteriosclerosis, cataract, prevention of malignancies, control damage on other tissues and enzyme systems.

In old age, because of the general decline in health, vitality and activity, there are changes in the mental state, which mark the onset of affective disorders such as depression and dementia among the aging individuals. Loss of appetite and therefore under-nutrition, along with other nutritional deficiencies has been found to be widely prevalent among aging individuals. The interaction between nutrition and aging could be probed from two different approaches: a) with the biological ageing and associated physiological and structural changes in the body, the food preferences, food and nutrition intake, and at the same time, the nutritional requirements undergo considerable change. These are the impact of the ageing process on the aging individuals, their food intake and their consequences; b) the second approach explores whether specific foods and their nutrients can either slow down the aging process or accelerate it.

Specific nutritional deficiencies of Vitamins B-12, Vitamin B-6, Vitamin C, Tryptophan as well as excessive alcohol abuse can cause well recognized central nervous system disorder.

A cross-sectional study on 880 elderly subjects, aged 74-79 years, to assess their mental status found that depression was more prevalent in these subjects and that higher plasma levels of certain vitamins and carotenoids were associated with lower risk of developing dementia (Haller et al., 1998).

Clinical deficiencies of B vitamins in the elderly have been implicated in brain related disorders inducing reversible dementia, depression and electrophysiological dysfunction, including convulsions.

A study conducted on 79 male subjects aged 54-81 years. They observed an association between lower plasma concentrations of Vitamin B-12 and folate and higher concentration of homocysteine with poor spatial coping skills and cognitive performance (Riggs et. al., 1996).

Recent evidence suggests that naturally occurring low cholesterol concentration are associated with depression. Suarez (1999) conducted a study on 121 adult women aged 18-27 years found significant association between low lipid and lipoprotein concentration with higher rates of depression and anxiety.

In 1993, Christensen and colleagues studied the relation between carbohydrate craving and depression and found that carbohydrate helped in improving the symptoms of depression. Also the anti-depressant effect of tryptophan via the production of serotonin has been revealed where the underlying notion is that because serotonin is synthesized from tryptophan and the brain tryptophan level is dependent on both the diet and uptake of tryptophan into the brain decreased the availability of tryptophan by restricting the dietary intake of this amino acid should therefore decrease the amount of serotonin that can be synthesized.

Several studies have been conducted in India to assess the dietary intake and nutritional status of elderly individuals living under different situations, but their impact on mental health and the extent to which subtle nutritional deficiencies can lead to a poor mental state is not yet clear.

By and large, most elderly individuals are vulnerable to nutritional deficiencies and their impact on health mostly due to the following reasons.

- Most of them are economically dependent on others. They select foods by considering the cost and not their nutrient contents.
- They consume diets served by others, as in old age institutions, which in most cases are unsatisfactory. Most of those who cater to clients of very low economic strata are not aware of the specific nutritional needs of the elderly and how to respond to individual needs given the economic constraints.
- Most elderly individuals are socially isolated. A significant proportion of the elderly population especially elderly females are patients of depression, and even various types of dementia. Loss of appetite and lack of interest in food are common features of such conditions.

Indian elderly, especially the aged women are at a high risk of chronic undernutrition (Gopalan et al., 1992). Malnutrition among the aged is caused by a number of factors such as conditioning of the family, poverty, ignorance, superstition, lack of food, poor environmental sanitation, increased incidence of disease and disabilities which lead to alteration in dietary intake, absorption and metabolism of nutrients, endocrine imbalances, inability to chew, physical handicaps that prevent adequate shopping or food preparation, loneliness and lack of interest in eating and misconception concerning diet, undesirable social customs and traditional prejudices, and frequent infection.

Hormonal factors

All women are at risk for emotional swings when they experience extreme hormonal shifts. The role of hormones in depression is not clear, but female hormones undoubtedly play some role in premenstrual dysphoria, postpartum depression, and seasonal affective disorder (SAD). These forms of depression recede or stop after menopause. Evidence for hormonal causes of depression is mostly based on observations of depression during specific stages in female development. Women constantly undergo hormonal change throughout their life cycle. Hormonal changes begin from a very young age – that of adolescence when the menstrual cycle starts. These changes continue through every month of the menstrual cycle and in later years during pregnancy, lactation and then to changes during pre and perimenopause and finally to menopause[1]. These fluctuations in hormone levels can cause depression in women.

Postpartum depression is relatively common with a prevalence rate approximately the same as that for depression in non-pregnant women. Between 30 percent and 75 percent of women experience mild postpartum 'blues', lasting for 4 to 10 days. Postpartum depression is characterized by labile mood, fearfulness, irritability, anxiety and sleep and appetite disturbance. If physical symptoms and depressed mood persist for two weeks, patients should be evaluated for postpartum major depression, particularly if they have a history of depression. The risk is increased in women depression during, with a history of pre-menstrual dependant depression, during pregnancy, pre-menopause state and experience of negative life events during pregnancy, and having inadequate social support system and marital problems.

The most common cause of depression in women due to hormonal fluctuation takes place after the fourth decade of life. Major endocrine changes occur in women around the age of 40-45 years. There is a marked decline in estrogen production that leads to a series of changes commonly known as menopausal changes.

In women, after the age of 35, the ovary begins to decrease in weight and size and contains fewer oocytes and follicular structures. Fluctuating estrogen levels accompany perimenopausal transition. Estrogen modulates neurotransmission at multiple points in the serotonin pathway. The serotonin pathway is known to contribute to the regulation of behavior and mood. Perimenopausal and menopausal women are also at a risk of developing breast cancer, endometrial cancer, venous thrombosis and cardio vascular disease.

Upadhyaya and Chaturvedi (1988) conducted a 3-month study on women aged 25-35 years and 40-50 years attending an outpatient clinic. A total of 24 women were in the group of 40-50 years and 24 were in 25-35 years age groups. Thirty three percent of the perimenopausal women had depression and 20 percent of them had physical diagnosis associated with their psychiatric problem, like hypothyroid features, hypertension, malignancy and diabetes.

A study conducted by Dennerstein and associates (1999) for a period of 6 years involving 354 women aged 45-55 years, found that negative mood scores decreased significantly related to the natural menopausal transition, Follicle Stimulating Hormone, estradiol, inhibition, age and education. At risk were those women who already reported depressed mood, had a history of premenstrual complaints, had negative attitudes to menopause and to aging, were current smokers, did little exercise and had no partner or had only one child.

Witteman and colleagues (1989) conducted a study on 294 premenopausal women and 319 postmenopausal women. It was observed that carotid arteriosclerosis was present in 3 percent of postmenopausal women which was 3-4 times greater than in premenopausal women. This research may suggest that when estrogen production stops, the risk of arteriosclerosis is increased. It has been studied that estrogen deficiency results in malabsorption of dietary calcium. Estrogens are known to increase the intestinal absorption of calcium. Hence menopausal women are at higher risk of osteoporoses.

Winner and associates (1989) in their study found an increase in risk of falling among women, but not men, from ages 45-49 up to 55-59, followed by a decrease till age 70. The study concluded that chances in the risk of falling interact with osteoporosis in perimenopausal age.

Martini and colleagues (1994) conducted a study on 18 pressure menopausal women (20-34 years) where a significant increase was observed in energy, protein, carbohydrate and fat intake in midluteal phase as compared to midfollicular phase. Intakes of vitamin D, riboflavin, potassium phosphorous and magnesium were also significantly higher during this phase. The results supported the regulation of food intake by menstrual cycle hormones. Women who lived through extended periods of economic hardship were also more likely to begin this physical transition earlier. According to a report published in the Journal of Epidemiology and Community Health, stress, nutrition or toxins such as lead and tobacco smoke accelerate the rate at which eggs are depleted. Egg depletion is known to trigger perimenopause.

Health factors

In India, women bear a high burden of reproductive ill health which is an outcome of their poverty, powerlessness, low social status, malnutrition, infection, high fertility, and lack of access to health care. These factors play a role in women's health seeking behavior: that is, what women do when they have a health problem. The community's health culture also reflects the traditional values and biases related to women's health. Also, the accessibility, quality and range of health services provided, which include unsuitable time schedule, distance to clinic, loss of wages, lack of time on part of women (Mulgaonkar et al., 1994), and major influences on whether women feel inclined to seek medical help. But the interrelationship between poverty and utilization of health services is not always understood clearly. Most health services run by the government are provided free of charge but they are seen as worthless in comparison with the services offered at high cost by the private sector. All association between the quality and cost of services is so ingrained in the minds of the lay public that costly treatment is synonymous with quality treatment.

Women going through the menopausal phase seem to be more at risk for conditions such as osteoporosis and various forms of health disease. Doctors are beginning to suspect a link between Alzheimer disease (more prevalent in women than in men) and the changes that the body undergoes during menopause.

Many other gynecological problems are found in postmenopausal women like neoplasms, cancer of cervix, genital prolapse, senile vaginitis, malignant ovarian tumor (Debnath et al., 1994; Banajee and Hallie; 1976; Gath et al.; 1987).

According to Griffith (2002) the number of depressive symptoms increases as the number of small areas of damage in basal ganglia increase. These small lesions could represent a breakdown in the connection between the basal ganglia and the cortex. The presence of small blockages could directly relate to the degree of depressive symptoms. The Cardiovascular Health Study examined people over 65 selected from Medicare lists living in 4 areas of USA. MRI scan was conducted on 3500 volunteers and a short questionnaire was administered. MRI scans revealed changes in certain areas of the brain suggestive of loss of blood supply. Depressive symptoms were more common in older people, women, those with high blood pressure, heart disease and some disabilities.

In current psychiatric epidemiology much emphasis is given to stressful life events. Hansen and Jacobsen (1989) conducted a cross sectional study on 13,704 people male and female 20-54 years of age. It was reported that marital status, financial condition during childhood and current lifestyle were found to be highly significantly associated with mental distress.

According to WHO (2001) psychiatric and neurological disorders account for nearly a third of the world's disability, measured in years lived disability. Comorbidity is another factor that increases the incidence of depression. The increasing comorbidity of cardiovascular and a cerebrovascular disease is due to depression, whereas depression is also secondary to conditions like cancer, diabetes mellitus, asthma and AIDS (Shah, 1999).

Immune failures may contribute to mental illness, as demonstrated in AIDS, as patients live longer and develop psycho-neurological complications. Almost all known auto immune diseases occur predominantly in females, rheumatoid arthritis, 2:1; multiple sclerosis, 2:1; diabetes and hypertension, which are also female predominant diseases producing changes in brain activity. Any clinical or serious illness that is life-threatening or out of a person's control can lead to depression.

Studies have reported a strong association between depression and headaches, including chronic tension type, and migraine. Some experts believe that a syndrome of migraine headaches, anxiety and depression is caused by common factors such as abnormalities in chemical messengers, particularly dopamine or serotonin.

Ross (1989), using data from a representative sample of 2020 adults – 18 years and older, found no direct effect of being overweight on depression in most groups. Overweight persons were more likely to diet and to experience worse physical health, both of which were associated with depression. However, being overweight could lead depression among the more educated (but not among the less educated).

Han and colleagues (1991) found no overall association between obesity and mental health functioning using the mental health measure from the SF-36 in a sample aged 20-59 years in the Netherlands. However, men in the highest percentile of obesity were likely to report not being happy and women in the highest percentile for obesity were more likely to report depressed mood.

Other factors to consider:

- *Medications:* a number of drugs taken for chronic problems cause depression. Among them are pain relievers for arthritis, cholesterol lowering drugs, medications for high blood pressure and heart problems, and bronchodilators used for asthma, and other lung disorders.
- *Smoking:* There is a significant association between cigarette smoking and susceptibility to depression. Smoking impairs blood flow to the head via its vasoconstrictive action and displaces carbon dioxide in the erythrocytes. It also uses up vitamins C and B6. People who are prone to depression face 25 percent chance of becoming depressed. When they quit smoking this increased risk persists for at least 6 months.

Poor health, decreasing ability to function are some of the factors responsible for depression in aging women. A nationwide

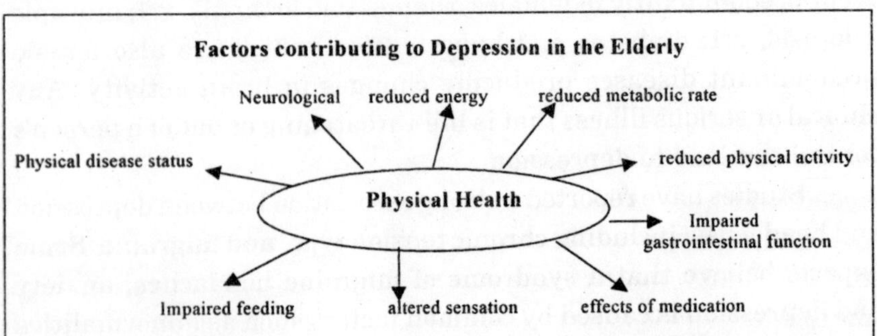

survey conducted by NSSO (1991) revealed that about 45 percent of elderly suffered from chronic illness. Socio-demographic factors not only influence the extent and severity of morbidity among the elderly but their quality of life as well (NSSO, 1991). Majority of the health problems among the aged are diet related and nutrition dependent (UNCAN). Nutritional assessment of the elderly plays a significant role in identifying those who are at "nutritional risk" (Anthony, 1993).

Morely and Silver (1998) found in their study that poor dentition, immobility, inability to feed oneself decreases food intake. Dormenual and associates in the same year carried out a study on elderly subjects aged 30 years and above and found that oral dryness and low salivary inflow were associated with loss of appetite and low body mass index among the elderly.

Smolen and Grosvenor (1997) found that the intake of medication for a long period alters appetite and decreases nutrient absorption.

Women, thus, in their entire life span face several stressful situations coupled with the physiological changes in the course of their physical development and reproductive age in the larger context of a patriarchal society. The complex web of these factors contributes to depression and its associated consequences in women's lives. The process of aging and resultant changes increase the vulnerability of women further. The increase in life span is associated with a variety of physiological problems that may affect dietary intakes and result in morbidity in the elderly.

Psycho-social and cultural factors

The diagnosis pattern extensively used in psychiatry is often criticized due to its failure to consider women's psychological needs and their social realities that differ from those of men. According to Taylor (1988) etiology of women's distress is different and psychology of women needs to be understood in the context of the patriarchal social relations. The exposure to stressful events, the nature of mental health problem, the manifestation of the disorder and even the social and familial response differ in the case of women from men. Mental disorders in women can be linked directly with alienation, powerlessness and poverty conditions most frequently experienced by women (Dennerstein, Astbury and Morse, 1993). Other potentially stressful factors affecting women's psychological well being are unequal work distribution, work overload, rigid role functions and stereotyping (Davar, 1995). Some of the most important factors related to depression in women are discussed below.

Socialization: Right from the birth through the entire life span there are considerable differences in the way men and women are socialized. From very early in life boys and girls get messages from their parents, families and society about approved and disapproved behaviours, roles and even expression of emotions. It is this difference in the socialization of men and women that largely makes women vulnerable to depression.

Contradiction in the image and expectations: Identity formation is an important factor in the process of personality development. Portrayal of women having dual image proves to be very stressful for women's mental health as it leads to more contradictory expectations from women. "Through our roles as wives and mothers, women largely act as the emotional caretakers and nurturers of society. Yet women are caricatured as dependent in the sense of being clinging, helpless and weak and it is this stereotype that women find difficult to assimilate (Taylor, 1990 as cited in Mane, 1993).

Another duality in the expectations that is emerging in recent times is about the traditional and contemporary roles of women. On one hand women are expected to be strong, independent, assertive, and be superwomen capable of handling both home and career efficiently. On the other hand, however, she is still expected to be "good girl" or "good wife" and "daughter-in-law" by being docile, obedient and passive. These dual expectations can cause immense distress and affect women's mental health.

Low self-esteem and self denial: Through various forms of discrimination, like preference to male child and denial of basic needs, like adequate food, clothing, attention, health care and education, women are made to believe that they are unwanted, inferior and a burden to the family. They are socialized to give importance to their family and social relations rather than fulfillment of their individual needs. A study by Rao Gupta (1985) showed that when faced with conflict and stress, women continuously sacrifice their personal needs and welfare for the needs and well-being of their families. When they were asked why they resorted to this behavior, they respond that they were taught in childhood to adjust to their circumstances without complaining. Being oriented towards passivity, submission and a life of self-denial, women develop traits connected with low self-esteem like depressive moodiness, over touchiness and morbid sensitivity (Kakar, 1988). According to Jack (1991) "Loss of self can result when in an effort to smooth and protect valued relationships, women develop habit of censoring their own expression and restricting their own initiatives. Over time, habitual self-censorship can lead to duplicity of experiences in which outer compliance is paired with inner confusion and frustration, often with ensuing depression".

Learned helplessness: Learned helplessness can be understood in the context of power and control. Seligman (1991) applied the researches on learned helplessness to explain depression. It was argued that people learn this behaviour in response to their inability to control events in their lives. This theory has been used to explain how the powerlessness that women experience in relationships and in the workplace can lead to reduced motivation and depression. Russo (1990) used this theory to explain why women who are low-income or single parent are particularly likely to be depressed. Wenegrat (1995) theorizes that women who have least power and control are most likely to develop depression, whereas women who have power and control are least likely to develop depression.

Factors related to social roles of women: The following are some of the factors which are said to be associated with depression in women.

Role accumulation/multiple roles: Women are more likely than men to suffer the stress of multiple roles, not only because they play many more roles than men but also because they play their roles simultaneously, while men more typically play their role sequentially (Harrington, 1983; and Rao Gupta, 1985). The role that marriage and children play in a woman's depression is complex. Women experience stress from juggling the demands of multiple roles, including that of employee, wife, mother, daughter-in-law and housekeeper. Fulfilling the responsibilities of multiple roles may account for why gender differences in depression are even greater among those individuals who are married than those who are unmarried (Gove, 1972; Radloff, 1975; Wu and DeMaris, 1996). The Report on women worldwide issued by the World Health Organization in 1996, indicated that married women with children had a higher risk for depression than did married childless women, single women or single or married men (Well-Connected Reports, 2002). The pressure of handling too many things at the same time causes stress, and failure to perform any of the roles may affect self esteem negatively, making women vulnerable to depression. This may lead to the assumption that women who do not have dual responsibilities may be less prone to depression. However this assumption also has been disproved. The perceived low status and isolation accompanying the role of housewife may lead to depression in a young mother. A European study reported that depression increased in men and fell in women between 1980 and 1995, a period coinciding with more women entering the workforce (Well-Connected Reports, 2002).

Role conflict: Multiple roles place greater burden on women and since most of the times the demands arising out of the roles are contradictory, they lead to role conflict. Being a working woman, a young mother and a daughter-in-law at the same time not only requires a woman to struggle with her limited resources but also requires her to play docile and nurturing as well as assertive roles at the same time. Not being able to handle these contradictory demands women may be criticized or feel guilty themselves. A study by Sethi and Dube (1982) suggested that there was a higher prevalence of guilt feelings in depressed women which could be attributed to a harsh and punishing super ego.

Deprivation or distortion of primary roles: Since marriage and motherhood are the primary status roles affecting a woman's identity, their absence, suspension or disruption in any form may cause serious threats to a woman's mental health (Mane, 1993). Khorana and Vyas have given a list of such circumstances which includes - being unmarried, divorced/separated, widowed, childless or having children who are handicapped (socially, physically, mentally), being deprived of the capacity to reproduce or loss of a child either prior to birth (miscarriage/abortion) or at birth (still birth), and sterilization. This explains the higher rates of depression in women who are widowed, divorced, and separated or women who face crisis in their married life.

Socio-economic status: Women as such are accorded lower status in their families and society. Low socio-economic status and the challenges associated with it increase the distress and increase the chances of women being depressed. The case studies of women from low income slums showed high rates of psychiatric morbidity in low-income slum dwelling and uneducated women (Blue et al; 1995) Women who are employed as agricultural labourers or with little education were most affected by mental illness (Vindhya, Kiranmayi and Vijayalakshmi, 2001).

Experience of violence and abuse: Experience of violence (physical or emotional) and sexual abuse in childhood or at any stage in life has severe repercussions on women's mental health. Feelings of shame, helplessness, vulnerability and depression are some of the long-term negative effects of sexual assault and domestic violence (Stewart and Robinson, 1995 as cited in Burt and Hendrick). The psychological dysfunctions associated with experiencing violence can also have fatal consequences like inducing suicidal behaviour. Battered women are four to five times more likely to require psychiatric treatment and five times more likely to attempt suicide than non-battered women (Purewal, 2003). Women with mental illness have reported experience of childhood sexual abuse and violence and/or discrimination within the marital home such as domestic violence, harassment by the in-laws, sexual coercion and reproduction related pressure or control (Purewal, 2003). Statistics on suicide indicate that female suicide due to harassment, dowry, and other problems related to women's familial roles is high in India. A one-year study of completed suicides in Delhi revealed that 56 percent of suicide cases were women. Most commonly reported reasons for suicide included marital discord and ill-treatment by husband and in-laws (Mullen, et al., 1998).

Industrialization and urbanization have led to socio-cultural changes at a large scale in society, and these have had adverse effect on the lives of older persons. Break down of joint families, increasing migration of the younger generation of the population, rising importance and utilization of new age modern technology compared to traditional wisdom – all these factors have collectively contributed in making older people feel alienated and adversely affected their well being. The variables such as, marital status, living arrangements, annual income, nature of family, family composition, satisfaction in social contacts, having friends, involvement in decision making, adjustment with old age, feeling of isolation, participation in leisure time activities, recreation, sufficiency of food, satisfaction of needs, savings and feeling secure are found to have significant association with geriatric depression (Sonar, 2004).

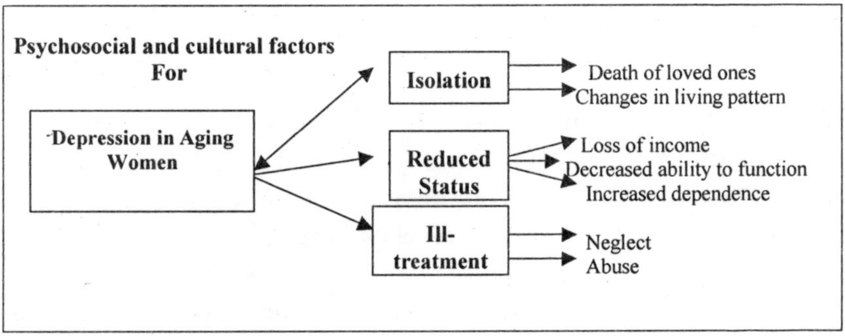

Isolation: The feeling of isolation can be caused by several factors, such as death of loved ones, changes in living patterns.

Death of loved ones: Depression is associated with the losses experienced at different times over the later life course, the most common being widowhood (Jaiprakash, 1997). A study by Jamuna, Lalitha and Ramamurthi (2004) suggested that with increasing age there was a gradual decline in self-esteem among widows. Psychological problems like feeling of self-worthlessness, loneliness, emotional inadequacies and economic dependency, which are brought on by widowhood make older women more miserable and vulnerable to negative changes in their self-perception and self-concept (Reddy and Jamuna, 1992 as cited in Jamuna, Lalitha and Ramamurthi, 2004). Loss of other significant relations, like death of friends and relatives of the same age adds to the distress of older people.

Changes in living patterns: According to the seven stages of family life by Duval, the stage when the couple is in their middle age is called 'empty-nest', i.e. when the younger generation leaves the house due to marriage, higher studies, careers and such reasons. Due to the prevalence of the joint family system in India, earlier this theory was not considered to be applicable, however, with the break-down of joint families and increased migration for higher education, better job opportunities and other advantages, older people are increasingly being left to live on their own. The social network being more central to women's lives compared to men, women may find it difficult to adjust when isolated. Several studies reveal that living alone and lack of social support causes reduced sense of well-being and depression (Rai, 1972; Ramachandran, 1980; Kaur and Kaur, 1987 as cited in Rikhi and Chadha, 2004).

In light of the socio-cultural changes discussed above, alternate arrangement for the care of older persons has become inevitable. The need for institutionalization is increasing day by day because of the breaking down of kinship and family organization. Studies have reported that long term residence in an institution leads to poor physical health, feeling of fatigue and depression, lower level of adjustment and dissatisfaction with life in older persons (Srivastava and Agrawal, 2002). Srivastava and Agrawal (2002) found higher rates of depression in older persons living in institutions than those living with their children.

Reduced status: Reduced social and economic status has adverse effect on the self-esteem of older women. Increased dependence and resultant low self esteem are considered to be related to depression. Kariguda (2001) reports that the problems of older women are not due to the aging process, but a result of their subordinate status throughout their life cycle.

Decreased ability to function: Deteriorating health restricts the mobility and ability to function in older women. They cannot contribute in the housework as before due to decreased physical capacity. Disabling health problems during old age makes them more dependent on others.

Loss of income: Along with physical dependence, economic dependence also a major cause for distress in older persons. Economic problems are the main source of stress, which increase with age (Vandana and Subramanyam, 2004). Retirement of self or spouse, both, directly or indirectly leads to loss of income and thus reduced status within the household. Besides loss of income, retirement also may create a void in the lives of working women. The feeling that one is no more a contributing member affects the self-esteem of older women. Patil (2000) reveals that low level of income is responsible for dissatisfaction, low health status and level of depression among older persons. Sonar (2004) in the study of Pensioners found that poor economic conditions increased the risk of depression among the old age pensioners.

Ill-treatment of older persons: There are studies showing increased incidents of abuse and neglect of older persons by the family members (Rao, 1995; Chakraborty, 2004; Khan, Vanlalhriatpuit and Gandotra, 2004). Studies indicate that more women than men experienced maltreatment like physical and verbal abuse (Rao, 1995; Srinivas, 1996; Chakraborty, 2004). Experience of abuse and neglect may leave older women helpless and depressed. Studies point towards a reciprocal relationship or a vicious cycle of ill treatment and depression. They suggest that ill treatment leads to depression and depression in turn makes older women more vulnerable to abuse and neglect. Khan, Vanlalhriatpuit and Gandotra (2004) found that older persons who are ill, disabled, mentally impaired or depressed are at a greater risk for abuse.

All the factors discussed above are essentially interlinked and thus it may be difficult to understand each specific factor leading to depression in old age separately from the others. The above discussion suggests that aging in a society that is in transition, from a traditional and collective society to a modernized, industrialized and individualistic one, poses several threats for older persons to develop depressive symptoms. Women, a group that is already disadvantaged in many ways, face additional challenges in old age, reinforcing the etiology of depression.

Background of the Project – 'Mental Health and Aging'

Mental health is an area long neglected in the public health discourse. As mental health is crucial for the overall well being of individuals, societies and countries, it must be universally regarded in a new light.

Among mental health disorders, depression is the most common. Referred to as the 'common cold' among mental illnesses, depression poses as a major public health challenge in the coming years. According to WHO estimates, within the next 20 years, recurrent depressive disorder will be the second most serious cause of morbidity in the world.

Available literature indicates women and older people being more at risk of depression due to physiological and socio-cultural reasons. The vulnerability of older women to depression is increased due to the process of aging, poor health, under nutrition, decreasing ability to function, loss of spouse, and other significant relations, feeling of isolation, insecurity, economic dependency, decreasing importance in the family, and so forth. The problem of depression in older women may be more complex due to the difficulty in recognizing depression in older persons and their double disadvantage of being women and elderly persons at the same time.

There is thus an urgent need for interventions to combat depression in women, particularly older women. For this, it is important to understand the role that various psycho-social, health and nutrition related factors associated with depression play in the onset of depression, and how women understand and cope with it. An understanding of the specific factors associated with aging would also help in the design of more appropriate and effective interventions to combat depression.

In view of this, the project 'Mental Health and Aging' was undertaken by the Women's Studies Research Centre (WSRC) of The Maharaja Sayajirao University of Baroda from Aug 2003 to Aug 2005.

The project had a research as well as an intervention component. As part of the research, conducted in two phases, two studies were conducted. The first study, conducted in the first phase of the project examined the prevalence of mental disorders as reported in the psychiatric units of private and public hospitals and private practitioners in six major cities of Gujarat state, India. The purpose was to assess the magnitude of depression in relation to the other psychiatric disorders. The second study, made an attempt to understand the prevalence of depression in women in the free-living population of Vadodara city, of Gujarat. The purpose was to carry out an in-depth study of the psychosocial and cultural aspects of their lives as well as their health and nutrition status, so as to understand the role of factors related to these aspects in depression in women.

As an intervention, several elderly women in the sample were provided Folic Acid supplementation to study its impact on depression in these women.

The present paper discusses the findings of the research and interventions carried out under the project.

Prevalence of Mental Disorders in Gujarat: Evidence from Retrospective and Prospective Data

To study the prevalence of mental disorders, in phase 1 of the project, retrospective and prospective (point prevalence) data were obtained from the medical records of cases of public hospitals and psychiatric wards of general hospitals, and clinics of private practitioners in six cities of Gujarat, namely - Ahmedabad, Bhavnagar, Jamnagar, Rajkot, Surat, and Vadodara.

The retrospective data were drawn from the records of the cases of mental disorders reported in the health facilities between October 2000 to October 2002. Though the focus of the study was on aging women, records of both males and females above the age of 40 were obtained. To ensure representation of all socio-economic groups, both public and private sector facilities were included. It was however found that none of the general hospitals maintained proper records of patients and finally, data were obtained primarily from mental hospitals and psychiatrists who had private practice.

The prospective prevalence data were obtained from the records of patients visiting the hospital or clinic in the period of one continuous week preceding the data collection from the six cities.

The study tool was a proforma that elicited information on age, sex, diagnosis of mental health disorder by the psychiatrists, precipitating factors for the disorder diagnosed, duration of illness and treatment administered, and hospitalization required.

In all, 17,710 records were obtained from public (4,775 records) and private hospitals and clinics (12,935 records), of which 10,908 were retrospective data and 6,802 were prospective data. The distribution of the retrospective and prospective data according to sex of the patients and their distribution by city were as follows:

Distribution of Retrospective and Prospective Data According to age of the patients and City

City	*Retrospective*				*Prospective*			
	Female	*Male*	*Sex not mentioned*	*Total*	*Female*	*Male*	*Sex not mentioned*	*Total*
Ahmedabad	1961	2301	1	4263	903	1103	7	2013
Bhavnagar	73	88	-	161	317	362	4	6831
Jamnagar	567	686	22	1275	219	214	22	455
Rajkot	430	534	7	971	489	644	10	1143
Surat	1008	1444	2	2454	647	855	12	1514
Vadodara	719	1063	2	1784	423	531	40	994
Total	**4758**	**6116**	**34**	**10908**	**2998**	**3709**	**95**	**6802**

Prospective and retrospective data collected from six major cities on clients of mental health services showed that:

- Depression and schizophrenia are the most prevalent mental health disorders, followed by anxiety disorder and bipolar disorders.
- Depression is included as either a cause or a symptom of other disorders, like mixed anxiety, somatoform disorders or generalized medical conditions.
- People in the age group of 26-40 years have the highest number of mental health problems. The reported cases of depression increase with increase in age, whereas the number of reported cases of schizophrenia drops in the age groups above 40 years.
- Some disorders are related with age; for example, mental retardation and seizures are reported more in the younger age group, whereas dementia is prevalent in older people.
- There are gender differences not only in the prevalence of mental health disorders but also in the utilization of mental health services. Bipolar disorder, anxiety and schizophrenia, sexual dysfunctions, substance abuse are found to be more prevalent in men, while depression is found to be significantly higher in women than in men. The fact that more men than women availed of mental health services indicates that mental health problems of women are underreported.
- There are differences in prevalence of various disorders across the six cities. The number of cases of depression is reported highest in Surat in both retrospective as well as prospective data, whereas schizophrenia is reported highest in Vadodara, in which women outnumbered men. The prevalence of schizophrenia is high in Jamnagar. However, interestingly, prevalence of depression is found to be much less here compared to other cities. Sexual dysfunctions are reported more in Surat compared to other cities. Substance use related disorders are found to be higher in larger cities, like Ahmedabad, Surat and Vadodara compared to other cities indicating the effect of stressful urban life on people, on men in particular, who turn to alcohol and other substances to cope with stress.

- In most of the cases, the medical records do not mention the precipitating factors for the particular disorder in the patients.
- The treatment options for mental disorders are mainly pharmacological, and in some cases, ECT is administered.
- There are systemic constraints which have affected the study of prevalence of mental disorders as well as the quality of service delivery. For instance, most of the civil hospitals did not maintain the records of OPD patients, though such information is critical for research, policy and program initiatives; the doctor-patient ratio was very poor in some of the cities. For example, in the OPD of the civil hospital in Jamnagar, there were only two doctors who attended to as many as 150 to 200 patients per day, all within a span of 3 hours!

Depression in Adult and Older Women

To study the prevalence of depression in adult and aging women from the free living population, in phase 2 of the project, in-depth interviews were conducted with women over 40 years of age in Vadodara city. The study design for this phase was both descriptive and experimental.

Vadodara city was divided into 25 areas, which were further classified into localities representing three income groups, viz. high,

Selection Criteria for In-depth Interview

inclusion criteria	*exclusion criteria*
1. Age: > 40 Yrs	1. Age: < 40 Yrs
2. Category of Depression Score on BDI: 20-28	2. Category of Depression Score on BDI: <20 & >28
3. Income Group: - Lower - Middle - Upper	3. Medical History - Cancer - Cardiac Disease - Dementia - Alzheimer's Disease - Parkinson's Disease - Post Operative
	4. Mental Illness - Psychosis - Mental Retardation

middle, and low income localities, on the basis of the socio-economic status of the pre-dominant population in each area. Using the snowball sampling method, subjects were identified from each locality of the city. The Beck's Depression Inventory (BDI) was used for screening women for depression. On the basis of their scores on the BDI they were identified as having 'minimal', 'mild', 'moderate' and 'severe' depression. The process of screening was continued till the sample of 180 women required for the in-depth interviews was reached.

After screening, the respondents for the in-depth interviews were selected based on the following criteria.

Those women who were selected according to these criteria were included for the in-depth study based on their consent and willingness to participate. A detailed structured interview schedule covering the psychosocial aspects and nutritional and health aspects of women's mental health was administered.

In all, 426 women were screened. Out of these, 180 women who fulfilled the inclusion criteria, i.e., were 40 and above years of age and had a moderate degree of depression, were selected for in-depth interview. In addition to the 180 women selected for in-depth interviews, 20 women over 60 years of age from the middle income group were selected as controls primarily to compare their nutritional status. For the purpose of analysis, women were categorized into two age groups 40-60 years and above 60 years, and into three income groups – low, middle and high.

The distribution of women with various grades of depression by their age and economic status is presented in Table 1.

Table 1: Distribution of the women screened for depression by age and income group

Level of depression	*Score range*	*40-60 yrs*			*>60 yrs*			
		LIG	*MIG*	*HIG*	*LIG*	*MIG*	*HIG*	*Total*
Minimal	0-12	12	66	41	4	37	13	173
Mild	13-19	5	20	8	8	19	2	62
Moderate	20-28	30	30	30	30	30	30	180
Severe	29+	2	0	1	4	2	2	11
Total	-	**49**	**116**	**80**	**46**	**88**	**47**	**426**

Psychosocial Profile of Women Identified as Moderately Depressed

There are several factors in a person's background that constitute a risk for depression, and life events which often bring about it. Counterbalancing these are factors which are protective, such as social support and security of the environment. It is usually the interplay of these that determine whether a person develops depression rather than one factor. This is why some people develop depression even in the absence of an adverse life and while in other a major life event does not lead to depression.

Precipitating factors can be stressful life events such as bereavement, acute physical illness of self or someone close, major financial crisis, negative interactions with family members or friends, etc. Other chronic stressors are declining health, dependence, socio-economic decline, marital difficulties, problems at work, retirement or loneliness and isolation.

Besides these risk factors and precipitating factors there are also factors which may protect against it, such as good nutrition, physical fitness, adaptive, integrated personality, capacity for confiding relationships, active coping styles to overcome adversity (as opposed to helplessness), besides a tangible social support and religious/spiritual beliefs.

Thus psycho-social aspects play an important role in determining rates and progression of depression in women. Living conditions, marital status, cultural factors, contradictions in the image and expectations, burden of fulfilling multiple roles, conflict in relationships, experience of violence, neglect or abuse, women's status within the power structure of the family, stressful life events – all these aspects have a bearing on the mental health of women. Therefore an attempt was made in the present study to collect information in this regard through in-depth interviews with 180 moderately depressed women age 40 years and above. The findings have been presented in this section.

Perceptions regarding various stages of life

In the in-depth interview, women were asked – "Which is the stage of life that you liked the most and the least and why? (Stages of life: childhood, adolescence, adulthood and middle age and old age). This question was specifically posed to the women because it reveals the kind of life they have led. It also gives an insight into their feelings and throws light on the precipitating factors of depression.

Table 2 presents responses of women regarding the most as well as the least preferred stage of life. As evident from the table, 'childhood' and 'adolescence' have been the most preferred stages of life for majority of the women. The reasons women gave for preferring childhood were: 'no responsibilities', 'fun filled life with friends', 'love and support of parents' and 'no health problems'.

Table 2: Preference for various stages of life by age and income level

Stage of Life	*40 – 60 yrs*			*>60 yrs*		
	LIG n=30	*MIG n=30*	*HIG n=30*	*LIG n=30*	*MIG n=30*	*HIG n=30*
	%	%	%	%	%	%
Most preferred						
Childhood	50.0	16.7	36.7	53.3	26.7	36.7
Adolescence	26.7	50.0	46.6	16.7	33.3	50.0
Adulthood	3.3	13.3	6.7	13.3	13.3	6.7
Middle Age	-	6.7	3.3	-	-	3.3
Old Age	-	-	-	-	3.3	-
No Response	20.0	13.3	6.7	16.7	23.4	3.3
Least preferred						
Childhood	3.3	-	3.3	3.3	6.7	10.0
Adolescence	6.7	-	3.3	10.0	6.7	-
Adulthood	33.3	26.7	36.7	13.3	3.3	16.7
Middle Age	36.7	53.3	46.7	26.7	20.0	20.0
Old Age	6.7	3.3	6.7	33.3	30.0	46.7
No Response	13.3	16.7	3.3	13.4	33.3	6.6

The responses of women indicate that love and support in relationships are among the most important factors for happiness, and therefore lack of it in later life becomes one of the causes of depression in women. The fact that women gave 'no responsibilities' as a reason for preferring 'childhood' or 'adolescence' over all other stages of life also indicates that perhaps inability to bear the burden of multiple responsibilities in later life can also cause mental distress (as can be seen later in this section, women have mentioned burden of responsibilities as a reason for describing adulthood and middle age as the 'least preferred' stage of life).

Four women stated 'middle age' and one woman stated 'old age' as their most preferred stage of life because they felt more confident about themselves at this age. One of them, a homeopathic doctor, had been sexually abused by her father-in-law and had an unsupportive husband, who had an extra-martial relationship with their maid servant. Although she could not break away from her marriage due to societal pressures all these years, now she felt in-charge of her life in her middle age.

Regarding the least preferred stage of life, as can be seen from Table 2, maximum number of women in the 40–60 age group have reported 'middle age' (i.e. the stage at which these women are at present) as being the 'least preferred' stage of life. Most of the women have given reasons like 'health problems', 'family problems', 'lot of work and responsibilities', 'financial problems' and 'loneliness'. More women from the low income group stated 'financial problems' as a reason for preferring middle age least.

Majority of the women aged above 60 years stated 'old age' and 'middle age' as the least preferred stages of life for reasons such as 'deteriorated health', '(increased) dependency or financial problem', 'loneliness' and 'death of husband'. Not only women in the low income group but also those in the middle and high income groups stated 'financial problem' as a reason for preferring old age least. This indicates that a woman may have financial dependence even if she belongs to higher income group.

'Adulthood' has also been described by many women (especially by those in the 40–60 age group) as the least preferred stage of life, mainly because of the 'financial problems' and 'increased work and responsibilities' that they have to face at this age. The other reasons given were 'problems with in-laws', 'death of husband / death in family', 'adjustment problems', 'health problems' or 'childlessness'.

Family composition and living arrangement

Living arrangements have a direct bearing on the relationships of a person. In joint families, despite greater likelihood of conflicts, the extended family also provides support in the time of crisis. Loneliness is seldom felt by a person in a joint family. Thus breaking down of the joint family system and proportionate increase in nuclear families is found to be associated with increased rates of depression due to lack of confiding relationships, support of elders and increased responsibilities (Sethi and Manchanda, 1978).

Figure 1: Number of members in the family of women with depression (n=180)

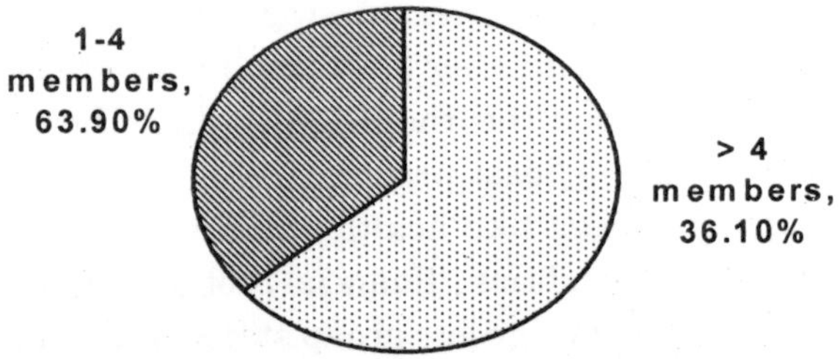

Figures 1 and 2 show that the nearly two thirds of the women with moderate depression belonged to small families or 1-4 members, while over one third were from families having more than four members. Thus majority of the women lived in small families.

Figure 2: Living arrangement of women with depression (n=180)

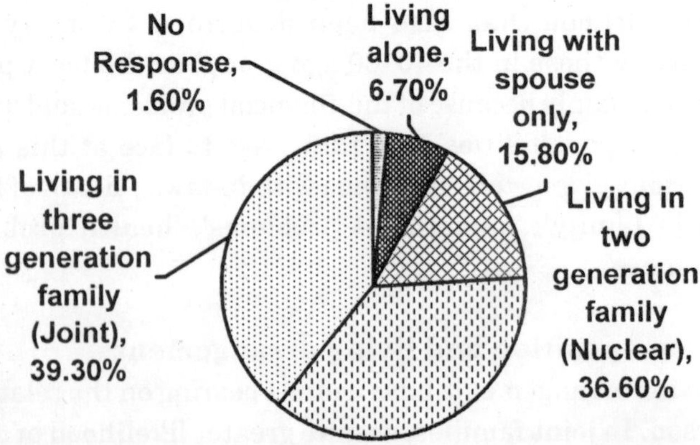

Over two thirds of women (36.6 percent) lived in nuclear families (two generation) and a slightly higher percentage of them (39.3 percent) lived in joint families (three generation). About 16 percent women lived with their spouse only (possibly affected by the 'empty nest syndrome'). There were a few women (6.7 percent) who lived alone (Figure 2).

Among those who lived alone, more of women belonged to low income and middle income groups and were found to be in the older age group of 60 years and above. Women who lived alone may find it harder to cope with loneliness and isolation. Moreover, women from low income groups were also facing financial difficulties. One of them was living in penury. She had been abandoned by her children and was surviving on the support offered by her neighbors.

Table 3: Living arrangement of women with depression by age and income level

Family composition	*40 – 60 yrs*			*>60 yrs*		
	LIG n=30	*MIG n=30*	*HIG n=30*	*LIG n=30*	*MIG n=30*	*HIG n=30*
	%	%	%	%	%	%
Alone	-	-	6.7	20.0	13.3	-
With spouse only	13.3	-	26.7	10.0	20.0	23.3
With spouse & children	33.3	60.0	20.0	13.3	6.7	23.3
With spouse & in-laws	6.7	6.7	-	6.7	-	-
Spouse, children and in-laws	6.7	10.0	16.6	6.7	3.3	13.3
Spouse, children & parents	-	-	-	-	-	-
Spouse, children & grandchildren	3.3	6.7	6.7	13.3	16.7	6.8
With children only	3.3	-	6.7	6.8	13.3	3.3
With children & grandchildren	16.7	6.7	3.3	10.0	16.7	20.0
With in-laws only	-	-	-	-	-	-
With in-laws & children	-	3.3	-	3.3	-	3.3
With parents only	3.3	-	3.3	3.3	6.7	3.3
With parents & children	-	-	3.3	-	-	-
With parents & siblings	3.3	6.6	-	-	-	-
With relatives	3.3	-	-	3.3	-	-
Others	6.8	-	-	3.3	-	3.4
No Response	-	-	6.7	-	3.3	-

Studies have found an association between marital status and depression. Married, divorced, separated women are more likely to be depressed than men (Radloff 1975). Being single (divorced, widowed) is also associated with depression (Amin, Shah and Vankar, 1998). Further, married women are likely to experience isolation if their spouse is living away from home, on account of being burdened with the extra household responsibilities and bringing up of children as a single parent. Lack of comfort and support of a spouse can also bring about depression. Similarly, women whose children or grandchildren are living away from home also experience loneliness and isolation because children/grandchildren are potential sources of companionship. Isolation is thus one of the key psychosocial risk factors, and can lead to or be a symptom of, depression.

In order to know further whether factors like living without the spouse or children or grandchildren, childlessness and child loss are probable causes of depression, married women in the sample were asked whether their husband, children or grandchildren were living away from home. They were also asked whether they were childless or had experienced the death of a child. Women's responses are presented in Table 4.

Table 4: Probable factors for depression in married women, by age and income level

Number of married women	*40 – 60 yrs*			*>60 yrs*		
	LIG n=24	*MIG n=27*	*HIG n=24*	*LIG n=18*	*MIG n=14*	*HIG n=23*
With husband living away from home	3	3	7	3	-	3
With children/grandchildren living away from home	8	5	12	12	13	10
Who are childless	3	1	3	2	1	2
Who have experienced death of a child	-	-	1	1	-	-

Table 4 shows that among 180 women with moderate depression, there were 19 married women (10.5 percent) who had spouses living away from home. There have been mixed responses about how these women felt about their spouse living away from home. Out of these 19 married women, 32 percent expressed being happy, whereas a much higher percentage (44.9 percent) reported feeling 'lonely' and 'unhappy' (23.1 percent) about it.

Out of 180, 95 women (52.8 percent) had children and grandchildren. Of these 60 women (63.1 percent) have children / grandchildren lived away from them. Again there were mixed responses regarding their feelings about their children/grandchildren living away from home. While some women (31.6 percent) reported 'feeling happy' as children had gone away for better career opportunities, others reported being 'unhappy' (21.1 percent) or 'lonely' (12.6 percent) in the absence of their children/grandchildren. However over a third of the women (34.7 percent) did not respond to the question.

Out of 180, 12 women (6.7 percent) were childless and 2 women (1.1 percent) reported death of a child. Childless women reported

Table 5: Profile of widowed women with depression, by age and income level

Particulars	*40 – 60 yrs*			*>60 yrs*		
	LIG n=6	*MIG n=2*	*HIG n=3*	*LIG n=9*	*MIG n=13*	*HIG n=6*
	%	*%*	*%*	*%*	*%*	*%*
Period of widowhood						
Less than 10 years	66.7	50	100	22.2	38.5	16.7
More than 10 years	33.3	50	-	77.8	61.5	83.3
Who took care of spouse during illness						
Self	66.7	50	-	55.6	23.1	16.7
Self and son	-	-	100	11.1	30.8	16.7
Self and son and grandchildren	-	-	-	-	-	50.0
No response	33.3	50	-	33.3	46.2	16.7
***Feeling about widowhood**						
Relief (from suffering)	50	-	-	22.2	30.8	16.7
Lonely	33.3	100	66.7	66.7	38.5	66.7
Helpless	-	-	33.3	11.1	15.4	33.3
Insecure	16.7	-	33.3	55.6	7.7	-
Dependent	16.7	-	-	11.1	7.7	33.3
No Response	-	-	-	-	23.1	-
Any other	-	-	-	-	-	16.7

* Percentages exceed 100 due to multiple responses.

that they had to bear the taunts of relatives and neighbors about their inability to have children. Except one, none of them had ever thought of adopting a child.

Table 5 shows that older women (above 60 years of age) had been widowed for more than 10 years while in the younger age group (40-60 years), more women had been widowed in the last ten years. Most of the women in the low and middle income group had taken care of their ill / bedridden husbands themselves or with the help of their son(s). More women in the high income group took care of their ill / bedridden husbands with the help of their son / grandchild.

Majority of women in all the three income groups and in both age groups reported experiencing loneliness after the death of their spouse. Some women also expressed that they felt relief after their spouse's death as the spouse was suffering. More women in the low income group reported feeling relieved after the death of their spouse because of the extra financial burden and work load that their spouse's illness was causing them and adding to their stress.

Women who were separated or divorced constituted only a small percentage (7 women, i.e. 3.9 percent) of the 180 women with moderate depression. Out of these 7 separated and divorced single women, 5 belonged to the low income group. There was a mixed response as to whether they are 'satisfied' or 'dissatisfied' with being divorced or separated and women were also equally divided in their response to whether they considered remarrying'. None of these women had remarried.

Women who were unmarried also constituted a small number, i.e., 11 women (6.1 percent) in the sample of 180 women with moderate depression. Among the reasons they stated for remaining unmarried were 'dowry' (inability to fulfill demand), 'no desire', 'no suitable partner' and 'family responsibilities'. Most of these women were either dissatisfied with their unmarried status or were not sure about how they felt being unmarried. Only one woman in the middle income group, age over 60 years expressed being 'satisfied' with her unmarried status.

Involvement in physical, social, and religious activities

It is commonly accepted that leading an active life result in better health than living a sedentary life which leads to poor health,

Table 6: Mean time (in minutes) spent by women with moderate depression in a day for physical, recreational/social and religious activities, by age and income level

Type of activity	*40 – 60 yrs*			*>60 yrs*			*f ratio*	* *p. value*
	LIG n=30	*MIG n=30*	*HIG n=30*	*LIG n=30*	*MIG n=30*	*HIG n=30*		
Physical								
Mean	344.50	*489.47	400.83	316.67	*243.33	243.33	3.1971	.0051
S.D.	198.68	325.27	215.92	269.47	164.29	164.29		
Recreational/Social								
Mean	482.63	647.13	706.80	417.80	601.53	535.97	2.0341	.0630
S.D.	383.59	386.43	482.90	447.43	438.26	412.80		
Religious								
Mean	158.43	86.17	135.83	93.47	165.67	139.43	.6585	.6832
S.D.	299.82	112.75	253.16	148.58	179.87	364.23		

* Significant P £ 0.05 level

Note: Physical activities include: dusting, sweeping/mopping, laundry, cooking, other indoor and outdoor chores, child care, shopping, gardening, yoga, going for walks, sports, etc. Recreational or social activities include: listening to music, watching TV, reading, visiting theatre/exhibition, arts and crafts, chatting with friends and neighbors, visiting friends and relatives, attending any association, going to clubs, kitty party/mahila mandal, etc. Religious activities include: visiting religious places, praying at home, reciting *mantras*, meditation, etc.

which in turn can result in depression. However, it is also true that too much of physical work can lead to chronic fatigue resulting in inability of women to take care of their nutrition and health. Some researchers suggest that aerobic exercises are effective as other forms of psychotherapy and that exercises have an antidepressant effect on patients with mild to moderate forms of depression. Physical activity has been found to enhance the self concept of women who are depressed. Social activities also reflect the support network of a person.

Recently it has been shown that social support and the availability of a confiding relationship can offset the negative effect of disability (Schoevers et al., 2000).

Religious affiliation has generally been observed to have a protective effect on proneness to depression (Helm et al., 2000)

Table 6 shows that in recreational/social activities and religious activities no two groups were significantly different (P< 0.5).

There was a significant difference between younger women (40-60 years) and older women (above 60 years) in the middle income group with regard to the time they spent on physical activities in a day. The younger women in the middle income group spent more time in physical activities in a day compared with the older women in the same group (489.47 minutes as compared to 243.33 minutes).

The type of physical activity though was different for women in the low income group and their counterparts in the high income group. Women in the high income group spent more time doing physical exercise, yoga, shopping, or sports, while women in the low income group spent more time in cleaning, cooking and doing other household chores. The types of physical activities carried out by women in the middle income group are a mix of both.

Younger women in the high income group spent more time in recreational/social activities as compared to other groups, particularly those from low income group, though the difference is not significant.

Most women across all income groups and both age groups were independent in their daily activities (Table 7). A greater percentage of older women in the high and middle income groups are not independent in their daily activities as compared to younger women in the same income group, which is as expected, because

Table 7: Ability of women with depression to carry out daily activities independently

Whether independent in daily / personal activities	*40 – 60 yrs*			*>60 yrs*		
	LIG n=30	*MIG n=30*	*HIG n=30*	*LIG n=30*	*MIG n=30*	*HIG n=30*
	%	*%*	*%*	*%*	*%*	*%*
Yes	83.3	86.7	80.0	86.7	76.7	63.3
No	16.7	13.3	20.0	13.3	23.3	36.7
Women who need help in	**n=5**	**n=4**	**n=6**	**n=4**	**n=7**	**n=11**
Cooking/domestic work	-	1	1	-	2	1
Climbing stairs	1	-	-	3	3	3
Lifting heavy objects	2	-	-	1	1	-
Walking/ going out	-	1	-	-	-	-
Any other	-	-	-	-	-	2
No response	2	2	5	-	1	5

with increasing age a number of physical health problems also develop. Moreover, as already mentioned earlier, about two fifths of the women (42.8 percent) had arthritis.

In contrast, the number of older women in the low income group who are independent in their daily activities is higher than that of younger women in the same income group (though the difference is small).

Among those who needed help in their daily activities 13.3 percent in both age groups needed help with domestic chores, 6.7 percent in the younger age group and 40.9 percent in the older age group needed help in climbing stairs, which is not surprising given the fact that a significant number of women had arthritis.

A small percentage of women, 13.3 percent in the younger age group and 9 percent in the older age group, needed help in lifting heavy objects and 6.7 percent of younger women needed assistance in going out.

Satisfaction of personal needs

Table 8 shows that with the exception of the older women in the middle income group, the emotional needs of most women were 'sometimes' or 'never' met. Both younger and older women in the low income group were a disadvantaged lot in comparison with their counterparts in the middle and high income groups with respect to fulfillment of or satisfaction with all needs whether emotional, physical, social, financial or religious. Regarding financial, it is not surprising that a large percentage of low income women of both age groups report that their financial needs are satisfied 'never' or only 'sometimes'.

Table 8: Level of satisfaction of personal needs of women with depression, by age and income level

Satisfaction Level	*40 – 60 yrs*			*>60 yrs*		
	LIG n=30	*MIG n=30*	*HIG n=30*	*LIG n=30*	*MIG n=30*	*HIG n=30*
	%	*%*	*%*	*%*	*%*	*%*
Emotional Needs						
Always	10.0	23.3	10.0	13.3	46.7	20.0
Sometimes	46.7	50.0	63.3	46.7	36.7	60.0
Never	43.3	26.7	26.7	40.0	16.6	20.0
Physical needs						
Always	26.7	50.0	46.7	30.0	56.7	40.0
Sometimes	36.7	33.3	26.7	33.3	13.3	36.7
Never	36.6	16.7	26.7	36.7	30.0	23.3
Social Needs						
Always	23.3	36.7	40.0	30.0	56.7	53.3
Sometimes	50.0	40.0	43.3	40.0	26.7	26.7
Never	26.7	23.3	16.7	30.0	16.7	20.0
Financial Needs						
Always	6.7	50.0	70.0	16.7	80.0	66.7
Sometimes	40.0	36.7	26.7	40.0	10.0	20.0
Never	53.3	13.3	3.3	43.3	10.0	13.3
Religious Needs						
Always	50.0	73.3	70.0	53.3	86.7	66.7
Sometimes	20.0	20.0	26.7	16.7	10.0	26.7
Never	30.0	6.7	3.3	30.0	3.3	6.7

Religious needs of most women were 'always' or 'sometimes' satisfied, perhaps because one is not dependent on others to satisfy this need. Yet there were a substantial number (30 percent) of younger and older women in the low income group who reported their religious needs 'never' being satisfied. This could mean that due to financial constraints or lack of time they were not able to visit religious places or engage in religious pursuits.

Table 9: Addiction(s) in women with depression to various substances, by age and income level

Addiction			*40 – 60 yrs*			*>60 yrs*		
			LIG n=30	*MIG n=30*	*HIG n=30*	*LIG n=30*	*MIG n=30*	*HIG n=30*
			%	*%*	*%*	*%*	*%*	*%*
1) Alcohol	Yes	Past	-	-	6.7	3.3	3.3	3.3
		Present	-	-	3.3	-	-	-
	No		100	100	90.0	96.7	96.7	96.7
2) Cigarette/Bidi	Yes	Past	3.3	3.3	-	3.3	-	-
		Present	-	-	3.3	-	-	-
	No		96.7	96.7	96.7	96.7	100	100
3) Tobacco Powder	Yes	Past	3.3	-	-	6.7	-	-
		Present	-	-	3.3	3.3	-	-
	No		96.7	100	96.7	90.0	100	100

(Contd.)

(Contd. Table 9)

Adiction		*40 – 60 yrs*			*>60 yrs*		
		LIG n=30	*MIG n=30*	*HIG n=30*	*LIG n=30*	*MIG n=30*	*HIG n=30*
		%	%	%	%	%	%
4) Tobacco Paste Yes	Past	3.3	3.3	-	6.7	-	-
	Present	-	-	3.3	3.3	-	-
No		96.7	96.7	96.7	90.0	100	100
5) Snuff Yes	Past	13.3	-	-	3.3	3.3	6.7
	Present	-	-	3.3	-	-	-
No		86.7	100	96.7	96.7	96.7	93.3
6) Coffee Yes	Past	10.0	-	3.3	-	6.7	-
	Present	-	-	3.3	-	-	-
No		90.0	100	93.4	100	93.3	100
7) Tea Yes	Past	23.3	36.7	23.3	23.3	40.0	6.7
	Present	-	-	3.3	-	-	-
No		76.7	63.3	73.3	76.7	60.0	93.3

(Contd.)

Addictions

Table 9 indicates that despite depression most women had not turned to any addictive substance. Among the few who had done so in the past most had given up the habit. There is a negligible percent (3.3 percent, i.e., only one woman) who consume alcohol, cigarette, tobacco, snuff or tea and coffee at present. The consumption of these substances was reported only among younger women in the high income group and among older women in the low income group (only tobacco powder and tobacco paste). Though several women had consumed tea in the past, currently only one of them consumed tea.

These findings show that women do not turn to substance abuse when faced with stressors or traumas in life but tend to ruminate over their problems (This is a different reaction from men who try to react to emotional distress by not thinking about it or turning to substance abuse). This increases the likelihood of their developing depression.

Women's Status and Responsibilities in the Family

The low status accorded to women within their families is said to be associated with depression, particularly in elderly women. In the present study an attempt was made to understand women's position in the existing power structure in their families. To measure the existing power structure, the main parameters were: a) households headed by women; b) their involvement in household responsibilities and their perceptions regarding the same; c) their involvement in decision-making on various important aspects (e.g. health, education, marriage of children and finance besides purchasing groceries, preparing meals and fulfilling other social obligations); d) their access to and control over the family's finances. Each of these parameters is discussed below.

Women-headed households

Among women age 40-60 years, the percentage of women who reported self as the head of their household was highest in the high income group (56.7 percent) followed by low income (46.7 percent). Among middle income women in the same age group, husband was the head of the household in the majority of the households (53.3

percent). Among older women, the percentage of women who reported self as the head of their household was the highest in the low income group (53.3 percent). Among middle income women in this age group, the head of the household was either the woman herself (36.7 percent), or her husband (33.3 percent), while in the high income group the head of the household was the husband (33.3 percent), followed by the women themselves (26.7 percent). A significant percentage of middle and high income women in this age group also mentioned their son being the head of the household (20 percent each).

Overall, more women from low income headed their households, although a substantial percentage of them are homemakers (with 46.7 percent in both age groups not working, i.e. earning) and are married (73.3 percent in 40-60 year age group and 50.0 percent in the 60 years and above age group respectively). One would have expected single women, widows and women having a source of income to be the head of the household.

Middle income women over 60 years of age also have the highest percentage for 'self' as head of household, but there is not much difference with the second most representative category, i.e. 'husband' (3.4 percent only). This could be due to the fact that a greater percentage of women in this group are widowed or single (53.3 percent combined) as compared to married (46.7 percent).

There is a difference in the power structure of middle income women of the two age groups. 'Husband' is the head of the household in the maximum number of younger middle income homes, while there is an almost equal distribution among 'self' and husband in the older middle income homes. It is expected that 'Husband' has more power, being the head of the household, in the middle income group, as most of the younger middle income women (i.e., age 40–60 years) are married (90 percent) and are homemakers (70 percent).

A higher percentage of women as head of the household is further supported by them as the decision makers (Table 11).

Son as head of households forms the third most representative category among older middle income and high income women (here widows constituted 43.3 percent and 23.3 percent respectively of middle and high income women age 60 years and above), thus reflecting the patriarchal character of Indian society where sons take charge of households after the father's death.

Majority of the women have expressed 'satisfaction' with the power structure in their homes.

Involvement in household responsibilities

Around 90 percent of the women across age and income group, responded in the affirmative when asked if they were taking part in household responsibilities.

Table 10: Power structure and involvement in household responsibilities by women with depression, by age and income level

Particulars	*40 – 60 yrs*			*>60 yrs*		
	LIG n=30	*MIG n=30*	*HIG n=30*	*LIG n=30*	*MIG n=30*	*HIG n=30*
	%	*%*	*%*	*%*	*%*	*%*
Household headed by						
1. Self	46.7	33.3	56.7	53.3	36.7	26.7
2. Husband	20.0	53.3	30.0	30.0	33.3	33.3
3. Mother-in-law	10.0	6.7	6.7	-	-	10.0
4. Father-in-law	6.7	-	-	3.3	-	-
5. Father	-	3.3	3.3	3.3	6.7	-
6. Mother	6.7	-	-	-	-	-
7. Son	6.7	3.3	3.3	3.3	20.0	20.0
8. Daughter-in-law	-	-	-	-	-	-
9. Son + Daughter-in-law	-	-	-	-	3.3	6.7
10. Husband +Mother-in-law	-	-	-	3.3	-	-
11. Other	3.3	-	-	3.3	-	3.3
Feelings about self/others heading household						
1. Satisfied	63.3	63.3	79.3	76.7	83.3	56.7
2. Unsatisfied	20.0	13.3	13.8	13.3	6.7	16.7
3. Not Sure	16.7	23.4	6.9	10.0	10.0	26.6
Whether taking part in household responsibilities						
1. Yes	90.0	93.3	96.7	90.0	86.7	93.3
2. No	10.0	6.7	3.3	10.0	13.3	6.7

Involvement in decision-making on family related matters

Table 11 shows the areas in which women are involved in 'decision making'. In health related aspects most women across all income categories and both age groups were taking decisions.

Table 11: Involvement of women with depression in decision-making on family related matters, by age and income level

Particulars		*40 – 60 yrs*			*>60 yrs*		
		LIG *n=30*	*MIG* *n=30*	*HIG* *n=30*	*LIG* *n=30*	*MIG* *n=30*	*HIG* *n=30*
Whether women take decisions in matters related to		%	%	%	%	%	%
1. Health	Yes	80.0	96.7	90.0	73.3	83.3	80.0
	No	20.0	3.3	10.0	26.7	16.7	20.0
2. Financial	Yes	40.0	30.0	50.0	50.0	36.7	36.7
	No	60.0	70.0	50.0	50.0	63.3	63.3
3. Charity / Donation	Yes	46.7	56.7	86.7	53.3	43.3	53.3
	No	53.3	43.3	13.3	46.7	56.7	46.7
4. Education of children	Yes	53.3	66.7	56.7	53.3	26.7	46.7
	No	46.7	33.3	43.3	46.7	73.3	53.3
5. Marriage of children	Yes	53.3	36.7	36.7	60.0	50.0	53.3
	No	46.7	63.3	63.3	40.0	50.0	46.7
6. Other matters relating to children e.g. buying clothes	Yes	36.7	53.3	50.0	43.3	23.3	43.3
	No	63.3	46.7	50.0	56.7	76.7	56.7

(Contd.)

(Contd. Table 11)

Particulars		40 – 60 yrs			>60 yrs		
		LIG n=30	*MIG* n=30	*HIG* n=30	*LIG* n=30	*MIG* n=30	*HIG* n=30
7. Purchasing	Yes	73.3	66.7	76.7	63.3	33.3	66.7
	No	26.7	33.3	23.3	36.7	66.7	33.3
8. Preparing Meals	Yes	76.7	83.3	80.0	66.7	50	66.7
	No	23.3	16.7	20.0	33.3	50	33.3
9. Social obligations	Yes	66.7	60.0	83.3	60.0	56.7	83.3
	No	33.3	40.0	16.7	40.0	43.3	16.7
10 Any other e.g. like going to a movie or restaurant etc.	Yes	20.0	3.3	26.7	30.0	10.0	16.7
	No	80.0	96.7	73.3	70.0	90.0	83.3
Whether others are consulted while making decisions		**n=22**	**n=27**	**n=23**	**n=15**	**n=14**	**n=21**
Yes		46.7	90.0	63.3	13.3	66.7	70.0
No		53.3	10.0	36.7	86.7	33.3	30.0

Regarding involvement in decision making on financial aspects, lesser percentage of women were taking decisions in most groups except high income women from the younger age group and low income women from the older age group, where the percentages of women saying 'yes' and 'no' were equal.

In matters relating to education and marriage of children there was divided involvement.

More women were involved in decision making related to purchasing, preparing meals and fulfilling social obligation across all groups with the exception of the middle income women in the older age group in matters related to purchase.

Middle income women in the older age group were found to be less involved compared to other groups in other areas also such as 'education of children', 'other matters, relating to children' and other decisions like 'going to a movie' or 'going out to eat', etc. This could be due to the fact that there were less number of women educated above secondary level among older middle income women as compared to the younger middle income women and high income women of both age groups. Also, this group (i.e., middle income women age 60 years and above), had the highest percentage of widows, many of them living in a joint family indicating that their sons may have taken over the 'decision making' process.

In spite of being involved in so many aspects of decision making a lesser percentage of women took decisions related to other aspects like 'going out to a movie' or going out to a restaurant, etc. This indicates that when it comes to social and entertainment activities, the preferences of women take a backseat to let the wishes of others (husband or sons or children) prevail.

Over all, low income women in both age groups seem to be more independent in taking decisions than others. This is evident in the high percentage of younger low income women (53.3 percent) and older low income women (86.7 percent) stating that they did not consult others while making decisions. A possible explanation for this could be that more women from this group were living in nuclear families as compared to joint families (56.6 low income women age 40-60 years and 53.3 percent low income women age 60 years and above). The percentage of women who take decisions independently was the highest among low income women over the age of 60 years, probably because, 20.0 percent women in this group were living alone. Yet this is relatively higher when compared with older low income women living in nuclear family (53.3 percent) indicating that low income women in joint families were also taking decisions independently. Majority of the women in the middle and high income groups consulted others when they made decisions, with as high as 90 percent middle income women age 40-60 years reporting the same, even though the percentage of high and middle income women living alone or in a nuclear family was higher than those living in a joint family (66.7 percent and 60 percent respectively for middle income women in the two age groups; 63.4 and 53.3 percent respectively for high income women in the two age groups).

Women, who consulted others for decision-making, across both age groups and all income categories, generally took their husband's advice in decision making in all aspects. Some took the advice of their son, even daughter-in-law.

Access to and control over financial resources

Except low income women in the age group of 40-60 years, across all income groups and both age groups, most women reported *not* being financially independent. This implies that even though women may belong to a higher income group, yet they may not be financially independent. Low income women age 40-60 years form the highest percentage of 'partially' independent women, when compared with all the other subgroups.

There is a marked difference between high income women in the two age groups who were financially independent, 42.9 percent of the older high income women were fully independent financially as compared to 21.4 percent of younger high income women, despite the fact that more high income women in the younger age group (26.7 percent) were retired and 13.3 percent working compared to 10.0 percent retired and 36.7 percent working (in younger low income group).

One of the reasons may be that older women were widowed and hence independent.

It is evident from Table 12 that even though lesser percentage of women were financially independent, a higher percentage of them had 'full' or 'partial' control over their family's finances. The percentage of women having full control over the family's finances was the highest among high income women in the 40-60 age group

Table 12: Control of women depression over their family's finances, by age and income level

Particulars	*40 – 60 yrs*			*>60 yrs*		
	LIG n=30	*MIG n=30*	*HIG n=30*	*LIG n=30*	*MIG n=30*	*HIG n=30*
	%	*%*	*%*	*%*	*%*	*%*
Whether women are financially independent						
Fully	10.0	19.0	21.4	18.8	27.3	42.9
Partially	50.0	14.3	7.1	31.3	9.1	14.3
Not at all	40.0	66.7	71.4	50.0	63.6	42.9
Whether women have control over family's finances						
Fully	33.3	30.0	53.3	46.7	26.7	30.0
Partially	43.3	53.3	33.3	30.0	50.0	46.7
Not at all	23.4	16.7	13.4	23.3	23.3	23.3
If not fully, family's finances are controlled by						
1. Husband	35.0	57.1	64.3	31.3	31.8	19.0
2. Father-in-law	10.0	-	7.1	-	-	-
3. Mother-in-law	5.0	4.8	-	-	-	4.8
4. Father	10.0	-	-	-	-	-
5. Mother	5.0	-	-	-	-	-
6. Son	10.0	14.3	7.1	25.0	36.4	14.3
7. Daughter-in-law	5.0	-	7.1	-	-	-
8. Son + Daughter-in-law	5.0	4.8	-	-	9.1	9.5
9. Others	-	4.8	-	-	4.5	4.8
10. No Response	15.0	14.2	14.3	43.8	18.2	47.6
Women's feeling about it						
Satisfied	25.0	61.9	50.0	43.8	72.7	47.6
Dissatisfied	50.0	23.8	21.4	43.8	9.1	28.6
Not Sure	25.0	14.3	28.6	12.5	18.2	23.8
Whether financial needs of their family are met						
Fully	5.0	47.6	85.7	12.5	63.6	76.2
Partially	40.0	47.6	14.3	68.8	36.4	23.8
Not at all	55.0	4.8	-	18.8	-	-
Whether women support others financially						
Yes	20	28.6	78.6	18.8	36.4	38.1
No	80	71.4	21.4	81.3	63.6	61.9

(even though only 6.7 percent of women in this group were living alone and 36.7 are working) followed by the older low income women (20 percent of these women were living alone and 40 percent were still working).

Most middle income women in both age groups had 'partial' control only. For the younger middle income group women, this was expected as 90 percent were married and only 23.3 percent were working. However, among the older middle income women, 43.3 percent were widowed and 10.0 percent were still working, indicating that control over family's finances had passed on from father to son. (36.7 percent live in a joint family and 60 percent in nuclear family and alone).

Among younger women, regardless of the income group, the control over the family's finances lie with their husbands. There is a difference in the percentage of husbands who had control over the family's finance in the middle and high income groups in both age groups of women. If one relates this to the power structure, one finds that women had not reported 'self' as head of households indicating that finances are more in the husband's hands or son's hands. In older middle income group women 'sons' as controllers of family's finances constituted the highest percentage. A substantial percent of older women in the low and high income groups have not responded to the question.

Regarding satisfaction with control of financial matters of the family, in both the age groups, a greater percentage of middle income women were satisfied with the control of financial matters in their family. More low income women in both age groups were 'dissatisfied' in both age groups, though more older low income women were satisfied than their younger counterparts.

In the high income group, women were divided according to their responses about the feeling of being satisfied, dissatisfied and were unsure about their feeling regarding the structure of financial controls in their families.

When asked the question 'Are financial needs of your family met?' most middle and high income women stated that they were fully met. As expected most low income women stated that their financial needs were either not met at all or were met only partially. There was a significant difference in percentage of low income women of the two age groups who stated that their family needs were not at all met (55 percent in the 40–60 age group and 18.8 percent in the age of 60 years and above). This could be because the younger low income women may be having more needs and aspirations, while the older low income women may have accepted their condition and learnt to live with the existing means (though 68.8 percent of older low income women reported their financial needs to be only 'partially met').

Most of the younger women in the higher income group supported others financially.

Overall the results of this section are indicative of women's empowerment across subsections. Further it indicates that in the present sample power is not associated with women's employment.

Women's Work

Women's work includes paid as well as unpaid household work. Those who are engaged in an occupation, either as dependent employees or as self-employed, have to bear the double burden of functioning well in their jobs and running a household. Thus balancing between the two may push them into stressful situations and affect their mental health. Further, those who retire after long years of service face several changes in their life. Besides causing loss of financial independence and increased financial dependence on others, retirement may result in a loss of sense of identity, value and importance as it can be profoundly unsettling to no longer be needed in familiar roles. Women's unpaid work is most undervalued. Being completely involved in the discharge of responsibilities of the family and household, many women find themselves having little else to be occupied with as they grow older. Those who may have put family before a career may find it difficult to adjust to not being needed by the family or household as they grow older. Therefore in the present study, an attempt was made to know from women whether they were satisfied with the work they were doing or had done as employees or self-employed, as retired persons, and as homemakers.

Majority of women in the present study were homemakers (58.9 percent), a little less than one third were currently working (30.5 percent), they were either self-employed or were salaried, and 10.6 percent of them were retired.

Women who were homemakers were asked whether they had ever felt that they should had taken up a job. As can be seen from Table 13, a significant percentage of women in both age groups and across income categories, had felt always or sometimes that they should have taken up a job. The percentage of women who had never felt that they should have taken up a job was the highest among low income women in the age group of 60 years and above (46.1 percent), followed by high income women in the age group of 40-60 years (38.9 percent). Overall, with the exception of high income women in the 40-60 age group the percentage of women who never felt that they should have taken up a job was highest among women age 60 years and above. The desire to take up a job was reported highest by younger women from the low income group. These women were probably motivated to think of taking up a job to supplement the family income.

Table 13: Views of homemakers among women with depression regarding their work, by age and income level

Particulars	*40 – 60 yrs*			*>60 yrs*		
	LIG	*MIG*	*HIG*	*LIG*	*MIG*	*HIG*
	n=13	*n=22*	*n=18*	*n=13*	*n=21*	*n=19*
	%	%	%	%	%	%
Ever felt they should have taken up a job						
Always	30.8	36.4	22.2	15.4	28.6	36.8
Sometimes	53.8	45.5	38.9	38.5	42.8	31.6
Never	15.4	18.1	38.9	46.1	28.6	31.6
Whether they expressed desire to take up job						
Yes	46.1	45.5	27.8	38.5	33.3	52.6
No	38.5	31.8	50.0	23.0	52.4	26.3
No Response	15.4	22.7	22.2	38.5	14.3	21.1
Whether they found themselves increasingly involved in children and family responsibilities						
Yes	100	95.5	88.9	100	95.2	100
No	-	4.5	-	-	4.8	-
No response	-	-	11.1	-	-	-
Feeling about increased involvement in family						
Satisfied	53.8	61.9	75.0	46.2	75.0	57.9
Dissatisfied	15.4	14.3	25.0	15.4	15.0	5.3
Not Sure	23.1	23.8	-	38.5	10.0	36.8
No Response	7.7	-	-	-	-	-

Women who reported that they had always or sometimes felt that they should have taken a job were further probed on whether and to whom they had expressed their desire to take up a job. As can be seen from Table 13, among women in the 40-60 age group,

Table 14: Views of employed and retired women with depression regarding their work, by age and income level

Employment status and level of satisfaction	*40 – 60 yrs*			*>60 yrs*		
	LIG n=6	*MIG n=0*	*HIG n=7*	*LIG n=2*	*MIG n=1*	*HIG n=2*
	%	%	%	%	%	%
Self employed						
Feeling about work/job						
Satisfied	33.3	-	100	50.0	100	100
Dissatisfied	50.0	-	-	50.0	-	-
Not Sure	16.7	-	-	-	-	-
No Response	-	-	-	-	-	-
Whether satisfied with income						
Fully	-	-	71.4	50.0	100	100
Partially	33.3	-	28.6	-	-	-
Not at all	66.7	-	-	50.0	-	-
No Response	-	-	-	-	-	-
Salaried employment	**n=10**	**n=7**	**n=4**	**n=13**	**n=2**	**n=1**
Feeling about work/job						
Satisfied	20.0	28.6	50.0	46.2	100	100
Dissatisfied	60.0	14.3	-	23.1	-	-
Not Sure	10.0	57.1	25.0	30.8	-	-
No Response	10.0	-	25.0	-	-	-
Whether satisfied with income						
Yes	10.0	42.9	75	30.8	50.0	-
No	80.0	57.1	-	69.2	50.0	100
No Response	10.0	-	25	-	-	-
Retired						
Feelings about retirement	**n=1**	**n=2**	**n=3**	**n=2**	**n=6**	**n=7**
Satisfied	-	-				
Dissatisfied	-	-	-		-	-
Not Sure	-	-	-	-	-	1
No Response	1	2	-	2	3	6
Impact of retirement						
Financial dependence	1	-	-	1	2	-
Boredom	-	-	2	-	2	6
Any other	-	1	1	1	1	1
No Response	-	1	-	-	1	-

over two-fifths of the low and middle income women had expressed their desire – mainly to their husbands, followed by family - to take up a job, whereas about half of the high income women in this age group had never mentioned their desire to anyone.

In contrast, among higher income women aged 60 years and above, over half of the sample (52.6 percent), as against 38.5 percent women in the middle income group and 33.3 percent women in the middle income group, had expressed their desire to take up a job mainly to their husbands or family. Some women in both age groups had expressed their desire to take up employment to their in-laws, very few older women had expressed the same to their children.

Almost all women in both age groups and across income categories have found themselves more involved in children and family responsibilities. Majority of the women expressed satisfaction with their involvement in family responsibilities. However, a significant percentage of older women in the low and high income group were not sure about their feelings in this regard. Further, except high income women over 60 years of age, at least 15 percent of women across all other age and income groups were dissatisfied with their increased involvement in family responsibilities.

Out of 30.5 percent women who were currently employed, 10 percent were self-employed and 20.5 percent had salaried employment. Table 14 presents the views of employed women regarding their work and their level of satisfaction with their income.

Middle income women who had salaried employment were divided in their views regarding their work and income.

As the number of retired women in the sample is very small, it is difficult to draw any conclusions regarding the association between their retired status and depression. As can be seen from Table 14, two women were satisfied with their retired life (one high income woman from the 40-60 age group and one middle income woman from the 60 years and above age group). Similarly two women, both middle income women from the older age group, were dissatisfied with their retirement. The remaining women either did not respond or were not sure.

Regarding the impact that their retired status had on their life, two low income women (one in the younger and the other in the older age group) reported increased financial dependence, whereas most high income women (8 out of 10 including both age groups) reported boredom. Five out of the 21 retired women stated that after retirement they could now spend more time in other activities, visiting relatives or just relaxing.

Existing Social Support

A strong network of social support is important for prevention and recovery from depression. It has been observed that social networks are more important to women than men (Bell, 1982; 1987). Besides family, friends and neighbors also form an important support network. The presence or absence of this support influences the way individuals cope with different stressful life situations, and it also affects the person's self-esteem. A good support network would also lead a person to be more open and capable of sharing/ confiding in others rather than repressing it within oneself.

In order to know the social support existing for women, they were asked if they confided in others (i.e. family, friends, relatives, neighbors) and whether others confided in them, and their feelings about it. "Confiding" here is in respect of sharing of personal, health, financial and social matters.

Table 15: Confiding/sharing of problems by women with depression, by age and income level

Particulars	*40 – 60 yrs*			*>60 yrs*		
	LIG n=30	*MIG n=30*	*HIG n=30*	*LIG n=30*	*MIG n=30*	*HIG n=30*
	%	*%*	*%*	*%*	*%*	*%*
Confiding in others						
Yes	60.0	70.0	83.3	76.7	60.0	80.0
No	40.0	30.0	16.7	23.3	40.0	20.0
Being confided in by others						
Yes	63.3	73.3	66.7	73.3	63.3	76.7
No	36.7	26.7	33.3	26.7	36.7	23.3
Feelings about confiding						
Satisfied	60.0	73.3	56.7	50.0	63.3	66.7
Dissatisfied	33.4	23.3	40.0	43.3	30.0	30.0
No Response	6.7	3.3	3.3	6.7	6.7	3.3

Majority of the women in both age groups as well as all three income groups do confide their problems in others. Among women age 40-60 years, ability to confide in others was highest among high income women (83.3 percent) and lowest among low income women (60 percent). A similar pattern was be observed in older women over 60 years of age, where ability to confide in others was highest in high income women, but lowest in middle income women (60 percent).

When asked if others confide/share their personal, health, financial and social matters with women, over 60 percent of the women across age and income groups replied in the affirmative. In the 40-60 age group being confided in by others was reported highest by middle income women (73.3 percent), while among older women, the same was reported by high income women (76.6 percent).

Women from both age groups were generally satisfied (50-73 percent) with the way they were able to the share with/confide in others. Dissatisfaction was higher among high income women and low income women age 40-60 years and among low income women age 60 years and above.

To know whether women have any support during crises, their absence from the family or during illness, or on major occasions, women were asked about who supported them in such circumstances.

As evident from Table 16, within the 40–60 age group, children were the main caretakers for low income (26.7 percent) and high

Table 16: Caretakers for women with depression during crises, absence or ill health, by age and income level

Persons who take care	*40 – 60 yrs*			*>60 yrs*		
	LIG n=30	*MIG n=30*	*HIG n=30*	*LIG n=30*	*MIG n=30*	*HIG n=30*
	%	%	%	%	%	%
Husband	6.7	30.0	20.0	3.3	6.7	26.7
Children	26.7	23.3	23.3	13.3	16.7	13.3
Daughter-in-law	16.7	10.0	13.3	13.3	40.0	20.0
No one	23.3	6.7	20.0	20.0	6.7	10.0

Note: Multiple responses.

income women (23.3 percent), while husbands were the main caretakers for middle income women (23.3 percent). In the 60 years and above age group, the daughter-in-law was the main caretaker for middle income women (40 percent), the husband was the main caretaker for high income women (26.7 percent) followed by the daughter-in-law (20 percent).

Looking at the living arrangements of women in the 40-60 age group it can be said that as majority of the women in this age group were living with their husbands and children, they were being taken care of by them in the time of crisis and or ill health. In older women, age 60 years and above, though most of the respondents were staying 'with husband only', husband is the caretaker for women in the high income group only.

Of particular concern is that a significant percentage of women, particularly those in from low income group (23.3 percent in the 40-60 age group and 20 percent in the 60 years and above age group), did not have any one to take care of them during illness or crisis, or their absence or ill health. A fifth of high income women age 40-60 years also reported that they had no one who would take care of them.

Social support and self esteem

Several studies suggest an association between social support available to individuals and their level of self-esteem. A person's support network is said to also affect their self esteem; the better the support network, the higher the person's self-esteem. Therefore, in the present study, an attempt was made to examine the association between women's satisfaction with their support network and their level of self-esteem. The same is presented in Table 17.

As evident from the table, most of the women were satisfied with the social support that they get and the also had high self-esteem.

Among women in the 40-60 age group, satisfaction with existing social support was highest in middle income (73.3 percent), followed by low income women (60 percent) and high income women (56.7 percent). Among women in the 60 years and above age group, level of satisfaction was the highest among high income women (66.7

Table 17: Level of satisfaction with existing support and its effect on self esteem of women with depression, by age and income level

Particulars	*40 – 60 yrs*			*>60 yrs*		
	LIG n=30	*MIG n=30*	*HIG n=30*	*LIG n=30*	*MIG n=30*	*HIG n=30*
	%	*%*	*%*	*%*	*%*	*%*
Support						
Satisfactory	60.0	73.3	56.7	50.0	63.3	66.7
Dissatisfactory	26.0	10.0	13.3	30.0	23.3	20.0
Undecided	6.7	13.3	26.7	13.0	6.7	10.0
No Response	6.7	3.3	3.3	6.7	6.7	3.3
Self-Esteem						
High	56.7	90.0	86.7	46.1	86.7	66.7
Low	43.3	10.0	13.3	56.3	13.3	30.0

percent), followed by middle income women (63.3 percent) and the least among low income women (50 percent). Corresponding to that, the level of self-esteem of older women in the low income group was also less, with only 46.7 percent women in this group having high self-esteem. A possible explanation for this could be that along with aging, this group also faces greater economic problems, low social status and failing health. Also, it may be noted that many of these women had no one to take care of them during illness or crisis. Therefore it is not surprising that older low income women were not satisfied with the social support that they had and this seems to have a negative effect on their self-esteem.

The availability of social support to women needs to be further examined in the context of the status of their relationships with significant others who were part of their social network, i.e., who are members of their family, their relatives, friends and neighbors. It is important to know the status of their relationship with these persons: weather their relationship changed for the better or the worse over the years. Do they bond well or is their relationship marred by conflicts? This information will help explain the extent of social support available to women.

Relationship and Conflicts

The status of relationships of women with people around them, i.e., their family members, relatives, friends and neighbors, has been presented in Figure 31.

Figure 3: Relationship of women with depression with family, relatives and neighbors

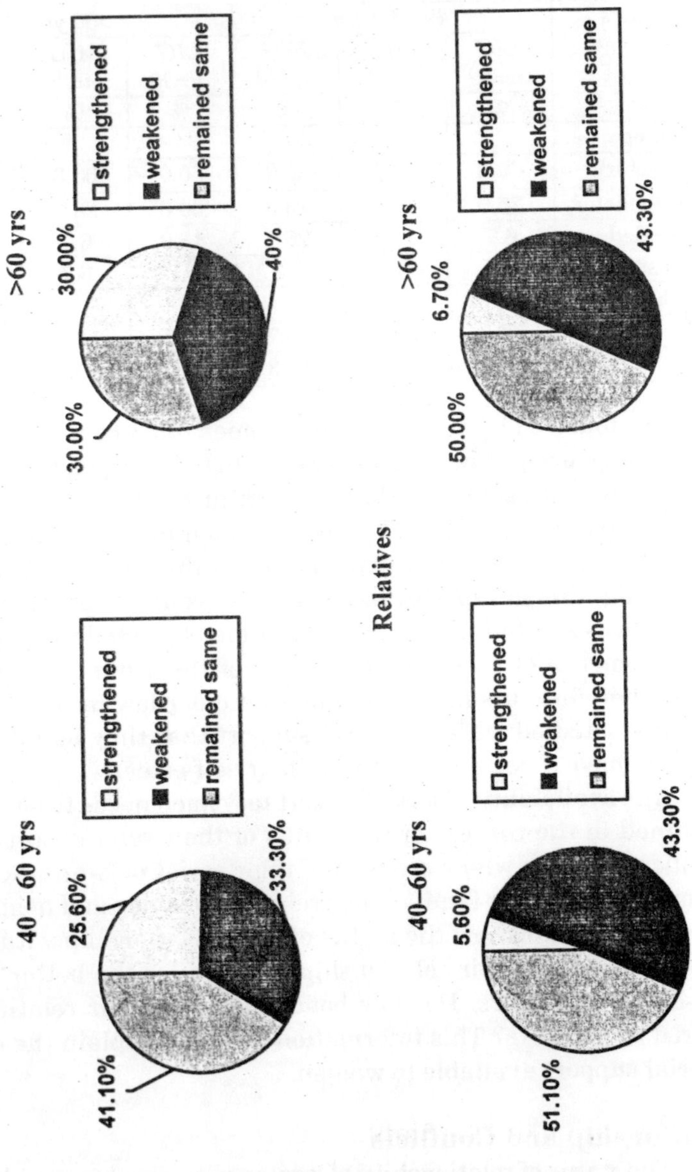

(Contd.)

(*Contd. Figure-3*)

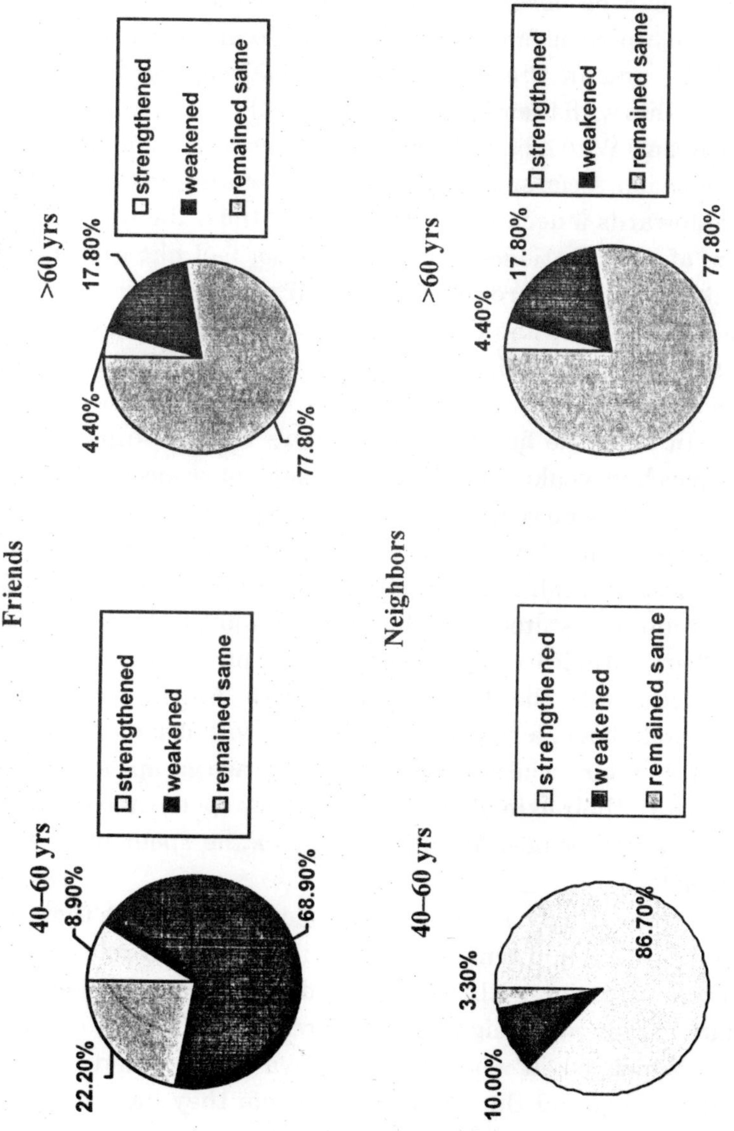

Women were asked whether their relationships with each of these groups of people have strengthened, weakened or remained unchanged over the years.

It can be observed that in the 40–60 age group women's relationship with family members had remained the same (41.1 percent) and in the 60 years and above age group, women's relationship with their family members had weakened over the years (40 percent).With advancing years, changes occur in family structure and available social support, and the social status of a person changes, more towards a decline. In the present study, the women over 60 years of age mentioned that they did not feel like a part of their family anymore. More so because their children were now leading independent lives and their importance or participation in various household or domestic activities was not recognized or welcomed as before.

In both the age groups, women's relationships with their relatives had weakened (51.1 and 50 percent respectively). Women in the age of 40–60 years did not seem to depend on or give importance to their extended family, i.e., relatives, as their lives revolved mostly around their children and their spouse. Some of the women in this age group also stated that they did not want to interact with the members of their extended family due to property related matters and also due to the distribution of work. Among women age 60 years and above, a similar phenomenon was observed. Due to the decline in their social status women in this age group did not interact much with their extended family, but they spent time in attending religious gatherings, or with friends, or the spent more time by themselves.

Interestingly, relationships of older women with their friends and neighbors had remained unchanged, whereas relationships of younger women with their friends had weakened and their relationships with neighbors had strengthened over the years.

When asked whether they have or have had conflicts in relationships and the person with whom they have or have had conflicts, majority of the women in both age groups reported having conflicts in their relationship with their husbands. Among women in the 40–60 age group, half of the women in all three income groups reported conflicts with their husbands. Conflicts with mother-in-law or father-in-law were reported more by middle income (40 percent) and high income women (30.4 percent) in the same age group.

Among women over 60 years of age, conflicts with husband was reported more by high income women (48 percent) followed by middle income women (35.3 percent) and the least by low income women (28 percent). The percent for the response 'husband' is high in all the income groups. Other than with husbands, conflicts with daughter-in-law were reported by a significant percentage of high income (32 percent), middle income (23.5) and low income (24 percent) women above 60 years of age. Conflicts with the son were reported by low income women age 60 years and above. A middle and low income women age 60 years and above also reported conflicts with relatives more than women in other age and income groups.

Table 18: Conflicts in relationships of women with depression, by age and income level

Relationship	*40–60 yrs*			*>60 yrs*		
	LIG n=30	*MIG n=20*	*HIG n=23*	*LIG n=25*	*MIG n=17*	*HIG n=25*
	%	*%*	*%*	*%*	*%*	*%*
Husband	50.0	50.0	52.2	28.0	35.3	48.0
Mother-in-law/Father-in-law	19.2	40.0	30.4	12.0	11.8	16.0
Relatives	7.7	10.0	0	23.5	23.5	12.0
Daughter-in-law	7.7	5.0	13.0	24.0	23.5	32.0
Son	11.5	5.0	4.3	28.0	0	12.0

Note: Multiple responses.

Thus overall it can be said that older women, over 60 years of age had more conflicts with their husband, relatives, daughter-in-law, while younger women in the 40-60 age group had more conflicts with their husband, mother or father-in-law.

Experience of Loneliness / Isolation

It can be gathered from the earlier section, over the years, most of the relationship of the women have either weakened or have remained the same and most of the women, especially women above 60 years of age, also had conflicts in their relationships. It is therefore not very surprising that majority of the women across age and income groups feel loneliness and isolation.

Table 19: Loneliness and isolation experienced by women with depression, by age and income level

Whether experience	*40–60 yrs*			*>60 yrs*		
	LIG n=30	*MIG n=30*	*HIG n=30*	*LIG n=30*	*MIG n=30*	*HIG n=30*
	%	*%*	*%*	*%*	*%*	*%*
Loneliness						
Yes	86.7	76.7	86.6	83.3	93.4	96.7
No	13.3	23.3	13.3	16.7	6.7	3.3
Isolation						
Yes	60.0	50.0	63.3	70.0	40.0	70.0
No	40.0	50.0	36.7	30.0	60.0	30.0

In the 40–60 age group, an equal percentage of low income and high income women (87 percent) reported of feeling lonely, whereas a comparatively lower percentage of middle income women in this age group reported the same. In women over 60 years of age, loneliness was reported highest by high income women (96.7 percent), followed by middle income women (93.4 percent) and low income women (83.3 percent).

As women age their status within the household diminishes. They are no longer considered active participants in the house. Also, age brings along with it failing health and other psycho-social set-backs such as widowhood, or separation from children due to break-down of joint families. Hence, lack of support within and outside the family, changing life style, break-down of joint family system, loneliness may be experienced more by elderly women.

With regard to feeling isolated, about two-thirds of low and high income women in the 40-60 age group and 70 percent low and high income women above the age of 60 reported feeling isolated. Isolation was comparatively less reported by middle income women in both age groups. Overall, the percentage of women reporting isolation was comparatively lesser than that of women reporting loneliness. This maybe so because, despite feeling lonely, they have a better support system, wherein they are able to confide in or share with others (friends, neighbors, etc.) their personal, health related or other general matters. As one of the respondents in the middle income women in the age of group of 40–60 years stated –

"I do feel lonely lately as my children have grown up and are able to take care of themselves. So, whenever I try to do or say something to them, they argue and don't listen to me. Hence, I feel that no one is bothered about me or listens to me. Even my husband does the same. But then I do know that when crisis come along, i.e. when I am sick, or have any other problems, these very people will be there to take care of me and they will not abandon me.

It may also be noted that experience of isolation was reported by a relatively less percentage of women compared to loneliness.

How copy strassed used for loneliness and isolation by the woman has been depicted in Table 20.

As it can be observed from the table, the most frequently used coping strategy used for loneliness by women age 40–60 years is to 'cry', as reported by 34.6 percent, 34.8 percent and 30.8 percent of low, middle and high income women respectively. Among women above the age of 60, crying was the most frequently used coping strategy by low income (36 percent) and high income women (37.9 percent). However, the most frequently used coping strategy of middle income women in this age group was 'diverting mind to other work" (39.3 percent).

Looking into the coping strategy for isolation, it may be said that a more or less similar pattern of response as that for loneliness emerged, with tolerance or crying as the main strategy used by low income (44.8 percent) and high income women (36.8 percent) age 40-60 years. Doing nothing (26.7 percent) was the coping strategy used more frequently by middle income women in the same age group. Similarly, among women age 60 years and above, the strategy used by low income and high income women to cope with isolation was to tolerate or cry (38.1 percent each).

It may be noted that 'find solutions' as the most frequently reported coping strategy by middle income women over the age of 60 (25 percent) which explains why women in this category feel least isolated as compared to women in the other groups. Also, tolerance or crying as coping strategy has been reported least by

Table 20: Strategies of women with depression to cope with loneliness and isolation, by age and income level

Strategy	*40 – 60 yrs*			*>60 yrs*		
	LIG n=26	*MIG* n=23	*HIG* n=26	*LIG* n=25	*MIG* n=28	*HIG* n=29
	%	*%*	*%*	*%*	*%*	*%*
To cope with loneliness						
Involvement in religious/spiritual activities	11.5	17.4	15.4	24.0	32.1	13.8
Meditation	0	8.7	0	0	3.6	3.4
Talking to others	23.1	13.0	15.4	28.0	14.3	17.2
Diverting mind to other work	34.6	26.1	30.8	8.0	39.3	24.1
Sleeping	3.8	8.7	3.8	32.0	3.6	17.2
Cry	34.6	34.8	30.8	36.0	25.0	37.9
Do nothing	11.5	8.7	0	8.0	17.9	20.7
Any other*	26.9	43.5	34.6	20.0	25.0	41.3
No Response	0	4.3	3.8	0	0	0
To cope with isolation	**n=18**	**n=15**	**n=19**	**n=21**	**n=12**	**n=21**
Tolerate / Cry	44.4	6.7	36.8	38.1	16.7	38.1
Meditation / Visit Temple	-	20.0	21.1	-	16.7	4.8
Music / T.V.	-	13.3	5.3	-	8.3	-
Go for walks	-	6.7	5.3	4.8	-	-
Visit relatives	-	6.7	-	4.8	-	-
Revolt	27.8	13.3	10.5	14.3	16.7	14.3
Divert mind to work	5.6	13.3	26.3	14.3	16.7	-
Find solutions	11.1	13.3	-	4.8	25.0	19.0
Do nothing	11.1	26.7	10.7	28.6	8.3	14.3
Any other**	22.2	6.7	10.5	23.8	8.3	28.6
No Response	5.6	6.7	-	-	-	4.8

Note: *'Any other' includes responses such as smoking, eating, reading, joining a social group, or a kitty party group. **'Any other' includes 'remember the past'/'husband', 'cursing self', 'daydreaming', 'going for walks', 'playing with grandchildren'.

middle income women in both age groups, whereas this strategy was most frequently reported by women in other income groups. 'Find solutions' means that women in this group tried to talk about the issues which led to conflicts or the engaged themselves in other creative work. Thus, middle income women in both age groups have a more action-oriented or practical approach to coping with isolation, hence the feeling of isolation is least among them.

Experience of Abuse or Neglect

Experience of abuse (physical, emotional and verbal) at any stage affects a woman's overall well being. Violence is a means by which coercive control can be gained over every aspect of women's functioning that affects her physically, sexually, emotionally, socially and economically. Abuse of any form can and does occur anytime over the lifespan. Any form or abuse or violence take place in a variety of settings, but is most likely take place at home, by one's own husband, family members or someone close. Several studies have shown that the perpetrator of violence is someone the woman usually knows. Violence in the home tends to be repetitive and to escalate in severity over time (American Medical Association, 1992).

Emotional and psychological abuse often includes manipulation, social isolation from family and friends, neglect by self and others as well as humiliation. All this consequently leads to self-blame, loss of sense of self, and damaged self-esteem. Abuse is not restricted to any particular age group. Studies show has that older women too face the same fate at the hands of their own children

Table 21: Abuse and neglect experienced by women with depression, by age and income level

Whether experienced	*40 – 60 yrs*			*>60 yrs*		
	LIG n=30	*MIG n=30*	*HIG n=30*	*LIG n=30*	*MIG n=30*	*HIG n=30*
	%	%	%	%	%	%
Abuse						
Yes	66.7	60.0	56.7	80.0	43.3	76.7
No	33.3	40.0	43.3	20.0	56.7	23.3
Neglect						
Yes	41.4	26.7	40.0	66.4	23.3	50.0
No	58.6	73.3	60.0	33.3	76.7	50.0

and other family members. The abuse and neglect faced by women pushes them into a state of depression. Hence it becomes important for the present study to know of the extent of abuse and neglect faced by the women as well as their strategies to cope with abuse.

As can be seen from Table 21, Majority of the respondents admitted to having been abused. The prevalence of abuse was highest in low income women of both the age groups, with 66.7 percent low income women in the age group of 40–60 years and as high as 80 percent low income women over the age of 60 reporting experience of abuse. A similar pattern emerged in the case of high income women in both age groups (56.7 percent in 40-60 year-old women and 76.7 percent in those above 60 years of age). A much higher percentage of middle income women in the younger age group reported experience of abuse (60 percent) as compared to those above 60 years of age in the same income group (43.3 percent), who incidentally had lowest prevalence of abuse among all women.

While experience of abuse was reported by a very high percentage of women, experience of neglect was reported by lesser number of women. Experience of neglect was highest among low income women age 60 years and above (66.4 percent), followed by high income women in the same group (50 percent). Neglect was experienced least by middle income women over the age of 60 (23.3

Table 22: Form of abuse experienced by women with depression, by age and income level

*Form of abuse**	*40 – 60 yrs*			*>60 yrs*		
	LIG n=20	*MIG n=18*	*HIG n=17*	*LIG n=24*	*MIG n=13*	*HIG n=23*
	%	%	%	%	%	%
Physical	55.0	22.2	47.1	54.2	38.5	39.1
Emotional	85.0	77.8	76.5	83.3	69.2	91.3
Verbal	15.0	11.1	-	12.5	15.4	13.0
Social	-	16.7	17.6	-	-	4.3
Financial	5.0	-	-	-	-	-
Sexual	10.0	-	-	12.5	-	-
No Response	-	5.6	5.9	-	7.7	-

Note: *Multiple responses

percent) and those age between 40-60 years in the same income group (26.7 percent). This could be due to the fact that women in this group were more practical in dealing or coping with the problems or conflicts that they faced in their relationships and had better social support available to them at the time of crisis or absence or ill-health.

'Emotional abuse was the most commonly reported form of abuse across all age and income groups and was highest among high income women over 60 years of age (91.3 percent) and lowest among middle income women in the same age group (69.2 percent). It may be recollected that feelings of loneliness and isolation were the highest among high income women over 60 years of age (refer Table 22).

Table 23 presents information on the persons who inflict abuse or neglect women. As can be clearly seen, women were neglected by their husbands the most, with 50 percent of low income women in both age groups reporting neglect by their husbands. Among women in the 40–60 age group, particularly middle income women, the persons who neglected them were 'other in-laws', who included the immediate and extended family of their husbands (sister-in-law, brother-in-law, even father-in-law's brother) or their own son-in-law. Interestingly, neglect by daughter-in-law was reported more frequently by women above the age of 60, especially those from high income group (33.3 percent). None of the women in the 40-60 age grip reported being neglected by their daughters-in-law. This could be so because, in women in this age group are mostly very much in command of the running the house and are still actively participating in it, taking upon themselves responsibilities of the household. Moreover, women in this age group are likely to have young daughters-in-law and they may be in the process of molding their daughters-in-law to adapt to the lifestyle of their family and household. Hence there was not much scope for feeling or experiencing neglect by the daughter-in-law. In contrast, women over 60 years of age may participate less in the running of the household due to declining physical fitness and thus making way for the daughter-in-law to take over the responsibilities of the household. In this manner, having lost control over household and family, they may begin to feel neglected by their daughter-in-law.

With regard to perpetrator of abuse, once again, 'husband' was the most frequent response obtained in all categories except in middle income women over 60 years of age, who reported daughter-in-law and other relatives as abusers. Husband as perpetrator of abuse was reported by 70 percent of low income women age 40-60 years followed by high income women (47 percent) in the same age group. Most of these women stated that they felt left out and ignored by their husband.

Table 23: Perpetrators of abuse and neglect of women with depression by age and income level

Relationship with perpetrator	*40 – 60 yrs*			*>60 yrs*		
	LIG	*MIG*	*HIG*	*LIG*	*MIG*	*HIG*
	%	%	%	%	%	%
Of abuse	**n=20**	**n=18**	**n=17**	**n=24**	**n=13**	**n=23**
Husband	70.0	27.0	47.0	37.0	15.4	39.1
Son	-	11.1	11.8	-	-	13.0
Daughter-in-law	30.0	27.8	22.5	25.0	23.1	8.7
Mother-in-law/ Father-in-law	15.0	38.9	23.5	8.3	7.7	17.4
Relatives	10.0	-	5.9	16.7	23.1	13.0
Of neglect	**n=12**	**n=8**	**n=12**	**n=20**	**n=7**	**n=15**
Husband	50.0	37.5	33.3	50.0	28.6	40.0
Other in-laws	16.7	50.0	-	10.0	28.6	6.7
Daughter-in-law	-	-	-	15.0	-	33.3
Mother-in-law/ Father -in-law	16.7	-	8.3	10.0	-	6.7

Daughter-in-law as perpetrator of abuse was reported by 23-30 percent women in across age and income groups, except by high income women over 60 years of age (8.7 percent). Though none of the middle income women in the 40-60 age group mentioned daughter-in-law making them feel neglected, a significant percentage (27.8 percent) felt they were being abused by their daughters-in-law. Incidentally, mother and father-in-law were also mentioned as perpetrators of abuse most frequently by women in this category.

Women who reported experience of abuse or neglect, were asked how they cope or deal with it. In the case of neglect, the most frequently mentioned coping strategies by women age 40-60 were: 'tolerate or cry' (50 percent of high income women), 'do nothing' (33.3 percent of low income women), be 'self reliant' (37.5 percent middle income women)

As can be seen, in the 40–60 age group, the second most frequently used coping strategy was 'becoming self reliant'. Even though there was a high percentage of women in this age group reporting 'tolerate or cry' as coping strategy, higher percentage of

Table 24: Strategies of women with depression to cope with neglect/abuse, by age and income level

Type of coping strategy	*40 – 60 yrs*			*>60 yrs*		
	LIG n=12	*MIG n=8*	*HIG n=12*	*LIG n=20*	*MIG n=7*	*HIG n=15*
	%	%	%	%	%	%
For abuse	**n=20**	**n=18**	**n=17**	**n=24**	**n=13**	**n=23**
Separated	25.0	11.1	5.9	4.2	7.7	-
Tolerate / Cry	60.0	27.8	52.9	58.3	46.2	65.2
God's name	5.0	-	-	8.3	15.4	-
Do nothing	25.0	22.2	11.8	16.7	30.8	17.4
Retaliate / revolt	40.0	22.2	11.8	16.7	23.1	13.0
Shared with others	-	-	-	-	-	8.7
Any other	10.0	11.1	11.8	29.2	-	13.0
No Response	-	27.8	23.5	-	-	13.0
For neglect	**n=12**	**n=8**	**n=12**	**n=20**	**n=7**	**n=15**
Separated	8.3	25.0	-	5.0	14.3	-
Self-reliant	16.7	37.5	16.7	15.0	28.6	6.7
Tolerate / Cry	25.0	12.5	50.0	35.0	14.3	26.7
God's name	-	-	-	-	-	6.7
Do nothing	33.3	-	-	10.0	42.9	33.3
Retaliate	8.3	25.0	16.7	20.0	-	6.7
Any other	-	-	8.3	5.0	-	20.0
No Response	-	-	8.3	10.0	-	-

middle income women in this age group stated 'being self-reliant' (37.5 percent) and even retaliation against the perpetrators (25 percent) and separation from the perpetrators (25 percent). Thus indicating that middle income women in the age group of 40-60 have a problem solving approach to the issue, and they are less tolerant of such behaviors in their relationships.

The most frequently mentioned coping strategy by older women above 60 years of age was 'tolerate or cry' (35 percent middle income women) and 'do nothing' (26.7 percent high income women), indicating helplessness.

For abuse, the most frequently used coping strategy by women in the 40–60 age group is once again 'tolerate or cry' as mentioned by 60 percent low income women, 52.9 percent of high income women and 27.8 percent middle income women. Interestingly, retaliation or revolt and separation from the abuser were mentioned more frequently as coping strategies by low income women in this age group.

The most frequently used coping strategy by women over 60 years of age was 'tolerate or cry'. Thus, overall the coping strategies for both neglect and abuse were more or less similar.

Experience of Stressful Events

Social, cultural or economic difficulties can cause stress to individuals. Events such as loss of job, social status, ending of a relationship, widowhood and for that matter even ill-health may trigger episode(s) of depression In today's world where there are multiple roles to be played a person, the pressure to meet the expectations of others, and the environment and living patterns all add up to stress to an individual leading to depression.

Hence, it becomes essential to know of the life stressful events that may have occurred amongst the respondents of the present study. The Gurmeet Life Event Scale was used for the same purpose. As seen from Table 25, in the 40–60 age group, the stress level is high for low and high income women (63.3 percent and 63.3 percent respectively) and it is moderate for middle income women (46.7 percent).

Looking into the event that were more stressful it may be said that among 40-60 year-old women with depression, "change in sleep pattern" was the most stressful even, while "fear of illness was the highest stressful event in women over 60 years of age.

Again in the 40–60 age group the highest percentage for the most stressful event in the low income group was for the event "illness of close family member" (73.3 percent), which was also true for 43.3 percent middle income women in the same age group. For high income women in this age group, 'family conflicts' was the most stressful event (70 percent).

Table 25: Level of stress in women with depression by age and income group, Chi square test

Level	*40 – 60 yrs*			*>60 yrs*		
	LIG n=30	*MIG n=30*	*HIG n=30*	*LIG n=30*	*MIG n=30*	*HIG n=30*
	%	*%*	*%*	*%*	*%*	*%*
Low	8.3	10.0	-	-	6.7	6.7
Moderate	33.3	46.7	36.7	16.7	43.3	13.3
High	63.3	43.3	63.3	83.3	50.0	80.0

Note: *d.f.*= 12; *p*. value = .0000

Table 26: Experience of stressful life events in women with depression by age and income level

Life event	40 – 60 yrs			>60 yrs		
	LIG n=30	MIG n=30	HIG n=30	LIG n=30	MIG n=30	HIG n=30
	%	%	%	%	%	%
Death of close family member						
Less stressful	10.0	3.3	6.7	3.3	-	-
More stressful	30.0	26.7	33.3	50.0	30.0	50.0
Neutral	6.7	3.3	-	-	-	3.3
N.A.	53.3	66.7	60.0	46.7	70.0	46.7
Illness of self						
Less stressful	-	3.3	3.3	6.7	3.3	6.7
More stressful	40.0	43.3	56.7	50.0	50.0	50.0
Neutral	3.3	3.3	10.0	10.0	10.0	6.7
No Response	56.7	50.0	30.0	33.3	36.7	36.7

(Contd.)

(Contd. Table 26)

Life event	40 – 60 yrs			>60 yrs		
	LIG n=30	MIG n=30	HIG n=30	LIG n=30	MIG n=30	HIG n=30
	%	%	%	%	%	%
Illness of close family member						
Less stressful	-	-	6.7	-	-	-
More stressful	73.3	43.3	40.0	63.3	46.7	23.3
Neutral	10.0	13.3	-	3.3	3.3	6.7
No Response	16.7	43.3	53.3	33.3	50.0	70.0
Not having male child						
Less stressful	-	3.3	3.3	-	6.7	3.3
More stressful	46.7	30.0	20.0	43.3	26.7	10.0
Neutral	6.7	-	-	3.3	-	3.3
No Response	46.7	66.7	76.7	53.3	66.7	83.3
Family conflicts						
Less stressful	-	3.3	3.3	6.7	-	3.3
More stressful	56.7	26.7	70.0	50.0	46.7	63.3
Neutral	10.0	20.0	-	16.7	13.3	10.0
No Response	3.3	50.0	26.7	26.7	53.3	20.0
Change in sleep patterns						
Less stressful	-	-	3.3	13.3	-	6.7
More stressful	46.7	50.0	63.3	43.3	56.7	46.7
Neutral	3.3	6.7	-	3.3	10.0	10.0
Not Response	50.0	43.3	3.3	40.0	33.3	36.7
Change in eating habits						
Less stressful	13.3	10.0	13.3	20.0	23.3	26.7
More stressful	36.7	50.0	46.7	43.3	33.3	26.7
Neutral	10.0	10.0	10.0	6.7	16.7	3.3
No Response	40.0	30.0	30.0	30.0	26.7	43.3

(Contd.)

(Contd. Table 26)

Life event	40 – 60 yrs			>60 yrs		
	LIG n=30	MIG n=30	HIG n=30	LIG n=30	MIG n=30	HIG n=30
	%	%	%	%	%	%
Fear of illness						
Less stressful	13.3	3.3	-	6.7	13.3	10.0
More stressful	43.3	53.3	50.0	50.0	50.0	73.3
Neutral	6.7	6.7	6.7	3.3	6.7	-
Not Response	36.7	36.7	43.3	40.0	30.0	16.7

Note: These events are among multiple events on the Gurmeet Life Event scale.

Among women with depression over 60 years of age, 'illness of a close family member (63.3 percent) was the most stressful event for low income women, while 'change in sleep patter (56.7 percent) was more stressful for middle income women and 'fear of illness' (73.3 percent) was more stressful for high income women.

It may be observed from the table that among women in the older age group, i.e. above 60 years of age, in all the income groups have experienced highly stressful events, whereas in the 40–60 age group, low income and high income women have experienced highly stressful life events, whereas middle income women in this age group had experienced moderately stressful life events.

Prevalence of medical illness and hypochondriasis

Accompanied with depression, women would tend to complain of more health problems than the others taking into consideration their lifestyles, stressful life events and other psycho-social as well as health factors. Hence, it would be helpful to know presence of any medical illness would mark the presence of hypochondriasis in women. A hypochondriasis scale had been used to asses its presence in women with depression in the present study.

Medical illness was reported to be present by majority of the women in both the age groups, and by as high as 90.0 percent women over 60 years of age. In the 40–60 age group, medical illness was

Table 27: History of medical illness and hypochondriasis in women with depression by age and income level

Particulars	*40 – 60 yrs*			*>60 yrs*		
	LIG n=30	*MIG n=30*	*HIG n=30*	*LIG n=30*	*MIG n=30*	*HIG n=30*
	%	*%*	*%*	*%*	*%*	*%*
History of medical illness						
Yes	76.7	86.7	80.0	90.0	83.3	96.7
No	23.3	13.3	20.0	10.0	13.3	3.3
No response	-	-	-	-	3.4	-
Hypochondriasis						
Yes	76.7	60.0	36.7	73.3	53.3	70.0
No	23.3	40.0	63.3	26.7	46.7	30.0

mostly reported by low income women (76.7 percent) and in the 60 years and above age group, it was reported mostly by middle income women (96.7 percent).

Simultaneously, hypochondriasis was present by most of the women. Among women in the 40-60 age group, it was most prevalent in low income women (76.7 percent) followed by middle income women (60 percent). In women age above 60 years it was once again most prevalence in low income women (73.3 percent) followed by high income women (70 percent) and less prevalent in middle income women (53.3 percent).

It may be observed that high income women 40–60 age group reported significantly less prevalence of hypochondriasis, i.e. only 36.7 percent, even though there was 80 percent prevalence of medical illness among them, probably because more of these women may be availing medical care for their illness.

It has been widely believed that hypochondriasis is common in the elderly population, but the prevalence of hypochondriasis may not be any greater among older adults than among others (Siegler and Costa, 1985). Longitudinal survey data indicate that concerns about health do not increase with age but remain fairly stable over the life span.

The reason why women in the low income group reported highest percentage of hypochondrias can be attributed to their lack of resources for better medical facilities. Also, as a whole, people tend to underreport medical illness symptoms, rather than overreport them and often fail so seek help for serious illness (Besdine, 1980), perhaps because of overriding concerns about the cost of health care or a belief that aches and pains are an inevitable part of aging.

Table 28 presents the most common medical illness prevalent in women with depression.

As can be seen from the table, the most prevalent medical illness in women age 40-60 years was arthritis, which was highly prevalent in all the three income groups. The other medical illnesses prevalent among women were tension, spondylitis, skin disease, and anemia to name a few.

Table 28: Prevalence of medical illness in women with depression by age and income level

Particulars	*40 – 60 yrs*			*>60 yrs*		
	LIG n=30	*MIG n=30*	*HIG n=30*	*LIG n=30*	*MIG n=30*	*HIG n=30*
	%	%	%	%	%	%
B.P.	43.3	36.7	36.7	36.7	46.7	53.3
Arthritis	53.3	43.3	46.7	36.7	43.3	33.3
Thyroid	-	-	-	3.3	20.0	6.7
Cardiac problems	-	-	-	3.3	16.7	10.0
Diabetes	-	10.0	16.7	-	-	-
Body ache/backache	16.7	13.3	10.0	16.7	3.3	13.3

Note: Multiple responses

In women age 60 years and above, the most prevalent medical illnesses were blood pressure and arthritis.

Thus, it may be said that the prevalence of medical illness was present and at the same time there was a high percentage of prevalence of hypochondrias amongst the women in the present study.

Unfulfilled wishes and desires

All humans have aspirations, hopes and desires which lead them to want or achieve things in life. However, inability to achieve these may contribute to lowering of self esteem and development of a feeling of being a failure, thereby affecting their mental health. Therefore in the present study an attempt was made to know from women whether they had any unfulfilled wishes or desires. Table 29 provides women's responses in this regard.

As can be seen from the table, over 80 percent of low and middle income women in the 40-60 age group has unfulfilled wishes or desires. Among older women, i.e., above 60 years of age, as high as 90 percent low and high income women had unfulfilled wishes or desires. Comparatively lower percentages of high income women in the younger age group (66.7 percent) and middle income women in the older age group (56.7 percent) reported having any unfulfilled wishes or desires.

When probed about their unfulfilled desires and wishes, majority of middle income women in the 40–60 age group responded that they wanted to 'do a job/better job', by which they meant taking a profession or work, as well as doing better in their domestic work or household responsibilities. About one fifth of them wished they had higher education.

Table 29: Unfulfilled desires and wishes reported by women with depression, by age and income level

Particulars	*40 – 60 yrs*			*>60 yrs*		
	LIG *n=30*	*MIG* *n=30*	*HIG* *n=30*	*LIG* *n=30*	*MIG* *n=30*	*HIG* *n=30*
	%	*%*	*%*	*%*	*%*	*%*
Whether women have any unfulfilled wishes or desires						
Yes	83.3	86.7	66.7	90.0	56.7	90.0
No	16.7	13.3	33.3	10.0	43.3	10.0
Type of unfulfilled wishes or desires*						
Do a job/better job	16.0	38.5	5.0	11.1	17.8	18.5
Higher education	20.0	19.2	10.0	18.5	17.6	7.4
Have more financial satisfaction	32.0	7.7	5.0	14.8	-	11.1
Better health of self/others	16.0	7.7	10.0	-	-	-
To have children	12.0	3.8	5.0			
Pursue hobbies	-	-	-	-	17.6	14.8
Better life style	-	-	-	11.1	11.1	-

Note: * Multiple responses.

Low income women in the 40-60 age group wished for greater 'financial stability', as mentioned by 32 percent of these women, followed by higher education (20 percent), and taking up a job (16 percent), better health for self and other family members (16 percent) and having children (12 percent).

Among women over 60 years of age, low income women wished they had higher education (18.5 percent), more financial satisfaction (14.8 percent), a better lifestyle and a job (11.1 percent each). For middle income women in this age group, besides doing a job/a better job and having higher education, opportunity to pursue their hobbies was an important unfulfilled wish. High income women also wished they had a job, could pursue hobbies and had more financial satisfaction. The desire for more financial satisfaction in higher income women may be understood as desire for greater decision making power in money related matters, which these women may not be given at this age. There were a few other responses by women in this age group, like 'to have a grandson', 'to resolve issues with relatives, death wish, and to have the company of their husbands.

Conclusion

Data on the psychosocial aspects of women showed that living arrangements are changing from joint to nuclear families, and increasingly women and couples have to live their lives away from their spouses and children, creating a feeling of loneliness in them. Among women who are widowed, death of the spouse is a major cause of loneliness besides creating a feeling of insecurity.

The emotional needs of many women are never or sometimes fulfilled, leading to feelings of sadness and neglect. A very high percentage of women have reported experience of abuse, mainly emotional abuse, at the hands of their husbands and in-laws, including daughter-in-law (reported mainly by women over 60 years of age). Experience of abuse was reported more than the experience of neglect. Women felt neglected by their husbands and daughters-in-law. Most women have conflicts with family members; mainly husbands, followed by mothers-in-law (for younger women) and daughter-in-law (for older women), and majority of the women have reported feeling lonely. Women cope with neglect and abuse mainly by crying or tolerating. The same coping strategy is used by many of them for dealing with feelings of loneliness and isolation.

It is observed that though isolated and lonely no women have reported developing hobbies, indicating that these women are emotionally dependent on others rather than creating a space for themselves.

Majority of women have reported weakened relationships with their relatives, besides friends and neighbors and they are mainly dependent on their husbands and children to take care of them in the time of crisis, or their absence or their illness. However, majority of the women were satisfied with the social support that they get. Most women had high self-esteem.

Women across age and income groups have experienced highly stressful life events, with perhaps the exception of middle income women age 40-60 years who have experienced moderately stressful life events.

As regards their status within the family, although many women report themselves as the head of the household and partaking in the decision-making on various family related matters, many of them do not take decisions independently, they generally consult their husbands in decision making. Decisions on financial matters are still taken by male members of the family.

A substantial percentage of women have perceived themselves as head of households and are involved in the decision making process indicating empowerment and yet these women are all depressed. This raises a question? Does the empowerment of women have any bearing on their mental health status?

There is a high prevalence of hypochondrias among women, besides high prevalence of medical illnesses such as arthritis and blood pressure.

Women's longing for a life free of care and responsibilities is amply evident in the fact that childhood and adolescence are the most preferred stages of life for many women, as these stages are considered to be the most fun-filled and care-free phases of one's life.

There is need to explore more about involvement in social and religious activities and their relationship with depression.

Health and Nutritional Status of Women with Moderate Depression

While the connection between nutrition and a physical disease state has been well understood and has been established, there is lack of awareness about the connection between nutrition and mental health. Although depression ranks second among the common mental health problems, it is more typically thought of as a strictly emotional or biochemical problem. Nutrition, however, can play a key role, both in the onset, severity, and duration of depression. Some studies have shown that the synthesis and release of neurotransmitters in the body can be altered to some extent by certain foods. Thus, one's diet can affect the way one feels and behaves. If the diet of depressed people were to be examined, one would find it far from adequate. Besides, people are making bad food choices and selecting foods (e.g. junk foods, processed foods, canned foods, etc.) that actually contribute, to development of chemicals leading to mental disturbances.

In elderly loss of appetite, fatigue, and under nutrition along with other nutritional deficiencies, have been found to be widely prevalent. Weight loss is known to be associated with depression and it has an adverse effect on nutritional status.

Therefore, besides an in-depth study of the psychosocial aspects, one of the objectives of the present investigation was to assess the health and nutritional status of depressed women. This information was collected from the 180 moderately depressed women through:

- a diet survey, which included questions on general dietary aspects, 24-hour diet recall, and food frequency;
- Anthropometric measurements (height, weight, mid-upper arm circumference, and body mass index) and measurement of blood pressure to asses their nutritional status.
- the use of an exhaustive checklist and free listing to study the major and minor health problems, as well as problems specific to menopause, prevalent among them.

In order to compare the nutritional status of depressed and non-depressed women, 20 women over 60 years of age from middle income group were selected as controls. These women were selected from among those who were classified as non-depressed, i.e., had a score of 0-2 points on the BDI scale during the screening. Appropriate statistical tests were applied on the data collected from the 180 women with moderate depression to find out whether there was any association between psychosocial and nutritional factors with respect to depression and to explore the interplay of these factors on each other. The findings have been presented under the following sub-headings:

- Dietary intake
- Nutritional status
- Prevalence of health problems.

Dietary intake

As mentioned above, the dietary intake of the women was assessed through a diet survey which included questions on general dietary aspects such as: water intake, meal pattern, fasting practices, skipping meals, intake of special health foods, craving for special food, reduction in food consumption, changes in food consumption pattern, food causing allergy, and food preference. The nutrient intake of the women was assessed through 24-hour dietary recall method and frequency of consumption of foods, using the food frequency questionnaire.

Majority of the women with depression in the 40-60 as well as the 60 years and above age group were vegetarians. The percentage of vegetarians was the highest among middle income women over 60 years of age (90 percent). The percentages of non-vegetarians and eggetarians were relatively higher among women in the high income group in both age groups. A comparison between middle income women in the depressed and non-depressed group showed that the percentage of vegetarians was much higher among depressed women (90 percent) as compared to those in the non-depressed group (65 percent).

As high as 75 percent of the non-depressed women age 60 years and above could not provide any information on their actual consumption of water in a day. Of those who did provide information on their daily water consumption, 20 percent reported consuming more than 10 glasses of water in a day. Though it is difficult to draw and conclusive comparison of the water intake of depressed and non-depressed women on account of high percentage of non-response, it may be said that non-depressed women had better water consumption compared to their depressed counterparts. An exploratory study among women of Boston has reported that depressed women have much lower water consumption (300ml per

Table 30: Meal pattern of depressed and non-depressed women, by age and income group

Meals	*Depressed*						*Non-depressed*
	40-60 yrs			*>60 yrs*			*>60 yrs*
	LIG *n=30*	*MIG* *n=30*	*HIG* *n=30*	*LIG* *n=30*	*MIG* *n=30*	*HIG* *n=30*	*MIG* *n=20*
	%	%	%	%	%	%	%
Breakfast							
(a) Always	33.3	51.7	**75.9**	33.3	**55.2**	**50.0**	**50.0**
(b) Sometimes	**26.7**	24.1	6.9	**50.0**	17.2	40.0	45.0
(c) Never	**40.0**	24.1	17.2	16.7	**27.6**	10.0	5.0
Lunch							
(a) Always	**100**	93.3	**100**	**100**	89.7	**100**	100
(b) Sometimes	-	**6.7**	-	-	**6.9**	-	-
(c) Never	-	-	-	-	3.4	-	-
Dinner							
(a) Always	86.2	**96.7**	96.6	73.3	**86.2**	80.0	**94.7**
(b) Sometimes	**13.8**	3.3	3.4	**26.7**	6.9	20.0	5.3
(c) Never	-	-	-	-	**6.9**	-	-
Any other							
(a) Always	21.4	25.0	**42.9**	-	**29.4**	16.7	**64.7**
(b) Sometimes	**50.0**	33.3	21.4	**81.8**	52.9	58.3	23.5
(c) Never	28.6	**41.7**	35.7	18.2	17.7	**25.0**	11.8

day) as compared to non-depressed women (80 ounces, i.e. 2272.8 ml, per day) (Benton, et al., 1997).

The most common reasons for limiting fluid intake was 'laziness', 'limited mobility', 'workload' and 'forgetfulness' in drinking water. These reasons clearly indicate that women tend to neglect their own needs while fulfilling the demands of their families. Further, women who are elderly and have limited mobility have low intake of water because they are dependent on their caregivers. Majority of the depressed women from both the age groups had fair meal pattern of lunch and dinner (80-100 percent).

Overall, as table shows, low income women did not follow the typical three-meal pattern. Majority of the low income women in the younger age group did not take breakfast, or any other meal, such as evening snacks, and some of them did not take dinner (13.8 percent) because they could not afford more meals in a day, had large families, or were not aware of the importance of following the three-meal pattern. A similar meal pattern was followed by low income women over 60 years of age. In fact a little over one-fourth of them (26.7 percent) did not take dinner regularly, probably due to health problems related to aging. A comparison of the meal patterns of middle income women over 60 years of age in both the depressed and non-depressed groups show that non-depressed women have more regular meal pattern than those who are depressed. Fewer non-depressed women never take breakfast or lunch or dinner and a substantial percentage of these women take evening snacks (64.7 percent) regularly.

Table 31 presents the fasting practices followed by depressed and non-depressed women. As can be seen from the table, among women with depression, fasting practices are followed more by women over 60 years of age than by women age 40-60 years. Among women aged 40-60 years, more women from middle income group (50 percent) followed by those from the high income group (43.3 percent) fast as compared with women from the low income group (39.3 percent). Also, more women in the depressed group (63.3 percent) than those in the non-depressed group (40 percent) fast.

The main reasons for fasting as cited by women were physiological changes due to age, health problems and inclination towards religion and rituals. Due to the declining capacity to digest, experience of digestive disorders, and other health problems like diabetes, hypertension, and cardiac probiems, women want to reduce their food intake, and they prefer to fast. Besides the above reasons, lack of choices in matters of food (their family did not take into consideration their choice of food), dependence on family members for food, loss of interest in food or development of aversion for food, loss of appetite and forgetfulness (sometimes women sit in prayer or other activities and forget to eat food on time and counted it as

Table 31: Fasting practices followed by depressed and non-depressed women, by age and income level

Fasting	*Depressed*						*Non-depressed*
	40-60 yrs			*>60 yrs*			*>60 yrs*
	LIG N=30	*MIG n=30*	*HIG n=30*	*LIG n=30*	*MIG N=30*	*HIG n=30*	*MIG n=20*
	%	%	%	%	%	%	%
Whether women fast							
Yes	39.3	**50.0**	43.3	60.0	**63.3**	**63.3**	40.0
No	**60.7**	50.0	56.7	**40.0**	36.7	36.7	**60.0**
Frequency of fasting							
Once in week	18.2	26.7	**36.4**	**47.1**	26.3	27.8	25.0
More than twice a week	**45.5**	40.0	27.2	23.5	15.8	**38.9**	**50.0**
Once in month	27.3	26.7	**36.4**	17.6	**52.6**	27.8	25.0
Twice in year	**9.0**	6.6	-	**11.8**	5.3	5.5	-
Meal pattern during fasting							
(a) Cereals	**30.0**	13.3	16.7	**50.0**	33.3	33.3	**50.0**
(b) Non- cereals	**20.0**	**20.0**	-	**44.4**	27.8	27.8	-
(c) Pulses/dals	20.0	**26.7**	8.3	**33.3**	26.3	16.7	**25.0**
(d) Green leafy vegetables	30.0	**53.3**	25.0	**44.4**	36.8	33.3	**75.0**
(e) Other vegetabl	20.0	**33.3**	-	**33.3**	31.6	22.2	**87.5``**
(f) Roots & tubers	40.0	**80.0**	50.0	61.1	33.3	**77.8**	**100**
(g) Milk & products	60.0	**73.3**	58.3	61.1	63.2	**88.9**	**87.5**
(h) Fruits	50.0	**93.3**	75.0	66.7	**84.2**	83.3	**100**
(i) Sweets	22.2	46.7	50.0	16.7	10.5	33.3	62.5
(j) Dry fruits	-	26.7	8.3	5.6	15.8	16.7	37.5
(k) Any other	-	-	-	-	-	7.1	-

fast), were reasons why older women fast. For younger women, i.e. 40-60 years of age, the reasons for fasting were mainly busy schedule of housework and being alone at home (no one at home to give company), due to which they either did not have the time to or they did not feel like cooking and preferred to fast.

With respect to frequency of fasting, among depressed women in the age group of 40-60 years, low and middle income women fasted more frequently, i.e. more than twice a week (40-46 percent). Non-depressed women fasted more frequently than depressed women, even though a lesser percentage of non-depressed women followed fasting practices.

With regard to meal pattern during fasting, among depressed women of both age groups, the majority showed higher preference for roots and tubers, milk and milk products and fruits. They preferred eating dry fruits, sweets and pulses the least.

Intake of cereals, non-cereals, pulses, green leafy vegetables, other vegetables is higher among low income women over 60 years of age, indicating that they may be taking a one time meal when they fast.

A comparison between meal pattern of depressed and non-depressed women shows that 75 – 87 percent of the non-depressed women consumed green leafy and other vegetables and all consume roots and tubers and fruits, while depressed women consume mostly fruits (84.2 percent) and milk and milk products (63.2 percent).

Skipping meals

Non-depressed women did not skip meals, the few who do, generally skip breakfast. The main reasons for skipping meals by depressed women were: busy schedule (completing household chores), low mood, digestive disorders or other complaints like headache, body ache, etc., inability to afford more meals in a day. Low income women cited their inability to afford more meals or unavailability of food as the main reason for skipping meals. It was also observed that feeling of isolation or loneliness, fatigue, resulting in lack of interest in preparing meals and undesirable or unfavorable environment in the family were also reasons why women in the younger age group skipped meals. Among older women age 60 years the reasons for skipping meals were: lack of support from the family, quarrels, arguments and conflicts in the family, lack of choices in matters of food cooked, physical disability or locomotor complaints impeding ability to prepare meals, financial dependence on other family members, and austerity practices on account of widowhood.

Overall the present study shows that women do not regularly take breakfast and it is also the meal that they tend to skip. The benefits of regular intake of breakfast are well known. A study has reported that eating breakfast regularly improves performance and leads to a more positive mood, better memory and feelings of calmness. Researchers who compared three studies involving breakfast, memory function and blood glucose levels concluded "Eating breakfast benefits memory". They found that a high blood glucose level after eating breakfast is one of the key reasons for the improvement in mental performance, particularly the speed of recalling new information. Skipping meals cuts calories, but all it does is to evoke a primal "fear of hunger response" that causes overeating later. Further it affects the brain functioning mechanism deteriorating the overall appearance (Kartz, 2004).

Among depressed women age 40-60 years, consumption of special health foods was highest in the high income group (62.1 percent), and lowest in the low income group (16.7 percent). The same is true for women with depression in the age of 60 years and above, except that intake of special health foods was much lower in women frcm the middle income group (35.7 percent) when compared with their counterparts in the 40-60 age group (44.4 percent) and also in comparison with their counterparts in the non-depressed category (55 percent).

The type of special health foods consumed by women were mainly multivitamin tablets, as reported by 42–54 percent of women in the 40–60 ag group, and ayurvedic supplements as reported by 30–78 percent of women over 60 years of age. While hardly any women consumed items like herbs or medicines, women reported that they used commonly available cooking ingredients as kitchen or home remedies for different ailments. For example they used garlic to control cholesterol levels, blood pressure, *methi* (fenugreek) seeds for arthritis and diabetes, ginger for respiratory problems, asofoetida for gastric troubles, clove for toothaches, and turmeric for cough.

The main reasons for not consuming any special health foods was that many of these women considered the decline in their physical health and fitness as a natural part of the process of aging, and therefore did not feel the need to consume any special health foods or medicines. Lack of family support, care and attention were also reasons for not consuming any special health foods. Not surprisingly, low income women did not consume any special health foods as they could not afford these.

Craving for special foods: Serotonin is responsible for the calming and relaxation states with a general sense of well-being. High levels of serotonin can cause a person to feel sluggish and drowsy. Low levels of serotonin will cause intense food cravings. Serotonin is released in the brain as a result of eating carbohydrates for e.g. foods such as fruits, bread and grains.

Women more commonly report food cravings than do men, and depressed mood appears to influence the severity of these cravings. Reports of food cravings are more common in the premenstrual phase, a time when total food intake increases and a parallel change occur in the basal metabolic rate. However, studies do not consistently show that carbohydrate-rich foods, thought to alleviate depressed mood, are preferentially chosen at this time. Restrained eaters, who suffer from premenstrual mood changes, are particularly prone to food cravings. Consequently, psychological factors are strong determinants of foods craved that tend to be high in fat and sweet tasting.

In the present study, women were asked whether they had any special craving for certain types of food. Table 32 presents the responses of women to this question. As can be seen from the table, craving for certain foods was most frequently reported by middle income women in the 40-60 age group (71.4 percent), followed by high income women (66.7 percent) in the same age group. Even among low income women, craving for certain food items was reported by a substantial percentage of women in both age groups (40-47 percent).

Craving for food items was reported less by non-depressed women (20 percent) than by depressed women (51.7 percent) than by). This could be attributed to more regular meal pattern, better care of health needs among non-depressed women.

Table 32: Craving for food items in depressed and non-depressed women, by age and income group

Whether women crave for any foods items	*Depressed*						*Non-depressed*
	40-60 yrs			*>60 yrs*			*>60 yrs*
	LIG n=30	*MIG n=30*	*HIG n=30*	*LIG n=30*	*MIG n=30*	*HIG n=30*	*MIG n=20*
	%	%	%	%	%	%	%
Yes	46.7	**71.4**	66.7	40.0	**51.7**	**50.0**	20.0
No	53.3	28.6	33.3	60.0	48.3	50.0	80.0

Overall most of the women with depression in both age groups had craving for foods like sweets, salty and crispy food items, and chocolates. When probed further, women reported that they experienced cravings for such foods when they felt lonely, neglected, or if they had skipped meals, or they had lost interest in other foods after menopause.

Reduction in food consumption: Reduction of food intake due to loss of appetite, low mood, and other psychological reasons has been associated with depression. To see whether women's depressed state has had any effect on their food intake, in the present study, women were asked whether there has been any reduction in food consumption as compared to the past few years due to any of the reasons such as lost appetite, no mood, development of aversion or dislike or any other reasons. Table 33 presents the responses of women. As can be seen in the table, reduction in food consumption due to any of the above reasons is greatest among low income women in the age groups of 40-60 years and above 60 years, with 80-87 percent women in both age groups reporting reduction in food consumption compared to the past few years due to any of the above reasons. For low income women, besides loss of appetite and low mood, inability to afford food of their choice, no choice in the matter of what to eat were reasons for reduction in food consumption.

After low income women, reduction of food consumption due to lost appetite and low mood is reported by a very high percentage of high income women, particularly those above 60 years of age (83 percent).

Nearly two-thirds of middle income women aged 40-60 years and those above 60 years reported reduction in food consumption due to lost appetite, low mood and aversion to food were also reported by 38-53 percent of the women.

Table 33: Reduction in food consumption as compared to past few years of depressed and Non-depressed subjects

Reasons	*Depressed*						*Non-depressed*
	40-60 yrs			*>60 yrs*			*>60 yrs*
	LIG n=30	*MIG n=30*	*HIG n=30*	*LIG n=30*	*MIG n=30*	*HIG n=30*	*MIG n=20*
	%	%	%	%	%	%	%
Lost appetite	**86.7**	60.0	66.7	**86.7**	60.0	83.3	25.0
No mood	**86.7**	53.3	63.3	**86.7**	37.9	83.3	-
Developed aversion/ dislike	**58.6**	44.8	46.7	**75.0**	50.0	63.3	10.0
Any other	**80.0**	100	100	**87.5**	22.2	87.5	50.0

It is interesting to note that an overwhelming majority of the women (80-100 percent), except middle income women over the age of 60, also stated other reasons such as isolation, loneliness, unpleasant situation/environment at home, lack of family support, loss of interest in cooking, lack of choice in what to eat, dominance of spouse/in-laws, etc., for the reduction in their food consumption.

In sharp contrast, only one-fourth of the non-depressed women reported reduction in food consumption due to lost appetite and an even lesser percentage reported reduction in food consumption due to development of aversion or dislike. As a matter of fact, half of the women stated other reasons such as advancing age, health consciousness, fasting, illness and major health problems, etc. for reducing their food consumption. Clearly, women who were non-depressed reduced their food intake due to health related reasons rather than psychological or social reasons as mentioned by women who were depressed.

Besides reduction in food consumption women were asked whether they had made any changes in the consumption of food over the past 5- 10 years. They were also asked to specify whether they had completely stopped, or decreased or increased the intake of foods read out to them. Nearly 80-100 percent of the women with depression across age and income groups have made changes in their food consumption in the past 5-10 years.

Between 48-52 percent of women in the age group of 40-60 yrs age group showed no change in consumption of cereals, pulses, *masalas*, sweet and sugars compared to 22.2 percent of women age 60 years and above. Further 43-60 percent of the subjects had decreased the consumption of milk and milk products, fried foods, ghee, pickles, citrus and other fruits. Reasons for decreasing consumption of these foods were: lack of awareness about the importance of milk and milk products and fruits, inability to afford these foods.

Similar findings also emerge for women in the middle income group. Among women in the high income group, more than half of the women over 60 years of age reported decrease in the consumption of various foods such as cereals, milk and milk products, fried foods, ghee, *masalas*, pickles, sweets, and sugar.

Overall a striking reduction in food consumption was reported by majority of women above age 60. The reasons given by them were lack of appetite, aging, indigestion, major health problems, disregard for their choice of foods by their family, and no power to decide what to eat.

Majority of the non-depressed women reported increased consumption of foods such as cereals, fried foods, ghee, *masalas*, vegetables and citrus fruits, whereas only 6-10 percent of depressed women reported an increase in the consumption of these foods. Complete omission of non-vegetarian foods was reported by the non-depressed women, whereas 14 percent of women with depression reported no change in the consumption of non-vegetarian food.

Food causing allergy: Studies have shown that prevalence of allergic manifestations from food is higher in people with depression because they become superstitious; they lose interest from the surroundings and become skeptical about eating and find problems.

In the present study women were asked whether there are foods they consume, which cause allergic manifestations. Those who responded in the affirmative were asked to specify the foods that they perceived were causing allergic manifestations.

Table 34: Experience of allergic manifestation caused by foods in depressed and non-depressed women regarding, by age and income level

Whether there are foods that cause allergic manifestations	*Depressed*						*Non-depressed*
	40-60 yrs			*>60 yrs*			*> 60 yrs*
	LIG n=30	*MIG n=30*	*HIG n=30*	*LIG n=30*	*MIG n=30*	*HIG n=30*	*MIG n=20*
	%	%	%	%	%	%	%
Yes	33.3	**51.7**	36.7	16.7	46.7	**50.0**	5.0
No	66.7	48.3	63.3	83.3	53.3	50.0	95.0

As can be seen from Table 34, allergic manifestations caused by food have been reported more by depressed women age 40-60 years from the middle income group (51.7 percent) and by high income women (50 percent) and middle income women (46.7 percent) in the age group of 60 and above years. Thus about half of the middle and high income women age 60 years and above are more prone to food allergy, whereas food allergy is reported least in by low income women. Also, while nearly half of the middle income women with depression (47 percent) reported allergic manifestations caused by food, the same was reported by hardly 5 percent of their non-depressed counterparts.

A study by Antonia (1999) conducted in the UK reports that although food allergy can have serious health consequences, little is currently known about people's perceptions. The study examined the differences in awareness and perceptions of food allergy and depression between young people with and without a food allergy. Out of the 162 participants of the study, 24 reported they were allergic to at least one food; these people perceived that their allergy had significantly less of an impact on their lives. Allergy status was found influenced by perceived health competence to affect anxiety leading to depression. People with an allergy and with high health competence reported the greatest depression levels. Very few of the subjects however, knew the meaning of the term 'allergy'.

Thus, food allergy signs and symptoms can also be very esoteric, and can impact the thought process and concentration, and this can change behavior or mood leading to depression, agitation or may even cause dizziness. Food allergy symptoms can also cause seemingly unrelated symptoms, making the diagnosis ever harder.

Food preference: To know the food preference of women, they were read out a list of foods and asked whether they liked eating any of them.

A comparison between the food preferences of depressed and non-depressed middle income women above the age of 60 shows that the majority of non-depressed women had greater preference for salted and baked items (53 percent each), milk based foods and fast foods (71 percent each), as well as dry fruits, processed items and instant mixes, when compared to their depressed counterparts, who showed greater preference for sweets and farsan.

Food choice is influenced by various physiological, social and cultural factors and is not determined solely by whether people consider a food to be healthy or not. Mood is just one factor that can impact on food preferences, food cravings, dietary behavior and short and long term responses to dietary intervention.

Nutrient intake: As stated in the beginning of this section, many people understand the connection between nutrition and a physical disease state, but fewer people are aware of the connection between nutrition and depression. Depression is more typically thought of as strictly emotional or biochemical.

A comparison between the food preferences of depressed and non-depressed middle income women above the age of 60 shows that the majority of non-depressed women had greater preference for salted and baked items (53 percent each), milk based foods and fast foods (71 percent each), as well as dry fruits, processed items and instant mixes, when compared to their depressed counterparts, who showed greater preference for sweets and farsan.

Food choice is influenced by various physiological, social and cultural factors and is not determined solely by whether people consider a food to be healthy or not. Mood is just one factor that can impact on food preferences, food cravings, dietary behavior and short and long term responses to dietary intervention.

Nutrient intake: As stated in the beginning of this section, many people understand the connection between nutrition and a physical disease state, but fewer people are aware of the connection between nutrition and depression. Depression is more typically thought of as strictly emotional or biochemical.

Nutrition, however, can play a key role, both in the onset, severity, and duration of depression, including daily mood swings. Many of the same food patterns that precede depression are the same food patterns that occur during depression. Being diet related or caused due to a deficiency of some nutrient, diet modification can help in mood change in depression, if depression is not a major one. For instance, folic acid is considered, as one of the key mood-related nutrients. Scientists say that many patients experiencing depressive behavior have been found to be deficient in folic acid and therefore increasing the amounts of folate (folic acid in foods) can make marked differences in depressive behavior. Repeatedly, diet for depression research has found that insufficient consumption of polyunsaturated fatty acids, antioxidant vitamins, folate, and Vitamin B12 is associated with depression. Moreover, Vitamin B12 works synergistically with other vitamins (namely folic acid) to lower homocysteine levels. Having elevated homocysteine levels is one of the most important markers for risk of unbalanced mental status, which can lead to depression and anxiety along with heart disease. Other functions and benefits include its role as an oxygen carrier, metabolizing fat and boosting the immune system.

The imbalance of levels of minerals such as magnesium and calcium has been found to be associated with depressed state. A study by Gudson (1998) measuring the level of magnesium and calcium in the cerebrospinal fluid of individuals who are depressed and suicidal, found higher levels of calcium in those who were depressed and lower levels of magnesium in those who were suicidal and depressed.

Selenium is known to have a marked effect in lifting depression. This mineral can be obtained by eating foods such as tuna and whole-grain foods. Large amounts of these foods are not required to get the benefits since only a small amount of Selenium is needed.

Tryptophan is an amino acid found in many high protein foods. When individuals who are depressed are put on a diet, the tryptophan levels decrease, which in turn increases depression. Therefore an attempt was made in the present study to assess the nutrient intake of women.

Nutrient intake was assessed using the 24-hour dietary recall method and the food frequency questionnaire, which had an exhaustive list of foods rich in nutrients that play an important role in depression. In order to assess deficiency, the frequency of consumption of these foods was also asked. All calculations of nutrient intake are based on the Recommended Dietary Allowance (RDA) which is standardized for all the nutrients involved. The assessment of nutrient intake was in terms of energy, protein, fat, iron, folic acid, isoflavone, Vitamins (C, B6, B12), minerals (Calcium, Choline, Potassium and Selenium), and Amino acids (Methionine, Phenylalanine and Tryptophan). The mean nutrient intake of depressed and non-depressed women is presented in Table 35.

As can be seen from the table, there was significant difference ($p \leq 0.05$) by income level in the nutrient intake of depressed women in both 40-60 and above 60 age groups. As expected, among depressed women, least nutrient intake was seen more among low income women above 60 years of age. A study by Boston (1999) involving 724 single, low-income women reported that those who did not have sufficient nutrients were more likely to have major depression.

Higher values of mean intake of all nutrients were seen in high income women age 40-60 years. Further, younger depressed women from the middle income group showed a higher significant difference ($p \leq 0.05$) and better nutrient intake with respect to energy, iron, folic acid and amino acids compared to older depressed women of the same income group.

There were marginal differences in the intake of nutrients like isoflavone, choline and Vitamin-C within the depressed group. The findings also reveal significant difference (p£0.05) with poor intake of folic acid, selenium, Vitamin B6 and Vitamin-B12.

There was also significant difference (p£0.05) in the nutrient intake of middle income older women with depression and their counterparts who were non-depressed, with the latter showing higher intake of all nutrients than the former.

The food frequency questionnaire included an exhaustive list of foods rich in isoflavone, folic acid, amino acids (tryptophan, phenylalanine, and methionine), Vitamin C, Vitamin B complex and Vitamin B12. The foods, which were included to evaluate the association between frequent intake of these nutrients and

Table 35: Mean nutrient intakes of depressed and non-depressed women, by age and income level

Nutrients	*Depressed*						*Non-depressed*	*f-value*	*p-value*
	40-60 yrs			*>60 yrs*			*>60 yrs*		
	LIG n=30	*MIG n=30*	*HIG n=30*	*LIG n=30*	*MIG n=30*	*HIG n=30*	*MIG n=20*		
Energy (Kcal)	1264 + 303	1832 + 369	1903 + 541	1012 + 357	1343 + 334	1305 + 337	1906 + 341	25.8717	*0.0000
Protein (gms)	22 + 10	35 +10	35 + 10	19+ 8	30+9	27+8	56+9	32.6112	*0.0000
Fat (gm)	18 + 7	28+ 8	29+ 11	18+ 8	23+ 8	28+ 8	45+ 9	27.2939	*0.0000
Iron (mg)	19 + 6	28+ 9	22+ 9	14+ 9	17+ 7	20+ 8	38+ 6	25.0492	*0.0000
Folic acid (ug)	83 + 37	102+32	80+39	59+29	53+17	70+37	141+23	20.7691	*0.0000
Vitamin B6 (mg)	1.47 +1.16	1.76+1.05	1.50+0.69	0.90+0.91	0.96+0.70	1.18+0.53	2.98+0.90	14.9898	*0.0000
Vitamin B12 (ug)	0.81+0.77	0.79+0.70	0.86+0.43	0.53+0.57	0.44+0.46	0.61+0.40	1.48+0.31	8.0870	*0.0000
Calcium (mg)	189 + 111	266+94	235+76	177+86	228+93	255+86	508+76	33.4221	*0.0000
Choline (mg)	23 + 10	24+12	28+11	20+8	18+9	27+9	46+11	20.0195	*0.0000
Isoflavone (mg)	35+ 14	40+13	41+10	31+12	31+11	40+11	73+9	34.6444	*0.0000
Tryptophan (mg)	120 +30	143+36	136+39	115+30	121+28	133+34	276+43	58.6545	*0.0000
Methionine (mg)	373 +127	481+116	387+150	343+136	409+115	443+118	657+45	16.7916	*0.0000
Phenylalanine (mg)	138 +54	148+44	130+44	110+37	125+36	113+34	249+26	29.7908	*0.0000
Vitamin C (mg)	22 +13	29+10	25+8	23+8	17+8	23+8	55+8	38.0134	*0.0000
Potassium (mg)	1720 +690	1826+882	1905+690	1990+690	1930+799	2016+1074	5219+855	46.6175	*0.0000
Selenium (ug)	8.09+10.51	6.79+8.14	8.53+9.00	7.33+7.09	7.47+9.86	6.89+6.40	42.75+12.15	45.7992	*0.0000

occurrence of the disease, were cereals, pulses, vegetables, fruits, nuts and oilseeds, isoflavone, folic acid, iron, amino acid and vitamin B6.

Consumption of milk and milk products was included to assess the role of folic acid, amino acid and Vitamin B12 with the occurrence of depression. Besides cereals, animal foods and sea foods were specially analyzed for minerals (choline and selenium) as it is known as "Good mood" minerals.

Consumption of fruits and vegetables were investigated to evaluate the relationship between these foods and Vitamin C. Craving for sweets and sugars stimulate the production of neurotransmitter and work as antidepressant therefore sugar dense foods were also included in the list of foods in the questionnaire. The consumption of all these food items was noted in terms of daily intake, once a week, twice a week, fortnightly, monthly, occasionally and never. The analysis is presented in Table 36.

Table 36: Food frequency of depressed and non-depressed women, by age and income level

Food groups	*Depressed*						*Non-depressed*
	40-60 yrs			*>60 yrs*			*>60 yrs*
	LIG n=30	*MIG n=30*	*HIG n=30*	*LIG n=30*	*MIG n=30*	*HIG n=30*	*MIG n=20*
	%	*%*	*%*	*%*	*%*	*%*	*%*
Cereals and grains							
(a) Non- Frequent	**13.3**	-	-	23.3	**6.7**	**23.3**	10.0
(b) Frequent	**86.7**	100	**100**	**76.7**	93.3	76.7	90.0
Pulses							
(a) Non- Frequent	70.0	36.7	**6.7**	60.0	43.3	**23.3**	15.0
(b) Frequent	30.0	63.3	**93.3**	40.0	56.7	**76.7**	85.0
Green leafy vegetables							
(a) Non- Frequent	**80.0**	33.3	-	**33.3**	33.3	10.0	15.0
(b) Frequent	**20.0**	66.7	100	66.7	**66.7**	90.0	85.0
Fruits							
(a) Non- Frequent	**70.0**	43.3	23.3	86.7	43.3	**36.7**	10.0
(b) Frequent	**30.0**	56.7	76.7	13.3	56.7	**63.3**	90.0

(Contd.)

(Contd. Table 36)

Food groups	*Depressed*						*Non-depressed*
	40-60 yrs			*>60 yrs*			*>60 yrs*
	LIG n=30	*MIG n=30*	*HIG n=30*	*LIG n=30*	*MIG n=30*	*HIG n=30*	*MIG n=20*
	%	*%*	*%*	*%*	*%*	*%*	*%*
Milk/Milk products							
(a) Non- Frequent	**76.7**	36.7	30.0	90.0	70.0	**60.0**	15.0
(b) Frequent	**23.3**	63.3	70.0	**10.0**	30.0	**40.0**	85.0
Spices							
(a) Non- Frequent	**20.0**	-	6.7	23.3	13.3	**23.3**	10.0
(b) Frequent	**80.0**	100	93.3	**76.7**	86.7	76.7	90.0
Roots and tubers							
(a) Non- Frequent	**26.7**	56.7	10.0	50.0	86.7	**30.0**	5.0
(b) Frequent	73.3	43.3	90.0	50.0	13.3	70.0	95.0
Other vegetables							
(a) Non- Frequent	**60.0**	23.3	-	**46.7**	40.0	16.7	5.0
(b) Frequent	40.0	76.7	100	53.3	60.0	83.3	95.0
Animal foods							
(a) Non- Frequent	**83.3**	**90.0**	76.7	**86.7**	90.0	86.7	80.0
(b) Frequent	**16.7**	10.0	23.3	13.3	10.0	**13.3**	20.0
Sea foods							
(a) Non- Frequent	**96.7**	100	86.7	96.7	93.3	**86.7**	85.0
(b) Frequent	**3.3**	-	13.3	3.3	6.7	**13.3**	15.0
Fats and oils							
(a) Non- Frequent	76.7	86.7	**3. 3**	100	**93.3**	86.7	55.0
(b) Frequent	23.3	13.3	**96.7**	-	**6.7**	13.3	45.0
Nuts and oilseeds							
(a) Non- Frequent	**83.3**	40.0	20.0	90.0	**60.0**	53.3	25.0
(b) Frequent	**16.7**	60.0	80.0	10.0	**40.0**	46.7	75.0
Sugar dense foods							
(a) Non- Frequent	**53.3**	36.7	20.0	66.7	**40.0**	53.3	20.0
(b) Frequent	**46.7**	63.3	80.0	33.3	**60.0**	46.7	80.0

Among women with depression in both age groups, non-frequent consumption of all food groups in the questionnaire was reported more by women from the low income group than by their counterparts in the middle and high income group.

A marked difference was seen among younger and older depressed women within the middle income group, with the former having more frequent intake of these foods compared to the latter. A similar trend was observed also among younger and older depressed women in the high income group.

Regardless of age or income level or depression status, animal foods and sea foods, were consumed less frequently by most women, indicating that important sources of "good mood" minerals such as choline and selenium were not being consumed by most women.

A comparison between frequency of consumption of various foods by depressed and non-depressed women age 60 years and above and belonging to the middle income group shows that a significantly higher percentage of non-depressed women consumed most of the food items, including animal foods, milk and milk products, more frequently than their counterparts who were depressed.

A number of studies have shown an association between low selenium intake and a significantly greater incidence of depression and other negative mood states. A UK study by Benton and Cook (2000) showed that a supplement of 100 mg/day of selenium significantly improved mood and decreased anxiety and depression. The beneficial effect of selenium was most marked in those consuming lesser amounts of dietary selenium. Older people may be particularly susceptible to depressed mood, so ensuring adequate intakes of selenium seems sensible. Rich dietary sources of selenium in the UK include Brazil nuts, kidney, liver and shellfish, particularly crab.

There is some evidence to support the various claims that the balance of protein and carbohydrate consumed in a meal can affect the synthesis and activity of the brain neurotransmitter serotonin that improves mood. However, other results suggest that the variations in protein and carbohydrate intake achieved by eating real foods are insufficient to affect brain serotonergic function significantly. Studies have shown that the ratio of fat to carbohydrate in a meal significantly affects mood, alertness and mental performance, albeit with optimal effects occurring when the composition of the experimental meals matched that of the participant's habitual diet. Similarly, studies on caffeine found that repeatedly pairing the consumption of a novel fruit juice drink with caffeine, improved mood and increased consumer's final preference for the drink. These results show that the mood effects of eating and drinking reinforce dietary preferences that benefit mood. In other words, the effects of food on mood help to shape food preferences.

The bottom line is that food plays a key role in maintaining mental health. In reality, the brain is basically a chemical factory that constantly produces dozens of neurotransmitters, such as serotonin and dopamine, which act as messengers to start, continue or stop biochemical processes. The raw materials or "building blocks" for these processes, the only ones, are vitamins, minerals, amino acids, fatty acids and other nutrients. If brain is given the wrong mix of nutrients, due to a) genetically determined imbalances that create excessive or insufficient levels of these nutrients in the brain, b) incomplete nutrition or c) both, the result will be the wrong mix of neurotransmitters leading to escalating levels of mental imbalances.

Hence from the above results of the present study and other studies reviewed here it may be concluded that there is significant difference in the mean nutrient intake of depressed women and non-depressed women. Vulnerability to depression is greater in the case of elderly women, who are found deficient in proper nutrient intake. This deficient intake is often associated with untreated and undiagnosed physical illnesses, which are commonly believed to be a natural part of the process of ageing, loss of spouse, dependence on others in food habits and dietary intake, lack of family support and isolation, all of which have affected the appetite and nutritional status of elderly women.

Nutritional status of women

Nutritional status was assessed in terms of anthropometric measurements and clinical parameters. Anthropometric measurements such as height, weight, mid-upper arm circumference (MUAC) and body mass index (BMI) were assessed using bathroom scale and measuring tape. The biochemical parameters included blood pressure assessment to know the prevalence of hypertension. Anthropometric and clinical parameters were analyzed using f-test. The mean levels of all the anthropometric and clinical parameters and *f*-values of depressed and non-depressed women are shown in Table 37.

Table 37: Mean anthropometric and clinical measurements of depressed group and non-depressed women, by age and income level

Parameters	Depressed						Non-depressed	f- ratio	f- value
	40-60 yrs			>60 yrs			>60 yrs		
	LIG n=30	MIG n=30	HIG n=30	LIG n=30	MIG n=30	HIG n=30	MIG n=20		
Anthropometric									
Height (cm)	153.0± 12.0	158.0± 11.0	159.2± 11.9	157.7± 8.6	154.8± 8.0	156.6± 12.4	154.4±10.4	0.83	0.54
Weight (kg)	57± 11	62±10	64±7	58± 13	61±10	61± 10	64± 7	1.98	0.07
MUAC (cm)	32± 12	40±15	33±8	32±9	39±11	31±8	43±9	4.12	0.007
BMI (kg/m²)	22.82± 7.09	25.16± 4.57	25.79± 5.55	23.26± 4.60	25.46± 3.72	25.10± 3.80	27.04± 3.87	2.18	0.046
Blood pressure									
Systolic MmHg	118 + 18	127 + 14	122 + 15	127 + 12	121 + 17	133 + 17	121 + 9	2.9297	0.0097
Diastolic MmHg	81 + 14	86 + 10	91 + 13	108 + 156	86 + 15	117 + 157	115 + 138	0.5318	0.7835

Volues are means ±S.E.

As the table shows, there was no significant difference (p£0.05) by income or age in the case of weight, height, MUAC and BMI in depressed women. In terms of BMI, except women from low income group, depressed women in both age groups as well as non-depressed women were overweight.

Further, no significant difference was found in the systolic and diastolic blood pressures in both age groups of depressed groups. A few women, but with marginal difference had hypertension. Similar results emerged for non-depressed women.

Prevalence of health problems

Using an exhaustive checklist and free listing method information was collected from the women on the prevalence of various major and minor health problems and diseases in them. Table 38 presents the morbidity profile of depressed and non-depressed women, the types of major health problems prevalent in them.

From the table it can be clearly seen that the prevalence of major health problems was higher in women over 60 years of age. Among them, prevalence was higher in middle income women.

Locomotor problems ranked first (52 percent) in all the income groups, followed by oral cavity problems (43.3 percent) and cardiovascular (31 problem) in middle income women above 60 years of age.

Neurological problems were reported least in depressed women of both age groups. Nearly one-third of depressed high income women age 40-60 years reported respiratory and gastrointestinal (23.3 percent) problems. Other problems were equally distributed in both the age groups of depressed women and there was only a marginal difference in prevalence.

In the non-depressed group, it was interesting to note that hardly 10 percent of the women reported locomotor problems and still fewer reported endocrine and respiratory problems (5 percent each) compared to their depressed counterparts. Other than these, non-depressed women did not have any major health complaints. A study by Sharma (1999) found that locomotor disability and amnesia/ senility (loss of memory) were also quite common among the aged.

Table 38: Major health problems in depressed and non-depressed women, by age and income level

Type of health problem	*Depressed*						*Non-depressed*
	40-60 yrs			*>60 yrs*			*>60 yrs*
	LIG n=30	*MIG n=30*	*HIG n=30*	*LIG n=30*	*MIG n=30*	*HIG n=30*	*MIG n=20*
	%	%	%	%	%	%	%
1. Oral cavity problems							
a. Yes	16.7	13.3	**26.7**	16.7	**43.3**	26.7	-
b. No	83.3	**86.7**	73.3	**83.3**	56.7	73.3	100
2. Gastrointestinal problems							
a. Yes	20.0	10.0	**23.3**	6.7	**26.7**	13.3	-
b. No	80.0	**90.0**	76.7	**93.3**	73.3	86.7	100
3. Respiratory problems							
a. Yes	13.3	16.7	**26.7**	16.7	20.7	**26.7**	5.0
b. No	**86.7**	83.3	73.3	**83.3**	79.3	73.3	95.0
4.Cardiovascular problems							
a. Yes	13.3	**20.0**	16.7	10.0	**31.0**	16.7	-
b. No	**86.7**	80.0	83.3	**90.0**	69.0	83.3	100
5. Genito-urinary problems							
a. Yes	**16.7**	6.7	13.3	6.7	-	6.7	-
b. No	83.3	**93.3**	86.7	**93.3**	100	**93.3**	100
6. Locomoter problems							
a. Yes	**46.7**	40.0	30.0	**53.3**	**51.7**	30.0	10.0
b. No	53.3	60.0	**70.0**	46.7	48.3	**70.0**	90.0
7. Neurological problems							
a. Yes	6.7	6.7	6.7	10.0	**10.3**	10.0	-
b. No	93.3	93.3	93.3	**90.0**	89.7	**90.0**	100
8. Psychiatric problems							
a. Yes	20.0	3.3	**20.7**	10.0	3.4	**20.0**	-
b. No	80.0	**96.7**	79.3	90.0	**96.6**	80.0	100
9. Endocrine problems							
a. Yes	3.3	**16.7**	3.3	6.7	**13.8**	3.3	5.0
b. No	**96.7**	83.3	**96.7**	93.3	86.2	**96.7**	95.0
10. Any other							
a. Yes	4.5	4.3	**10.0**	8.3	**16.7**	13.0	-
b. No	95.5	**95.7**	90.0	**91.7**	83.3	87.0	100

The prevalence of locomotor disability among the aged was as high as 11,107 per 100,000 in rural areas, while it was 8,781 per 100,000 in urban areas. The elderly females are more likely to have suffered from this problem than elderly males.

In a study conducted by Deoki (1999) in Agra district, it was found that the aged constituted 6.5 percent of the total population, and 79 percent had some morbidity, with an average prevalence of 1.6 morbidities per person. The most common morbidities were locomotor, gastrointestinal, respiratory and musculoskeletal problems (48.8 percent, 29.5 percent, 23.3 percent and 10.2 percent respectively). A similar study carried out on the health care of the aged in rural areas by Guha Raj (1994) in the district of Madurai, Tamil Nadu, reported that out of the 1910 elderly screened, 88 percent had vision related complaints, 40 percent had locomotor problems, followed by symptoms of nervous system (19 percent), cardiovascular disease (17 percent), respiratory problems (16 percent), gastrointestinal (10 percent) and psychiatric (9 percent) problems.

Depressed people often complain of more of minor illnesses, therefore an attempt was made to assess the prevalence of minor health complaints in women. As can be seen from Table 38.

Prevalence of psychological complaints and complaints related to the digestive system was reported in most of the women. Complaints like acidity, indigestion, flatulence, constipation and lack of appetite is mainly reported by depressed women in the older age group compared to those in the younger age group.

Most of the women in the younger age group reported loss of interest, fluctuation in blood pressure, lack of sleep, low mood and lethargy - all psychosomatic complaints. Low mood was highly prevalent in the entire group of depressed women.

Also, physical complaints like body ache ulcers, headache and dryness of skin are more prevalent in older depressed subjects, which reflect result of combination of ageing and depression. Conversely, in younger group acidity, psychosomatic problems, dizziness and headaches were reported more, which may be due to menopausal problems, anxiety, and isolation that women face at this stage.

Among women in the non-depressed group the prevalence of all minor complaints was ranged between 5-35 percent. Only cough and cold was reported by 50 percent of these women. This shows that prevalence of minor health problems is lesser in non-depressed women as compared to those who are depressed.

Findings of similar study done by Mehta and Desai (2004) showed that the prevalence of feeling of tiredness ranked highest in women who were depressed (85 percent). Problems like acidity (60 percent), backache (55 percent), headache (45 percent) and difficulty in doing daily activities (45 percent) were also more prevalent in this group of women. In the non-depressed group, the only complaints were headache (40 percent) and feeling of tiredness (40 percent), but their prevalence was much lower than that in the depressed group.

Correlation between Psychosocial and Nutritional Aspects in Women with Depression

As mentioned earlier, statistical tests were applied on the data collected from the 180 women with moderate depression to find out whether there is any association between psychosocial and nutritional factors with respect to depression and to explore the interplay of these factors on each other.

The psychosocial parameters selected for studying the association were: power structure, isolation, life events and self esteem. The nutrition related parameter selected for studying the association was: general nutrient intake or by and large calorie intake, i.e. the standard RDA calorie intake.

Tables 39, 40, 41, and 42 show the correlations between the psychosocial parameters - power structure, feeling of isolation, experience of stressful life events and self-esteem - and nutrient intake of women with depression.

Table 39: Correlation between power structure and calorie intake of depressed women (N=180)

Power structure	*Calorie intake Mean value±S.E*	*f- ratio*	*f- value*
Satisfied (n= 30)	1433± 501	0.6028	0.5484
Dissatisfied (n=100)	1393 ± 491		
Not sure (n=50)	1530 ± 470		

It can be seen from Table 39 that none of the categories of satisfaction with existing power structure showed significant difference with the calorie intake of depressed women. In other words, women who were satisfied with the existing power structure within the family had better calorie intake.

While screening for depression using the BDI, it was found that the prevalence of loss of appetite and feeling of isolation were high, therefore an attempt was made to see whether low calorie intake had any relationship with feeling of isolation.

Table 40: Correlation between isolation and calorie intake of women with depression (N=180)

Isolation	*Calorie intake Mean value ± S.E*	*t- value*	*p-value*
Always + sometimes (n=130)	1077 + 107.5	4.41*	0.000
Never (n=50)	1112 + 101.1		

*Significant at $p<0.05$

As can be seen from Table 40 the association of isolation and calorie intake were significant ($p \leq 0.05$) in depressed women, which means that women who ranked higher for isolation on the BDI also had lower calorie intake. Here it needs to be mentioned that when women were being interviewed on the psychosocial aspects they were asked what they do when they feel isolated. Their response was loss of appetite, no mood to eat. This explains the low calorie intake by women who experience feelings of isolation.

Stress is a major factor which affects the maintenance of overall health status as it leads to reduction in food intake, loss of appetite, reduction in weight, etc. Stresses that are chronic or severe can have far-reaching effects. Stress is epidemic and silent killer of the twentieth century. It is both, a physical and an emotional response to a triggering event; coping with it also involves lifestyle changes that many individuals resist in favor of their usual routines.

As can be seen from Table 41, there is a significant difference ($p \leq 0.05$) between the levels of stress caused by life events on calorie intake in depressed women. In other words, women who ranked higher on the Gurmeet Singh stress scale had lower calorie intake.

Table 41: Correlation between experience of stressful life events and calorie intake of women with depression (N=180)

Life events causing stress	*Calorie intake Mean value ± S.E.*	*t- value*	*p- value*
Mild + Moderate (n= 155)	1275.9 +263.8	2.31*	0.000
High (n=25)	1227.8 + 277.8		

*Significant at p<0.05

Stress can cause weight gain as well as weight loss. A study of 45 lean women aged between 65-75 years, found that women gained weight in response to stress and were unable to manage the stressful condition. The study concluded that release of cortisol, a major stress hormone, appears to promote abdominal fat and may be the primary connection between stress and weight gain in those subjects (Daniell, 2000).

Self-esteem can have a positive or negative impact on mental health and also possibly lead to reduced or increased food intake. Therefore an analysis was done to find the impact of self-esteem – both positive and negative - on calorie intake of depressed women as. As Table 42 shows, there is a significant difference (pe" 0.0005) between the positive self esteem level and negative self esteem level and calorie intake of the depressed subjects.

Table 42: Correlation between self-esteem and calorie intake of women with depression (N=180)

Self esteem	*Calorie intake Mean value ± S.E.*	*t- value*	*p- value*
Positive (n=130)	1494.9 + 507.36	-0.02	*0.0004
Negative (n= 50)	1308.1 + 431.7		

* Significant at pe" 0.0005

Women with positive self-esteem had better calorie intake compared to those who had negative self-esteem. Thus the analysis indicates that self-esteem of a person does affect the behavior and consumption of food.

Impact of Folic Acid Supplementation on Depression in Elderly Women

Ageing is associated with decline in physical and mental health. Though biological ageing varies among individuals, with advancing years there is a gradual slowing down of their intellectual functioning, their memory deteriorates and the speed in performance of many tasks also decreases. The physical and social environments have an impact on biosocial aspects of ageing for each individual. Alteration in or loss of social functions performed within the family or community network can change person's self-concept and affect their sense of self-worth. Because of the general decline in health, vitality and activity, there are changes in the mental state, which marks the onset of affective disorders such as depression. It has been found that a significant proportion of the aging population, are depressed.

Symptoms of depression however, are often mistaken for other illnesses or mere "signs of aging." For some reason, depression in most of the elderly people remains diagnosed and untreated. In many cultures, mental illness carries a social stigma. In addition, many administrators with tight budgets reduce services for the elderly.

As age advances, the health problems tend to increase, and often the problems are aggravated due to neglect, poor economic status, social deprivation and inappropriate dietary intake which often result in multiple nutritional deficiencies (Kumar, 1997).

The nutrients we obtain from food enable us to function. But because it is difficult to quantify and measure people's behavior and feelings in response to specific nutrients, researchers are not sure what effects different nutrients might have on our brain.

Though the role of nutrition in preserving mental function in the elderly still remains unclear, recent research has pointed to the role of folic acid[1] in depression. A study of 50 persons with depression, it was found that 31-35 percent of the subjects were deficient in folic acid. Some depressed persons non-responsive to anti-depressant medications became responsive with the addition of folic acid. The doses of folic acid used in the studies for treating depression were very high, ranging from 15-50 mg, which is 15,000-50,000 micrograms (Ross, 2002). Probably the most clinically useful finding so far is that people who are deficient in folate may not respond to drug therapy as well as those with normal folate status.

Several studies in India have assessed the dietary intake and nutritional status of elderly individuals living in different circumstances, but there is no clear or consistent evidence on the impact of eating habits, diet, and nutritional status on mental health. There is also no clear evidence on the extent to which subtle nutritional deficiencies can lead to a poor mental state or on the impact of dietary supplements in individuals with mental disorders. Hence, in view of the existing evidence on the role of folic acid supplementation in depression, it was thought worthwhile to include folic acid supplementation as an intervention in the present study and to evaluate its impact.

Among the 180 women with moderate depression who were selected for in-depth interviews, 90 women were above the age of 60. From among these 90 elderly women who were moderately depressed, 30 women from the middle income group were selected for the intervention, i.e., provision of folic acid supplementation. Elderly women were selected for the intervention as reviews have indicated that advancing age leads to reduction in folic acid levels, which in turn affects cognition. Low folic acid levels also leads to decline in the immune status and increase in the number of physical ailments or complaints. Serum estimations of blood samples showed that women in this age group were more deficient in folic acid than women in the age group of 40-60 years. Elderly women from the middle income group were selected mainly for two reasons: blood serum estimations as well as the calculation of nutrient intake based on the 24 hour recall showed that they were deficient. Women in this age and income group were also found to have more health and psychosocial problems than those in other age and income groups. Lastly, but most importantly, these women readily consented to participate in the intervention, unlike younger women.

The 30 women selected for the intervention were provided folic acid supplementation for a period of two months, which is the minimum period of intervention required to observe improvement in nutrition status.

The impact of folic acid supplementation was evaluated by comparing the pre and post intervention data on the following:

- depression status: severity of depression measured on the Beck Depression Inventory (BDI) Scale;
- nutritional status: estimation of blood hemoglobin and folic acid, measurement of blood pressure to asses the prevalence of hypertension;
- dietary intake: assessment of nutrient intake using 24-hour dietary recall after intervention;
- prevalence of minor health complaints.

Effect on depression status

The BDI scale was used to assess the impact of the intervention, i.e. folic acid supplementation, on the severity of depression. Table 43 shows the BDI scores of the 30 elderly (above 60 years) women, from the middle income group, who were provided folic acid supplementation for a period of two months.

Table 43: Severity of depression in elderly women before and after folic acid supplementation (N= 30)

Parameter	*Mean*		*t-Value*	*p- Value*
	Pre-intervention	*Post-intervention*		
Beck Depression Inventory Score	45.96 ± 3.49	6.131 ± 2.59	81.04	*0.000

*Significant at p£0.05

As can be seen from the table, there was a significant difference (p£0.05) in the severity of depression in elderly women after the intervention.

The level of depression decreased to a greater extent after supplementation from a moderate range of score 45 to 6, which is mild level of depression. Similar finding has also been reported by a study (Desai, 2004) on 20 depressed subjects. The study reported a significant difference in depression levels on BDI scores, where 60 percent of the subjects in moderate category of depression were reduced to 10 percent after intervention.

Effect on nutritional status

The effect of folic acid supplementation on the nutritional status of the 30 elderly women was assessed in terms of clinical (levels of hemoglobin and folic acid in blood and blood pressure) and anthropometric (height, weight, mid and upper arm circumference and body mass index) parameters. Table 44 shows the mean levels of all the clinical parameters and paired t-values of biochemical and clinical parameters.

Table 44: Levels of hemoglobin, folic acid and blood pressure in depressed elderly women before and after folic acid supplementation (N= 30)

Parameters	*Mean*		*t-Value*	*p-Value*
	Pre-intervention	*Post-intervention*		
Hemoglobin (gm/dl)	11.53±0.8	11.22±0.8	3.58	0.0097
Folic Acid (mg) (3-20) range	3.819 ± 1.54	16.13 ± 2.62	- 31.06	*0.0000
Blood pressure (mmHg)	121 ± 17 /86±15	118 ±18 /81± 14	1.57 1.18	0.7835

*Significant at p£0.05

As can be seen from the table, there was a marginal change in the hemoglobin levels. A slight reduction in blood pressure was seen but no significant difference was observed. Marked significant difference (p£0.05) was seen in folic acid levels after intervention. The serum values increased from 3mg to 16mg after intervention.

A study by Mary (1995) found from her study that, depressed patients were found to be deficient in folate, while others did not show statistically significant differences in folate levels between people with and without depression. It was still unclear which came first—the deficiency or the depression. Many depressed people tend to eat poor diets, which can lead to deficiencies of many vitamins and minerals, not just folate.

Further, no significant difference was obtained between the pre- and post-intervention estimates of the height, weight, mid and upper arm circumference (MUAC) (Table 45). However a marginal increase, albeit not significant, is observed in the body mass index (BMI).

Table 45: Anthropometric measurements of depressed elderly women before and after folic acid supplementation (N= 30)

Parameters			
	Mean Values	*f- Ratio*	*f- Value*
Height (cm)	154.8± 8.0	0.83	0.54
Weight (kg)	61±10	1.98	0.07
MUAC (cm)	39±11	4.12	0.007
BMI (kg/m²)	25.46± 3.72	2.18	0.046

Effect on dietary intake

To assess the effect of folic acid supplementation on the dietary intake of the elderly depressed women, pre- and post-intervention

Table 46: Nutrient intake of depressed elderly women before and after folic acid supplementation (N= 30)

Sr. No	*Parameters*	*Mean*		*p-Value*
		Pre-intervention	*Post-intervention*	
1.	Energy	1269	1701	*0.000
2.	Protein	28.03	62.93	*0.000
3.	Fat	24.49	29.62	*0.000
4.	Iron	18.19	36.54	*0.000
5.	Folic acid	59.29	148.40	*0.000
6.	Vitamin B6	0.93	2.35	*0.000
7.	Vitamin B12	0.54	2.18	*0.000
8.	Vitamin C	20.32	45.31	*0.000
9.	Calcium	236.75	611.03	*0.000
10.	Isoflavone	35.22	35.28	0.604
11.	Tryptophan	124.6	484.42	*0.000
12.	Methionine	416.45	630.08	*0.000
13.	Phenylalanine	120.8	293.5	*0.000
14.	Potassium	1941	3087	*0.000
15.	Selenium	7.6	9.4	0.177
16.	Choline	21.81	21.89	0.650

*Significant at p£0.05

data on their nutrient intake (collected using the 24-hour dietary recall method) was compared and is presented in Table 46.

As can be seen from the table, there was a significant difference in the intake of the majority of nutrients. Increased intake of folic acid, iron, vitamin B12, calcium and amino acids is seen after intervention. This shows that supplementation improved the appetite, reduced complaints like 'no mood' or 'aversion', and thereby resulting in reduction in the level of depression. No significant difference is observed in the intake of selenium, choline and isoflavone, the "good mood" minerals.

Effect on health status

In order to see the impact of folic acid supplementation on health status and its interplay with depression, data on disease profile were also analyzed with respect to minor health complaints reported by depressed elderly women after the intervention. The same is presented in Table 47.

Table 47: Minor health complaints reported by depressed elderly women after folic acid supplementation (N= 30)

	Parameters	*Mean*		*Chi-square Value*	*Degree of freedom*	*p- Value*
		Pre-intervention	*Post-intervention*			
1.	Cold & cough	55.7	16.4	20.47	1	*0.00001
2.	Viral fever	19.7	18.0	0.053	1	0.81695
3.	Malaria	6.6	0.0	4.135	1	0.04199
4.	Infections	27.9	11.5	5.187	1	0.02276
5.	Vomiting	6.6	0.0	4.135	1	0.04199
6.	Diarrhea	21.3	9.8	3.054	1	0.08051
7.	Constipation	60.7	23.0	17.82	1	*0.00002
8.	Acidity	57.4	18.0	20.10	1	*0.00001
9.	Indigestion	52.5	16.4	17.57	1	*0.00003
10.	Gas/ flatulence	59.0	16.4	23.59	1	*0.00000
11.	Chest pain	62.3	19.7	22.90	1	*0.00000
12	No interest	73.8	0.0	71.29	1	*0.00000
13	Psychosomatic problems	27.9	4.9	11.72	1	*0.00062

(Contd.)

(Contd. Table 47)

	Parameters	*Mean*		*Chi-square Value*	*Degree of freedom*	*p- Value*
		Pre-intervention	*Post-intervention*			
14	Ulcers	47.5	21.3	9.295	1	*0.00230
15	Body aches	54.1	18.0	17.20	1	*0.00003
16	Pain in joints	49.2	23.0	9.100	1	*0.00256
17	Dizziness	49.2	8.2	25.04	1	*0.00000
18	Dryness of skin	49.2	19.7	11.76	1	*0.00060
19	Trembling of limbs	29.5	3.3	15.30	1	*0.00009
20	Sleep disturbances	72.1	0.0	68.82	1	*0.00000
21	Fluctuation in BP	59.0	23.0	16.40	1	*0.00005
22	Low mood	77.0	11.5	53.15	1	*0.00000
23	Lethargy	55.7	0.0	47.13	1	*0.00000
24	Lack of appetite	77.0	0.0	76.45	1	*0.00000
25	Fluctuation in mood	60.7	18.0	23.21	1	*0.00000

*Significant at $p \leq 0.05$

As can be seen from the table, a highly significant difference ($p \leq 0.05$) was observed in majority of the minor health complaints reported by depressed elderly women. A marked difference was observed in complaints related to digestion, like acidity, constipation, ulcers, flatulence and indigestion. Along with psychosomatic complaints, like low mood, loss of interest, lack of appetite and sleep disturbances, physical complaints related to advancing age, like body aches, fluctuation in blood pressure, and pain in joints, also reduced.

Thus folic acid supplementation proved to be beneficial in lowering the depression levels. If supplementation is extended for a longer period of time, it can definitely prove to be effective against heavy antidepressants.

Conclusion

Depression is not a disease but a serious illness with biological, psychological and social aspects relevance to its cause, symptoms and treatment. This disease is more common in women (1 in 6 seek help for depression at some time in their lives) than in men (1 in 9) and is four times more likely to affect the elderly than the young. However, in case of elderly symptoms of depression are often mistaken for other illnesses or mere "signs of aging". Most depression in older people remains undiagnosed and untreated for several reasons. There are many causes of depression amongst which environmental factors play very important role. Nutritional status is one of the important determinants of health status or on the other hand poor mental health also affects nutritional status. The bottom line is that food plays a key role in maintaining mental health.

Correct testing and understanding of deficiencies and overloads can pinpoint the causes of many severe mental symptoms, thus opening the door to hope and recovery. The relationship between nutrition and mental illness is a relatively new area of research. Ayurvedic medicines are sometimes better accepted by people, as taking medicines from psychiatrists becomes stigma. Therefore intervention or treatment in the form of nutritive supplements or herbal medicines at the onset of illness is very essential.

From the findings of the present study, the following remarks can be made:

- Change in the dietary habits like skipping meals, increased cravings for sweets and salty items, seem to reduce food consumption in both the age groups of depressed women.
- Non-frequent consumption of animal foods and sea foods, green leafy vegetables, fats, oils and nuts in depressed group might be responsible for the deficiency of key nutrients like selenium, choline, omega-3 fatty acid, Vitamin B6 and vitamin B12. Therefore such dietary deficiencies may be considered as risk factor for depression.
- Poor nutritional status has a profound impact on the mental health of the majority of older women compared to younger depressed women and the picture deteriorates more in women from low and middle income groups.
- Depressed state leads to perception of poor health as shown by the findings where health problems were present to greater

extent in depressed women. A similar trend can be noted also in menopausal women.

- Folic acid supplement intervention showed beneficial effects. It has effected a marked change in the symptoms of depression by lowering the severity of depression, improving general health and nutritional status in elderly depressed women.

There is a need for future research on the use of herbal medicines for the treatment in depression that could show pronounced benefits in improving health status.

References

Amin, G. (1998). *Depression in primary care*. Unpublished dissertation, Department of Psychiatry, Medical College, Baroda.

Amin, G., Shah, S. and Vankar, G.K. (1998). The prevalence and recognition of depression in primary care. *Indian Journal of Psychiatry, 40*(4), 364-369.

Antonia, F. P. (1999). Food allergy and its impact on mental health. *Journal of Food Science and Nutrition, 47*, 147-157.

Austin, J. (2000). Psychological aspects of nutrition and aging. *Australian Medical Journal, 60*(12), 476-479.

Ayyar, S. (2000). *Nutritonal status, dietary habits and disease profile of elderly men and women aged 70 years and above belonging to high and middle income groups of urban Baroda*. Unpublished masters'dissertation, Department of Foods and Nutrition, The Maharaja Sayajirao University of Baroda, Vadodara, India.

Ballinger, B.C. (1997). Psychiatric morbidity and the menopause: Clinical features. *British Medical Journal, 1*, 1183-1185.

Baracat, E. C., Soares Jr., M. D, and Bang, A. (2002). Benefits of soy isoflavone therapeutic regimen on menopausal symptoms. *Obstetrics and Gynecology, 99*, 389-394.

Benton, D. and Cook, R. (2000). Facts about dietary supplements. *Journal of National Institutes of Health. Food And Nutrition Information Center, U.S. Department of Agriculture, 24*(1), 144-158.

Benton, G. (1997). Effective treatments for mental illness not being used WHO says. *British Medical Journal, 769*, 323-326

Blacker, C.V.R. and Clare, A.W. (1987). Depressive Disorders in Primary care. *British Journal of Psychiatry, 150*, 737-751.

Blue, I., Ducci, M., Jasswal, J., Ludumir, A. and Harphan, T. (1995). The mental health and low-income urban women: Case studies from Bombay, India; Olinda, Brazil; and Santiago, Chile. In: T. Harphan and I. Blue (Eds.), *Urbanization and mental health in developing countries* (pp.75-102). Brookfield, VT: Ashgate.

Broadhead, E., Blazer, D., George, L., Tse, C. (1990, November 21). Depression, Disability Days Lost From Work in Prospective Epidemiological Survey. *JAMA, 264*(19), 2524-2528.

Brown, G.W., and Harris, T.O. (1978). *Social origins of depression: A study of psychiatric disorder in women.* London: Tavistock Publications.

Chakraborti, P. (2004). *Elder abuse in rural West Bengal: An exploratory study*. Paper presented at the 12th Biennial Conference of Indian Aging Congress, New Delhi.

Coppen, A. and Bailey, J. (2000). Folic acid helps in depression. *Journal of Affective Disorders 60*(2), 121-30

Davar, B.V. and Dandekar, D. (2002). *Women and Mental Health – A Beginning.* Pune: Centre for Advocacy in Mental Health.

Debnath, S., Gita, S., Arora, R., and Rajaram, P. (1994). A study of gynaecological problems in post-menopausal women. *Journal of Obstetrics and Gynaecology of India, 44*(2), 286-289.

Dennerstein, L., Astbury, J. and Morse, C. (1993). *Psychosocial and mental health aspects of women's health.* Geneva: WHO.

Deoki, N. (1999). *India's Population – The Future*. Workshop on India's Future: Population, Environment and Human Development, India International Centre, New Delhi, January 14 – 15, 2002.

Desai, M. (2004). *A study on diet, health and nutritional status of adult depressed women (40-50yrs) with and without soya isoflavone supplementation*. Unpublished dissertation, Department of Foods and Nutrition, The Maharaja Sayajirao University of Baroda, Vadodara, India.

Desjarlais, R., Eisenberg, L., Good, B. and Kleinman, A. (1995). *World Mental Health: Problems and priorities in low-income countries*. New York: Oxford University Press.

Diane, M.E. and Susan, G. (2003). Gender differences in depression and response to antidynenant treatment. *Psychiatric Clinics, 26,* 581-594.

Dutta Ray, S. (1993). The field of mental health in India: A contemporary and futuristic viewpoint. In: P. Mane and K. Y. Gandevia (Eds.),

Mental Health in India (pp. 327-345). Bombay: Tata Institute of Social Sciences.

Gath, D., Osborn, M., Bungay, G., lles, S., and Day, A. (1987). Psychiatric disorder and gynaecological symptoms in middle aged women: A community survey. *British Medical Journal, 294*, 213-218.

Gore, W.R. (1972). The Relationship between sex roles, marital status and mental illness. *Social Forces, 51*, 34-44.

Gudson, L. (1998). Epidemiological findings on prevalence of mental disorders in India. *Indian Journal of Psychiatry, 42*(4), 14-20.

Hay, A., Bancroft, J., and Johnstone, E. (1994). Affective symptoms in women attending a menopause clinic. *British Journal of Psychiatry, 64*, 513-516

Hodgkinson, B., Evans, D. and Wood J. (1995). Maintaining oral hydration in older adults. *Systematic Review, 274*(19), 1552-6.

Indira, S.N. (1979). Midlife crisis: A psycho-social study of menopause. Unpublished doctoral dissertation, Department of Clinical Psychology, National Institute of Mental Health and Neurosciences, Bangalore, India.

Jack, D.C. (1991). *Silencing the self: Women and depression.* New York: Harper.

Jai Prakash, I. (1997). Women and Aging. *Indian Journal of Medical Research, 106*, 396-408.

Jamuna, D., Lalitha, K. and Ramamurthi, P.V. (2004). Psychological contributants to self-esteem among older widows. *Indian Journal of Gerontology, 18*(2), 151-158.

Kariguda, Z.K. (2001). Socio-economic-psychological problems of aged women in India. *Man in India*, 81(3 & 4), 291-300.

Karp, J. and Frank. E. (1995). Combination therapy and the depressed woman. *Depression, 3*, 91-98.

Kartz, P. (2004). Prevalence of obesity among psychiatrically ill patients. *Indian Journal of Psychiatry, 43*(2), 138-146.

Kaufman, S.A. (1967). Limited relationship of maturation index to estrogen therapy for menopausal symptom. *Obstetrics and Gynecology, 30*, 399-407.

Kaw, D., Khunnu, B., and Vasistha, K. (1994). Factors influencing the age at natural menopause. *Journal of Obstetrics and Gynaecology of India, 44*(2), 273-277.

Kendler, K.S., Kessler, R.C., Waltus, E.E. Maclean, C., Neale, M.C., Heath, A.C. and Eaver, L.J. (1995, June). Stressful life events, genetic liability and onset of an episode of major depression in women. *American Journal of Psychiatry, 152*(6), 833-842.

Kessler, R. C., McGonagle, K. A. Zhao, S. et al. (1994). Lifetime and 12-month prevalence of DSM-III-R psychiatric disorders in the United States: Results from the National morbidity survey. *Arch Gen Psychiatry, 51*, 8-19

Khan, A.M., Vanlalhrialpuit Gandotra. (2004). *Different facts of elderly abuse: Some interventions.* Paper presented at the 12th Biennial Conference of Indian Aging Congress, New Delhi.

Kuh, D.L., Wadsworth, M., and Hardy, R. (1997). Women's health in mid life: the influence of menopause, social factors and health in earlier life. *British Journal of Obstetrics and Gynecology, 104*, 923-933.

Kumar, V. (1997). Ageing in India- an overview. *Indian Journal of Medical Research, 106*, 340-348

Lewis, G. and Araya, R. (2001). Classification, Disability and the Public Health Agenda. *British Medical Bulletin, 57*, 3-15.

Mane, P. (1993). Mental health of Indian women: Realities and needed response. In: P. Mane and K. Y. Gandevia (Eds.), *Mental Health in India: Issues and concerns.* Bombay: Tata Institute of Social Sciences.

Mankodi, D. (1989). *Self-others' perception of aging women in a tribal area of Gujarat.* Unpublished master's thesis, The Maharaja Sayajirao University of Baroda, Vadodara, India.

Mary, C. (1995). Neurological, mental development, and aging. *Indian Journal of Neuroscience, 107*, 369-380

Matthews, K. A., Wing, R. R., Kuller, L. H., Meilahn, E. N., Kelsey, S. F., Costello, E. J., and Caggiula, A. W. (1990). Influences of natural menopause on psychological characteristics and symptoms of middle-aged healthy women. *Journal of Consulting and Clinical Psychology, 58*, 345-351.

Mehta P. and Desai, M. (2004). *A study on diet, health and nutritional status of adult depressed women (40-50) years with and without soya isoflavone supplementation.* Unpublished masters' dissertation, Department of Foods and Nutrition, The Maharaja Sayajirao University of Baroda, Vadodara, India.

Mehta, P. and Ray, S. (2005). *Study on thirst, fluid intake and urine excretion pattern of older adult and elderly females residing in Vadodara city.*

Unpublished masters' dissertation, Department of Foods and Nutrition, The Maharaja Sayajirao University of Baroda, Vadodara, India.

Mehta, P. and Vasavda, T. (2003). A study on assessment of diet, nutrition and health profile of elderly (60 years and above) from religious order in Vadodara city. *Indian Journal of Gerontology, vol. 3 & 4,* 283-289.

Miller, K. (2002). Estrogen treatment for depression in perimenopause. *American Academy of Family Physician*, 1-2.

Mukherjee, P., Nayak, A., and Mullick, J. (1996). Physical and psychological symptoms – comparative study of effects of estrogen replacement and psychometrics in menopausal distress. *Journal of Obstetrics and Gynaecology of India, 46*(2), 244-249.

Mulgaonkar, V.B., Parikh, I.G., Taskar, V.R., Dharap, N.D., and Pradhan, V. P. (1994). Perception of slum women regarding refusal to participate in a gynecological health program. In: J. Gittelsohn, M. E. Bently, Pelto, P. J., M. Nag, S. Pachauri, Harrison, A. D., and L. T. Landman (Eds.), *Listening to women talk about their health. Issues and evidences from India*, (pp. 145-167). New Delhi: HarAnand Publications.

Mullen, P.E., Reamns-Clarkson, S.F., Walton, V.A. and Herbison, G.P. (1998). Health impact of violence against women. In: *Women of South East Asia: A Health Profile.* New Delhi: WHO-SEARO.

Murthy, S. R. and Burns, B.J. (1992). *Community Mental Health: Proceedings of the Indo-US Symposium* (pp. iii-vi). Bangalore: NIMHANS Publication.

Murthy, S.R and Wig, N. N. (1993). Evaluation of the progress in mental health in India since Independence. In: P. Mane and K. Y. Gandevia (Eds.), *Mental Health in India* (pp. 17-42). Bombay: Tata Institute of Social Sciences.

Nolen–Hocksema, S. (1995) Gender differences in coping with depression across the life span. *Depression, 3*, 81-90.

Nolen-Hocksema, S. (1990). *Sex differences in depression.* Palo Alto: Stanford University Press.

Notman M.T. (1995). Reproductive and clinical transition in the lifespan of women patients with focus on menopause. *Depression, 3*, 99-106.

Patel, V. and Thara, R. (2003). *Meeting the mental health needs of developing countries.* New Delhi: Sage.

Patil, P.B. (2000, October). Active Aging: Psychosocial problems of the retired. *Social Welfare*, 13-17.

Porter, M., Penney, G.C., Russel, D., and Templeton, A. (1996). A population based survey of women's experiences of menopause. *British Journal of Obstetrics and Gynaecology, 103*, 1025-1028.

Prabhu, G.G. and Raghuram, A. (1987). Mental Health in India in India. *Encyclopaedia of Social Work in India, 2*, 188-189 (published by Ministry of Welfare, New Delhi).

Purewal, J. (2003). Gender violence, sexuality and health: Redefining the matrix. In: V. R. Patel and R. C. Thara, (Eds.), *Meeting the mental health needs of developing countries: NGO Innovators in India*. New Delhi: Sage.

Ramamurthy, I. (1997, October 12). Understanding menopause. *The Hindu*, p. VII.

Rao, V. (1992). Mental Health of the elderly in the Community. in Murthy, R.S. and Burns, B. (Eds.), *Proceedings of the Indo-U.S. Symposium on Community Mental Health*, pp 459-471. Bangalore: NIMHANS Publication.

Rao, V.A., Vasudevan, P.M., and Madhavan, T. (1982). Psychosocial aspects of geriatric population: A community study in rural area near Madurai. In: A. Kiev and A. Venkoba Rao (Eds.), *Readings in Transcultural Psychiatry* (pp. 23-30). Madras: Higginbothams.

Reader, E. (2000). *Our voices: Psychology of women*. California: Wordsworth.

Rikhi, M. and Chadha, N.K. (2004). The status of empirical research in issues related to the social support of the elderly. *Indian Journal of Gerontology, 18*(2), 237-264.

Ross, J. (2002, September/October). Mental health and protein nutrition. *Well Being Journal, 11*(5), pp. 1319-1328.

Roy, A. (2003). *Women in power and decision making*. New Delhi: Rajal Publication.

Russo, N.F. (1990). Overview: Forgoing research priorities for women's mental health. *American Psychologist, 45*(3). 368-373.

Sehgal, S. (1988). *Self perception of health and economic situation of aging women in Gujarat*. Unpublished master's thesis, The Maharaja Sayajirao University of Baroda, Vadodara, India.

Sethi, B.B. and Dube, S. (1982). Guilt in India. *Indian Journal of Psychiatry, 24*(2), 1010-107.

Sethi, B.B. and Manchanda, R. (1978). Socio-economic, demographic and cultural correlates of psychiatric disorders with special reference to India. *Indian Journal of Psychiatry, 20,* 199-211.

Shah, A. (2001). Gender issues in mental health: A clinical psychology perspective. In: B. Davar (Ed.), *Mental health from a gender perspective* (pp. 61-81). New Delhi: Sage.

Sharma, S. (1987). The Indian perspective on depression. In: S. M. Channabasavanna and S. A. Shah (Eds.), *Affective Disorders: Recent research and related Development: Proceedings of an Indo-U.S Symposium* (pp.171-181). Bangalore: NIMHANS.

Sharma, S. (1999). Elderly in India: Their mental health problems. In: P. Arun Bali (Ed.), *Understanding Greying People of India* (pp. 15-18). New Delhi: Inter-India Publication.

Sonar, G.B. (2004). Old age pensioners: A socio-psychological study. *Indian Journal of Gerontology, 18*(2), 187-200.

Srivastava, S.K. and Agrawal, S. (2002). Effect of living arrangement and gender differences on emotional states and self-esteem of the old aged persons. *Indian Journal of Gerontology, 16*(3 & 4), 312-320.

Turner, W. (1959). Under eating and undernutriton in old age: integrating bio-psychosocial aspects. *Age and Ageing 4*(27), 207-216.

Vandana, K.V. and Subramanyam, V. (2004). Counseling needs of the elderly. *Indian Journal of Gerontology, 18*(2), 219-226.

Vindhya, U., Kiranmayi, A. and Vijayalakshmi, V. (2001, October-November). Women in psychological distress. *Economic and Political Weekly, XXXVI*(43), 4081-4087.

Vishvanathan, N. and Wetzel, J. W. (1993). Concepts and Trends in Mental Health: A Global Overview. In: P. Mane and K. Y. Gandevia (Eds.), *Mental Health in India* (pp. 43-69). Bombay: Tata Institute of Social Sciences.

Note : Folic acid is one of the B complex vitamins. Folic acid deficiency is one of the most common nutrient deficiencies in the world. Deficiencies are associated with smoking, drug or alcohol abuse, strict dieting, birth control pills, poor eating habits, pregnancy, illness, old age, malabsorption, diarrhea, some antibiotics, and anti-convulsants, and infections.

SECTION - I
Aging Women and Mental Health: Issues and Concerns

3

Mental Health and Aging: A Gender Perspective

Archana Sinha

Introduction

Health is a multi-dimensional phenomenon. The levels and distribution of income, social and cultural practices and perceptions regarding health and illness, and the choice of technology, do influence the physical and mental health status of a society. In addition, people's perceptions of sickness and health, which in turn are based on several social, economic and cultural factors, and the role of the state in shaping health services are all instrumental in determining the health status of people.

The patterns of reporting of morbidity reveal important pointers not only to the health status of various groups, but also to inequalities in status and autonomy among various groups of individuals. Achieving better health care therefore cannot be based on an exclusively biomedical approach to human suffering, but has to involve an awareness of social factors impinging on health status and in the larger context, a struggle for equitable social relations.

Women's health is a crucial component of general health in a developmental approach. The world over, a tendency of public health policies and programs has been to link the well-being of women to that of children and the family, and, legitimately, to the health of society overall. This perspective is well founded given that the health of women is well documented to have a positive impact on the general health of all members of a society. And efforts to improve the health of women through programs are laudable. However, as feminist theorists have argued, women's well being is "not solely determined by biological factors and reproduction, but also by the effects of workload, nutrition, stress, war, migration." The origins of much of the pain and suffering particular to women can be traced to the social circumstances of many women's lives. Understanding the sources of ill health for women means understanding how cultural and economic forces interact to undermine their social status.

Mainstreaming a gender perspective into the health sector requires a broad-based definition of health for women as well as men that addresses well being across the life cycle and in domains of both physical and mental health. Mainstreaming a gender perspective needs to be coupled with mainstreaming mental health issues as well, because women disproportionately suffer from mental health disorders and are more frequently subject to social causes that lead to mental illness and psychosocial distress.

This paper seeks to discuss the issues of mental health and ageing from a gender perspective. It also discusses the available literature and existing policies and programmes related to mental health and aging.

Women and Mental Illness

Mental disorders are not randomly distributed throughout a population, but rather subgroups differ in the frequency of various disorders. Knowledge of this uneven distribution can be used to investigate causative factors and to lay the groundwork for programs of prevention and control.

It is more women than men, the world over, who are said to suffer from mental disorders. Both community surveys and hospital-based studies indicate that women are disproportionately affected by mental health problems and that their vulnerability is closely associated with their marital status, work and roles in society. Women's mental health cannot be considered in isolation from social, political and economic issues. Examination of women's position in society reveals that there are sufficient causes in current social arrangements to account for the surfeit of depression, anxiety and distress experienced by women. Consideration of women's mental health therefore requires recognition of the impact of social factors on mental health, a position that challenges traditional intrapsychic, biomedical approaches to mental illness.

Mainstream psychological approaches to mental disorders, for their part, have largely been gender-blind and gender-insensitive. Viewing mental illness from the biomedical model, these approaches usually consider somatic and psychological factors in their diagnostic efforts, overlooking the impact of social – cultural factors. On the other hand, feminist psychological research that has pointed out that consideration of women's mental health requires recognition of the impact of social factors on mental health. It is feminist research rather than mainstream psychological research, that has demonstrated the ways in which social inequities and social assumptions about womanhood influence different aspects of women's lives, and thereby their physical and emotional health.

Current research has demonstrated the impact of social circumstances upon women's private experiences and actions. Whether it is denial of economic resources, education, legal and health services deprivation, lack of physical and mental nurturance, exhaustion from overwork, or sexual and other forms of physical and mental abuse across the life span, research corroborates that it is women who are at the greatest risk. These issues not only fall within the purview of human rights, but also are those which understandably affect mental health. In addition, the routine of women's lives renders them at risk to experience more stress than men. This reflects the greater number of social roles women fulfill as wives, mothers, daughters, caregivers and as employees. Furthermore, women's reproductive role as bearer and nurturer of children, produces unique potential for stress related effects. Thus, the well documented higher morbidity in women's health across the life span has clear biosocial underlying causes.

Further, there is accumulating evidence that links mental disorders with poverty, powerlessness and alienation, conditions most frequently experienced by women. In fact, three of the five priority areas outlined in the document of the National Institute of

Mental Health, USA namely – violence, multiple roles and poverty, focus specifically on the ways in which women's actual experience and their subordinate position in society contribute to problems in their mental health.

There are two main routes through which women's position in society might contribute to poor mental health outcomes, one indirect and the other more direct and extreme. The first is concerned with role related stressors including multiple role strain, role overload and role conflict. The second includes actual sexual victimization whether through brutal stressors like rape, battering, or other forms of violence against women. While experiences of gender oppression – ranging from employment discrimination and sexual violence to trivialization of women's work – occur with regularity, the accumulation of such experience help account for mental heath risks that disproportionately affect women, such as depression, anxiety and phobic disorders. However, frequencies and patterns of mental disorder have been found to be vastly different for men and women.

Patterns of gender differences in prevalence rates has indicated that major depression, phobias, dysthmia and obsessive-compulsive disorder were the most common diagnoses for women. Men on the other hand, predominated in alcohol abuse/dependence. This pattern of gender differences in diagnoses has also been found to vary by marital status and class. In India however, in addition to the higher frequency of illness in married women, a higher frequency has been found in single women as well, when compared to single men. While the potential stressors associated with marriage are reported to be applicable to women, the social stigma and related tensions attached to single status have more adverse effects on women once again.

The findings underscore the importance of understanding complex relationships among gender, ethnicity, sex roles and mental health if effective mental health policies and programmes are to be developed. Furthermore, the psychosocial nature of these variables points to the need to go beyond narrow biomedical approaches in building the research knowledge base.

In the Indian context, although epidemiological investigations of mental health have been conducted since the 1960s, albeit in a scattered manner, studies on mental health needs of women are meagre, if not altogether lacking. There have scarcely been any focused studies on gender differences in the prevalence of disorders or access and utilization of mental health services, and on the specific vulnerabilities of women in various age, occupational, and socio-economic groups.

It was only recently that a gender – sensitive analysis, possibly the first of its kind in the country, of the data gathered in these epidemiological studies was made, which questioned the gender-biased assumptions of earlier research and highlighted the psychosocial stressors associated with women's position and roles in society. Drawing on the data gathered by epidemiological studies conducted in our country since the 1960s, Davar in her critique of these studies, pointed out that despite their methodological shortcomings and politically misleading inferences, the data converged qualitatively on some significant dimensions of being a woman with mental distress in India. While no marked gender difference has been seen in the case of severe mental disorders that have a biological basis, women were found to be at least twice as frequently ill as men in the case of common mental disorders which have a psychosocial etiology. In other words, where mental illness has a biological etiology, as in the case of severe mental disorders, frequency of illness is the same across gender. On the other hand, where mental illness has a psychosocial basis, more women have been found to be mentally ill than men. Therefore, a bio-medical approach to women's mental health is inadequate, since a larger part of mental disorder Epidemiology in women is constituted by the common mental disorders whose causes are located in psychosocial factors. This underscores the necessity of adopting a different and exclusive approach to women's mental health concerns.

Psychiatric disorders

Comparative analysis of empirical studies of mental disorders reveals a consistency across diverse societies and social contexts: symptoms of depression and anxiety as well as unspecified psychiatric disorder and psychological distress are more prevalent among women, whereas substance disorders are more prevalent among men. The disability-adjusted life-years data tabulated by the World Bank reflect these differences.

Depressive disorders account for close to 30 per cent of the disability from neuropsychiatric disorders among women, but only 12.6 per cent of that among men. Conversely, alcohol and drug dependence account for 31 per cent of neuropsychiatric disability among men, but account for only 7 per cent of the disability among women. These patterns for depression and general psychological distress and substance disorders are consistently documented in many quantitative studies carried out in societies across the world (Desjarlais et al., 1995).

There is evidence that poor women experience more and more severe life events than does the general population (Brown et al. 1975; Makosky 1982); they are more likely to have to deal with chronic sources of social stress such as low quality housing and dangerous neighborhoods (Makosky 1982; Pearlin and Johnson 1977); they are at higher risk for becoming victims of violence (Belle 1990; Merry 1981); and they are especially vulnerable to encountering problems in parenting and child care (Belle et al. 1990). Poverty also erodes intimate and other personal relationships (Cherlin 1979; Wolf 1987). In fact, social networks can represent additional stress for poor women as well as sources of support (Belle 1990). This gender difference has led some to contend that men tend to externalize their suffering through substance abuse and aggressive behavior, resulting in an under-reporting of psychological distress. Women, in turn, more often suffer distress in the form of depression, anxiety, "nerves," and the like.

Psychosocial distress

Ethnographic research and case descriptions enrich the quantitative findings of these prevalence studies of psychiatric morbidity, elaborating on the social context of depression, dependency and hopelessness and on the gendered dimension of these epidemiological clusters of social and psychological distress. Das (1994), recounts events in the life of an Indian woman following the loss of her husband and three sons in an ethnically charged riot, showing how her husband's family's subtle communication of the responsibility for the disaster converged with her own guilt to culminate in despair and eventual suicide.

Poverty, domestic isolation, powerlessness (resulting, for example, from low levels of education and economic dependence), and patriarchal oppression are all associated with higher prevalence of psychiatric morbidity in women. In short, a considerable body of evidence points to the social origins of psychological distress for women. Issues of hunger, poverty and overwork, sexual and reproductive violence, domestic, civil and state violence on the mental health and general well-being of the majority of women. Malnutrition in many parts was found more frequently among girls than boys, manifesting sex bias also found in traditional patterns of infanticide and newly practiced sex choices of fetuses, through selective abortion.

Employment may bring self-esteem and independence; however, low paid or unpaid labor may contribute to oppression rather than independence. Many women work a "double day" maintaining households, raising children, carrying out economically productive activities in marketing and agriculture and in household-based industries. Numerous studies document that women "work" more hours than do their husbands given their widely diverse economic and household responsibilities. Overwork may lead to exhaustion and stress leading to high rates of mental illness.

Women are the traditional care givers and are expected to provide care to parents, parents-in-law, and spouse. Women report lower life satisfaction and higher psychological distress (Prakash, 1997).

Sexual and reproductive violence, as well as rape, target women disproportionately. Severe and on-going domestic violence has been documented in almost every society in India. It is estimated that the consequences of familial and communal abuse account for approximately five percent of the global burden of disease for women during the reproductive years. Such abuse is often associated with depression, dissociative disorders, and suicide.

Mental Illness and Mental Health Services in India

Mental health problems currently are said to constitute about eight per cent of the global burden of disease and more than 15 per cent of adults in developing societies are estimated to suffer from mental illness. According to the new concept of measuring disability called Disability Adjusted Life Years (DALY), mental disorders constitute a significant part of total disability adjusted life years, more than the disability caused by several well recognized disorders such as cancer and heart diseases. Mental disorders may not produce high mortality rates but do give rise to high morbidity, which implies debility or disability. The seriousness of the problem in India is indicated by the fact that the estimated overall prevalence rates of mental illness vary from 9.5 / 1000 to 102.5 /1000. It is further estimated that nearly 30 million suffer from mental illnesses every year and that 175,000 new cases are added every year.

It was commonly believed that the prevalence of mental illness in India was much less than in the western countries, citing the 'oriental philosophy of life', the limited urbanization and industrialization, and the strong family ties as factors responsible for the 'low prevalence' of mental illness. Representative surveys of mental morbidity were also not taken up till the 1960s. Since then however, the accumulated evidence based either on hospital data or community surveys, points out that the prevalence rate of mental illness in India is not significantly less than that in the West. However, much of the work in the area of mental health continues to be directed at treatment of illness, rather than towards preventive or promotion efforts.

The mental health services in India consist of specialized mental hospitals, psychiatric units in general and teaching hospitals, private mental health clinics and nursing homes, voluntary sector services, traditional services ranging from homeopathy and ayurveda to spiritualism, and the National Mental Health Programme introduced in 1982. The conditions in the state mental hospitals have been pointed out to be dismal in terms of treatment, care, accommodation and nutrition. In India, moreover, most of the hospital beds are in urban areas, thus excluding the vast majority of the rural population from easy access to mental health facilities. The dominant modes of treatment are chemotherapy and electrotherapy; the availability of other modes such as child guidance clinics, occupational therapy units, detoxification centres and follow-up clinics, is secondary and varies considerably across institutions. Another serious lacuna of the mental health programme in India has been the lack of medically trained psychiatrists with adequate para-professionals such as psychotherapists and counselors, and psychiatric social workers. There is a shortage of psychiatrists as well, with only two psychiatrists per 10 lakh population (as against 150 per 10 lakh population in USA, for instance).

The picture that emerges from these findings is the gross inadequacy of facilities for mental health care. It is also important to know whether health care is equitable across gender, whether as many women receive treatment for their mental illnesses as they are suffering. Particularly, in view of the fact that gender bias in several aspects of society including health care is an accepted reality, it is a legitimate concern whether such bias exists in mental health care as well.

A critical analysis of women's mental health reveals that firstly, a large amount of mental distress among women remains unrecognized and untreated. Secondly, a number of mental disorders, which disproportionately affect women, are related to their work and position in society, rather than to biological factors alone. Thirdly, due to social and gender inequity, women receive less than their share of benefits of mental health services.

Mainstreaming a Gender Perspective in the Mental Health Policy

Epidemiological and anthropological data point to different patterns and clusters of psychiatric disorders and psychological distress among women than among men.

Women's mental health is greatly impacted by their access to employment, food, education, health care, and resources for economic development. When denied access to these services and resources, women become more vulnerable to physical and sexual violence, psychiatric disorders, and psychological distress. Women are more likely to live in poverty, be illiterate, and be victimized by partner violence than are men. Hence efforts to improve women's mental health should consider the social, biological, educational, and cultural aspects of their lives.

The National Mental Health Programme (NMHP, introduced in 1982) does not have a women's mental health agenda, despite its stated objective of "ensuring availability of minimum mental health care for all particularly to the most vulnerable and under-privileged sections of the population". Furthermore, adverse implications for women follow from the focus of the NMHP on the mental illness categories that it has chosen for intervention, namely-epilepsy, mental retardation, and the psychoses, which are severe disorders.

Just as important as an understanding of the social origins of women's ill health is a recognition of what can be done and is being done to improve women's status and well-being. The development of policies and programs consistent with broader definitions of health require listening to the women whom such programs are designed to serve and giving voice to their concerns, at all stages of planning, implementation and management. Listening to women who will use and staff programs maximizes the likelihood that services provided will fit well in local settings, and as a result be acceptable and used. The myth that poor women cannot or will not speak for themselves must be dispelled.

Building on local movements and enhancing grassroots strengths offer pathways through which the status of women and women's health may be improved. Numerous local initiatives abound, from adult literacy programs in India to grassroots movements throughout the world's local communities of women, to resist oppression and to organize and reshape community health programs.

Efforts at both the international and local levels are crucial, but to be maximally effective the two must connect. For women, this means being partners in the process of mainstreaming gender perspectives in health policy and development programs. International support for local initiatives is another connecting mechanism.

Recommendations for Initiatives in Mental Health Services

Health policies that incorporate mental health into public health and address women's needs and concerns from childhood to old age can be developed in numerous ways to further mainstreaming of gender perspectives. Ethical considerations and competence of practitioners are central to the formulation of integrated health programs capable of redressing the trauma of rape, the stigma of sexual or domestic violence, the depression of isolation or gender oppression, and the anxiety of scarcity. The following recommendations do not propose formulas for the development of specific solutions, but suggest ways that recognize the complexities of creating mental health policies, and ultimately, mainstreaming a gender perspective in the health sector that recognizes the concerns of the very people most affected by the problems in question.

1. *Upgrade the quality of mental health services*

Mental health services have a crucial role to play in alleviating suffering associated with psychiatric illnesses, emotional distress, psychological disorders, and behavioral pathology. Abused women, those who have attempted suicide and especially those who suffer acute or chronic mental illnesses can be helped substantially by competent mental health care.

Mental health services in most societies are inadequate. Well-trained practitioners are scarce, drugs and psychosocial interventions are unavailable or of poor quality, and even where expertise and resources exist, they seldom reach into the communities where the needs are greatest. The human rights of the mentally ill are often severely compromised, and mental health care is too often associated with abusive social control. Financial investment is required for sustainable programs, and creativity is needed to build programs that join local resources with professional knowledge.

2. *Mainstreaming a gender perspective in the mental health sector*

Educating women at all levels of society about the possibilities of mental health interventions and the potential for services and programs - is central to the success of mental health program development. The development of community-based programs may build upon the engagement of many women to their local communities and their commitment to community and family health.

3. *Encourage systematic efforts*

To upgrade the amount and quality of mental health training for workers at all levels, from medical students to graduate physicians, from nurses to community health workers.

Mainstreaming a gender perspective may build on the interests of many women professionals who have entered the field of mental health care as psychiatrists, psychiatric nurses, counselors and social workers.

4. ***Promote efforts to improve state gender policies***, toward interdicting violence against women, and toward empowering women economically, and to make women central in policy planning and implementation of mental health services. Research should evaluate the mental health consequences of these programs for women, and for men.

5. ***Direct efforts specific to primary prevention of mental disorders, and behavioral, psychosocial and neurological disorders.***

Such efforts would survey the scientific knowledge base, examine primary prevention activities around the world, address the cross-cultural relevance of prevention programs, and define training needs and related activities. Successful prevention programs call for the integration of biological and psychosocial factors, and the active promotion of proven preventive programs. In addition, prevention programs require an understanding of indigenous protective factors, such as the activities of caretakers of those who are ill and those local practices that enhance the mental and physical health and well-being of individuals and of communities. Listening to women, professional and lay, should help in identifying these factors.

What is Ageing

In most gerontological literature, people above 60 years of age are considered as 'old' and as constituting the 'elderly' segment of the population, and considered 'senior citizens' of the State. Arbitrary as it may seem, the age limit of 65 is the almost universal benchmark in any analysis of what is called ageing. In India, considering the retirement ages for government jobs (58 years) and universities (60 years), the chronological age of 58 or 60 are considered as beginning of old age.

The concept of 'ageing' has three dimensions: biological, psychological and social. Biological aging is characterized by a progressive, irreversible decline in physiological function with age, which makes the individual more susceptible to disease and death.

Sociologically speaking, ageing is a series of transition from one set of social roles to another, which is structured by the social system rather than mere biological one. In the traditional Indian culture, a human life span is one hundred years, divided into four life stages or *ashramas*. Old age began with the third life stage, when the individual had fulfilled all this worldly duties (marrying, begetting children, maintaining a household, and marrying off children) and was expected to detach himself from the worldly, engage in spiritual pursuits and finally renounce the world and live the life of an ascetic until his death. Thus a person whose children were married and had grandchildren was considered as old. Marriage of a son and arrival of a daughter-in-law (i.e. handing over of household responsibilities), menopause and arrival of grand-children usually marked old age for women. It is also common for women to consider themselves old at a younger age than men. Most women perceive themselves as 'old' by the time they are 50 years old. This perception of self as old is based on the presence of grandchildren, widowhood, shrinkage of social roles and post menopausal status (Prakash, 1997).

Ageing and Gender in India

India's demographic contours suggest a steep rise in the elderly population in the coming decades as a result of declining fertility, increasing expectation of life at birth and (partly) at later ages. Although the proportion of the elderly population in 2001 may be low, India ranks second in the world in absolute numbers. There are about 77 million elderly people in India; one out of every twelve persons was estimated to be aged 60 years or more in 2001.

Analysis of the data drawn from the 42nd Round of the National Sample Survey, has shown that, among population over 60 years of age, 10 per cent suffer from impaired physical mobility and 10 per cent are hospitalized at any given time, both proportions rising with increasing age. Of the population over 70 years of age, more than 50 per cent suffer from one or more chronic conditions.

This phenomenon, coupled with rapid social changes resulting in the gradual breakdown of the traditional joint family system and ever-increasing financial constraints at the national level, is likely to pose serious problems for the elderly.

Two-thirds of the elderly males and 90-95 per cent of the elderly females are illiterate and a large number of them, particularly females, are single. Thus, the level of economic dependency is quite high. It has been estimated that about 18 million elderly males and 3.5 million elderly females would need jobs in 2001. These figures are based on the proportion currently working. This means that a huge amount of resources would be needed in order to create jobs for them in the future. Moreover, finances will also be required to maintain the 55 million not working, the majority of whom probably will not have adequate savings nor family assistance.

It has also been estimated that about 27 million elderly people would be ill at any given point of time in the year 2001 and thus need specialized medical care. In the absence of such medical facilities, large expenditures on infrastructure would be required to meet their needs. The occurrence of physical disabilities is another important aspect of the aging process.

There will be about 17 million disabled elderly persons in India in 2001, half of whom are likely to be visually disabled. The great majority of these would not be able to work and thus would be economically dependent. In the absence of family support, they would expect help from the Government.

Gender is a very important variable that influences quality of life at all ages. India is one of the few countries in the world where men outnumber women at all ages till about 70 years. Only in the very old age group, 80 and over (Dandekar, 1996) are there more women in the population than men.

In most of the developed world, women live longer than men by four to eight years. That is not so in India; in 1991, for instance, life expectancy at birth for females was 59.8 compared to 60.1 for males. The reasons for this have to be sought in India's patriarchal social system and the generally low status of women.

Widowhood often lowers the socio-economic level of women. Older women are either illiterate or poorly educated. Only 8 per cent of older women were literate in 1981 and they were unlikely to have had remunerative jobs during adulthood. Their work as home-makers and carers is never monetized. Urban widows sometimes get the pension and life insurance money of their deceased spouse. Rural women rarely have this advantage. Nor are they likely to hold property exclusively in their names. These factors increase the dependency of women on others in old age. All this contributes to women's total dependency on the family for mere survival.

Older women's health is less than satisfactory. The proportion of women physically immobile due to various health problems is higher than for men of the same age. Low social status, discriminatory practices, early marriage, food taboos, multiple pregnancies and poor attention to health are responsible for the poor health of older women. There is an accumulation of disadvantages that make them vulnerable.

Older women have more problems with activities of daily living (ADL), but get less help from others.

Policies and Programmes for Welfare of Aging Population

The Constitution of India (Article 41 of the Directive Principles) directs the state to take effective measures to provide public assistance in old age, sickness and disability. It also speaks of the welfare of the aging population by way of old age pension, social security, social insurance (item 9 of State list and items 20, 23, 24 of the Concurrent List). In addition to these constitutional provisions, retirement benefits are provided to those serving the Government and public undertakings. Economic security of workers and their families is provided for in the Employees Provident Funds and Miscellaneous Provisions Act 1952. The National Social Assistance Programme (1995) has a National Old Age Pension Scheme being implemented through the Panchayats and municipalities of all state governments and union territories.

However, the amount of such pensions is very meager, ranging from only Rs. 30 to 60 per month. Moreover, owing to the paucity of funds available, the pensions cover only a fraction of the persons eligible. The very limited support provided to older persons by Goverment is brought out by the fact that even in Karnataka, one of the states with the most generous provision, only 15 per cent of persons over 65 years of age receive any type of pension.

The National Policy on Older Persons, 1999, focuses on financial security, health care and nutrition, shelter, welfare and other needs of the senior citizens and provides protection against abuse and exploitation (Mishra, undated). The challenge is to monitor the implementation and impact of this policy.

Recommendations for the Welfare of Aging Population

In India, the old have traditionally been honoured and respected. Even today, in India, old parents live with sons and their families. Living with the eldest son and his family is the most common living arrangement. While this tradition has assured that old people would have younger in-laws and grandchildren to care for them, today the extended family system is gradually breaking down, yielding place to the nuclear family system. Forces of modernization, technological changes and social mobility have changed people's lifestyles and values. These changes have adversely affected traditional respect as well as attitudes of empathy and care for the aged. Therefore state intervention is imperative.

The major problems faced by older people in India are: income generation, health, use of free time, social security, social participation, and dignity and respect. Further, the living conditions of older people in India are influenced by several factors such as caste, religion, education, health condition, dependence on the chief earner of the family, living standard of the adult members of the family and the process of migration (Raju 2002 and Mishra 1987, as cited in Mishra, undated).

Therefore policies for the welfare of the aging population should be inclusive to benefit the poor, vulnerable and neglected segments of the society. Such policies should aim to provide equal opportunities for basic amenities like food, shelter, health care facility, etc.; ensure access to these opportunities by removing all forms of discriminations and barriers; put in place institutional and regulatory mechanisms to remove discrimination; and mainstream marginalized sections of the society (Farah, 2004).

The first step towards this would be the institution of a social security system that covers every old person, irrespective of his or her class, caste, religion, residence in rural or urban area. The State should make itself responsible for ensuring a minimum standard of material welfare to all its citizens.

The public health care system should be improved and strengthened to cater to the specific health care needs of older persons. Another important measure is to provide opportunities for income generation to older persons so as to decrease their dependence and improve their economic condition. Those among the aged who still have the capacity to work after retirement must be encouraged to continue in alternative employment, so that they can increase their bargaining power in the contemporary competitive society.

Older people must be encouraged to organize themselves in the form Self-Help Groups (SHGs). Such groups would be best placed to identify and provide for the needs of older persons.

Public-private partnership is another strategy to address the needs of the aging population. Voluntary agencies should be involved in advocacy, research, training activities in gerontology.

Institutional support is required to address the structural problem of ageing. An institutional set up can deliver training programmes, orientation courses, conduct research on aging, and carry out mass campaigns for attitudinal changes against ageism.

Elderly women constitute a large segment of the aged population, they are among the poorest of the poor, and those least able to fend for themselves. The problem of their marginalization should find special recognition in policies and programmes. The policies and programmes should aim to alleviate their situation, ensure their physical and social autonomy.

The fact remains that the problem of old age is basically a problem of society. Among the positive factors which have been sustaining the elderly in India is the strong attachment of family members to the elderly. Social pressure continues to be placed on persons who fail to discharge this responsibility to their elderly family members. Thus it is important to strengthen these values and the capacity of families to cope with the problems of caring for the elderly. The elderly should be considered as human resources and their rich experience and residual capacities should be put to optimum use for the benefit of national development. Their ability to lead healthy and fruitful lives should be ensured by the Government.

References

Angra, S. K., Murthy, G. V. S., Gupta, S. K. and Angra, V. (1997) Cataract related blindness in India and its social implications. *Indian Journal of Medical Research, 106*, 312-324.

Ara, S. (1996) Old age among slum dwellers. New Delhi: South Asian Publishers

Bali, A. (1997) Socio-economic status & its relationship to morbidity among elderly. Indian Journal of Medical Research. 106, pp 349-360

Belle, D. 1990. Poverty and Women's Mental Health. American Psychologist 45:385-389.

Bhatla, P.C. (ed.). "Proceedings on Care of the Elderly - A Round-Table Discussion", 6-8 December 1986, New Delhi.

Biswas, A.K. "Demographic Profiles of the Aged in India," presented at the Eighth Annual Conference of I.A.S.P., New Delhi.

Boivin, G., Dupuis, J. and Meunien, P.J.: Fluoride and osteoporosis. In: Simpoulos, A.P. and Galdi, C., Osteoporosis: nutritional aspects. *World Rev Nutr Diet*, Basel Kargerr, 73:80-103, 1993.

Brown, G. W., Bhrolchain, M., and Harris, T. 1975. Social Class and Psychiatric Disturbance among Women in an Urban Population. Sociology 9:225-257.

Chanana, H.B., & Talwar, P.P. (1987) Ageing in India: Its socio-economic and health implications. Asian Pacific Population Journal 2 (3) pp 24

Chanana, H.B., P.P. Talwar, "Implications of Demographic Goals in 2000 AD for the Aging Population in India", presented at the World Congress on Sociology, 18-20 August 1986, New Delhi.

Cherlin, A. 1979. Work Life and Marital Dissolution. In Divorce and Separation: Context, Causes and Consequences, edited by G. Levenger and O. Moles, pp. 156-166. New York: Basic Books.

Cummings, S.R., Kelsey, J.L., Nevitt N.C. and O'Dowd, K.J.: Epidemiology of osteoporosis and osteoporotic fractures. *Epidemiol Rev*, 7:178-208 1985.

Dalal, P.M. (1997) Strokes in the elderly: prevalence, risk factors and the strategies for prevention. Indian Journal of Medical Research. 106, pp 352-332

Dandekar, K. (1996) The elderly in India. New Delhi: Sage publications.

Das, Veena. 1994. Moral Orientations to Suffering: Legitimation, Power and Healing. In Health and Social Change in International Perspective, edited by L. Chen, A. Kleinman and N. Ware, pp 139-170. Boston: Harvard Series on Population and International Health.

Desjarlais, Robert, Kleinman, Arthur, Eisenberg, Leon, and Good, Byron, (Eds.) (1995). World Mental Health: Problems, Priorities, and Responses in Low-Income Countries. Oxford University Press.

Dey, A.B. & Chaudhury, D. (1997) Infections in the elderly. Indian Journal of Medical Research. 106, pp 273-285

Expert Committee on Population Projections. All India Projections for 1991-2001, New Delhi, 1985.

Farah, F. M.2004. 'Population and Social Development Policies', *Health*, Vol.29(06).

General Economic Tables, Part II-B (ii), Census of India, 1971, Series I.

General Economic Tables, Part II-B (ii), Census of India, Vol. I, 1965.

Ghosh, P.S. (1998) Illegal Immigration from Bangladesh, I & II The Hindu, August 11th & 12th, p 12.

Gilsanz, V., Roe, T.F., Mora, S., Costin, G. and Goodman, W.G.: Changes in vertebral bone density in black girls and white girls during childhood and puberty. *N Engl J Med* 325(23):1597-1600, 1991.

Gopalan, C., Rama Sastri. B.V. and Balasubramanian, S.C: Nutritive value of Indian foods. (Revised and edited by Narasinga Rao, B.S., Deosthale, Y.G. and Pant, K.C.) NIN, Hyderabad, 1991.

Government of India (1998) Ministry of Health and Family Welfare. Family Welfare Programme in India year book, 1986-87. New Delhi.

Government of India, Ministry of Social Welfare, "The Aged ln India," country paper for World Assembly on Aging, 26 July- 6 August 1982, Vienna.

Goyal, R.S. (1997) Implications for the elderly of the demographic transition: An illustration from India. BOLD quarterly journal of INIA (UN), 7 (2), 2-10.

Growth of affluent Indian girls during adolescence. *NFI Scientific Report No 10*, 1989.

Guha Roy, S. (1994) Morbidity related epidemiological determinants in Indian aged. An overview. In Ramachandran C.R. & B. Shah, (eds) Public health implications of ageing in India. New Delhi: Indian Council of Medical Research, pp. 114-125.

Gutteridge, D.H., Price, R.I., Nicholson, G.C., Kent, G.N., Retallack R.W., *et al*: Fluoride in osteoporotic vertebral fractures — trabecular increases, vertebral protection, femoral fractures. In: Christiansen, C., Arnoud, B., Nordin, B.E.C., Parfitt, A.M., Peek, W.A., Riggs, B.L. (Eds), Osteoporosis, *Proc Copenhagen Int Symp*, June 3-8, Aslborg, Stiftbogtrykkery, 705-707, 1984.

Hand Book on Social Welfare Statistics, 1916, New Delhi.

Hens, B. B., Markson, E. W. and Stein, P. J.1998. *Sociology*. New York: Macmillan Publishing House.

Holbrook, T.L., Barrett-Connor,. E. and Wingard, D.L.: Dietary calcium and risk of hip fraiture: 14-year prospective population study. *Lancet ii*, 1046-1049, 1988.

Horsman, A., Gallagher, J.C., Simpson, M., *et al*: Prospective trial of estrogen and calcium in post-menopausal women. *Br med J*, ii:789-792, 1977.

Jai Prakash, I. (1999). *Ageing in India*. Prepared for WHO.

Johnston, C.C., Miller, J.Z., Slemenda, C.W., Reister, K.T., Siu Hui, M.S., Christian. J.C. and Peacock, M.: Calcium supplementation and increases in bone mineral density in children. *N Engl J Med*, 327:82-87, 1992.

Kacker, S.K. (1997) Hearing impairment in the aged. Indian Journal of Medical Research 106, pp 333-339.

Kalache, A. & Sen, K. (1998) Ageing in developing countries. In Pathy ** (ed). Principles and practice of geriatric medicine, 3rd ed, vol II, New York: John Wiley & Sons. Pp 1561-1574.

Key Population Statistics Based on 5 Per Cent Sample Data, Census of India, Paper-2, 1983.

Khan, M.Z. (1995) Services for the elderly in India. Research and Development Journal, 1 (2) pp 30-37.

Kinsella, K. & Taeuber, C.M. (1992) An Aging World II. International Population Reports pp 95, 92-3. US Department of Census. US Government Printing Office, Washington, DC

Krishnakumari, K. & Sudev, P.B. (1996) Population ageing in Kerala. In Kumar V (ed) Aging; Indian perspective and global scenario. New Delhi: All India Institute of Medical Sciences. Pp 32-35.

Krishnamachari, K.A.V.R. and Krishnaswamy, K.: *Lancet*, 2:877, 1973.

Kumar, V. (1997) Ageing in India – an overview. Indian Journal of Medical Research, 106, pp. 257-264.

Kurup, A.M. 'Welfare Progammes for the Aged," presented at the Seminar on Programmes and Services for the Aged, 28-30 October 1986, New Delhi.

Lakshmaiah N. and Srikantia, S.G.: Flouride retention in humans on sorghum and rice-based diets. *Ind J Med Res*, 65(4):543-548, 1977.

Makosky, V. 1982. Sources of Stress: Events or Conditions? In Lives in Stress: Women and Depression, edited by D. Belle, pp. 35-53. Beverly Hills, CA: Sage Publications.

Matkovic, V., Kostial, K., Simonovic, I., *et al*: Bone status and fracture rates in two regions of Yugoslavia. *Am J Clin Nutr*, 32:540-549, 1979.

Melton, L.J. and Riggs, B.L.: Epidemiology of age-related fractures. In: Avioli, L.V. (Ed), The osteoporotic syndrome: detection prevention and treatment. Second ed, Orlando, Fla Grune and Stration, 1-30, 1987.

Merry, S. 1981. Urban Danger. Philadelphia: Temple University Press.

Mishra Aditya Keshari. The process of ageing in India: A Sociological Inquiry. Department of Sociology, School of Social Sciences, University of Hyderabad, Hyderabad-500 046

Mishra, S. 1987. *Social Adjustment in Old Age*. Delhi: B. R. Publishing Corporation.

Narasinga Rao, B.S.: *Nutrition News 8*, No 5, NIN, Hyderabad, 1987.

National Sample Survey - 28th Round, Report on Morbidity, October 1973-January 1974, Report No. 292, Department of Statistics, New Delhi. 36th Round, Report on Survey of Disabled Persons, July-December 1981, Report No. 305, Department of Statistics, New Delhi.

National Sample Survey Organization. Socio-economic profile of aged persons. Sarvekshana, (1991) XV, Nos. 1-2, Issue No. 49.

Nilas, Lisbeth. (1993). Calcium intake and osteoporosis. In: Simpoulos, A.P., Galli., C. (Eds), Osteoporosis: Nutritional aspects. *World Rev Nutr Diet*, 73, 1-26,.

Nordin, B.E.C., and Polley, K.J.: Metabolic consequences of the menopause. A cross-sectional., longitudinal, and intervention study on 557 normal post-menopausal women. *Calcif Tissue Int 41* (suppl 1): IS 59S, 1987.

OECD (1979). (organization for Economic Co-peration and development) Socio-Economic Policies For the Elderly. Paris.

Osteoporotic Fractures: An Emerging Public Health Problem In Asia? Author: C. Gopalan October 1993 NFI

P.H. Reddy *Population Centre, Malleswaram, Bangalore, India The health of the aged in India 235 Supplement to Health Transition Review Volume 6, 1996*

Pearlin, L. I., and Johnson, J. S. 1977. Marital Status, Life-Strains and Depression. American Sociological Review 82:652-663.

Pollitzer, W.S. and Anderson, J.J.: Ethnic and genetic differences in bone mass. A review with a hereditary vs environmental perspective. *Am J Clin Nutr*, 50:1244-1259, 1989 [Erratum. *Am J Clin Nutr*, 52:181, 1990].

Prakash, I.J. (1997) Women and Ageing. Indian Journal of Medical Research. 106, pp 396-408.

Raju, S. S. 2002. Health Status of the Urban Elderly: A Medico-social Study. Delhi: B. R. Publishing Corporation.

Rao, M.S.A. (ed) (1986) Studies in Migration. Delhi: Manohar Publications.

Recker, R. R., Saville P.D. and Heaney, R.P.: Effect of estrogens and calcium carbonate on bone loss in post-menopausal women. *Ann Intern Med*, 67:649-655, 1977.

Reckor, R.R. and Heaney, R.P.: The effect of milk supplements on calcium metabolism, bone metabolism and calcium balance. *Am J Clin Nutr*, 41:254 263, 1985.

Registrar General of India, General Population Tables, Part II-A, Census of India, 1961, Series 1. General Population Tables, Part II-A, Census of India, 1971, Series 1. Key Population Statistics Based on 5 Per Cent Sample Data, Census of India, 1981.

Riggs, B.L., Baylink, D.J., Kleerekoper, M., Lane, J.M., Melton, L.J., *et al*: Incidence of hip fractures in osteoporotic women treated with sodium fluoride. *J Bone Miner Res*, 2(2):123-126, 1987.

Sathyanarayana, K. & Medappa, N. (1997) Editorial: care of the aged – a long haul ahead. Indian Journal of Medical Research 106, pp I-II.

Shah, B. & Prabhakar, A.K. (1997) Chronic Morbidity profile among elderly. Indian Journal of Medical Research, 106, pp 265-272.

Sharma, S.P. & Peter Xenos. Ageing in India: demographic background and analysis based on census materials. Occasional paper no. 2 of 1992, Office of the Registrar General and Census Commissioner, India, New Delhi, 1992 (4).

Shatrugana, V., Soundarajan, N., Sundaraiah, P. and Raman, L.: Back-pain. the feminine affliction. *Economic and Political Weekly* April 28, 2-6, 1990.

Srivatsava, M., Kapil, U., Kumar, V., Dey, A.B., Nagarkar, K.M., Sekaran, G. (1996) Knowledge, attitude and practices regarding nutrition in patients attending geriatric clinic at the AIIMS, In Kumar, V. (ed) Ageing-Indian perspective and global scenario. New Delhi: All India Institute of Medical Sciences, pp 407-409.

Subrahmanya, R.K.A. (1994.) Income security for the elderly in India. Quarterly Journal of INIA (UN). 4 (2), PP 28-29.

Venkoba Rao, A. & Madhavan, T. (1983) Depression and suicide behaviour in the aged. Indian Journal of Psychiatry, 25. Pp 251-259.

Venkoba Rao, A. (1985) Suicide in the elderly. Indian Journal of Social Psychiatry. 1, pp 3-10.

Venkoba Rao, A. (1997) Psychiatric morbidity in the aged. Indian Journal of Medical Research. 106, pp 361-369.

Wadhwa, A. Sabharwal, M. & Sharma, S. (1997) Nutritional status of the elderly. Indian Journal of Medical Research. 107, 340-348.

Wolf, B. 1987. Low-Income Mothers at Risk: The Psychological Effects of Poverty-Related Stress. Unpublished dissertation, Harvard Graduate School of Education, Cambridge, MA.

4

Adjustment Problems of Aging Women

Dipti Oza

Introduction

Like childhood and adolescence, old age is also a critical phase of life. This period of life is characterized by a markedly greater need for care and attention for both physical and mental well-being.

Aging has three dimensions: biological, social and psychological. Biological aging deals with bodily changes after the age of physical maturity. It is an involuntary process, which operates cumulatively with the passage of time and is revealed in different organs as inevitable modification of cells, tissues and fluids. There are structural alterations also due to infections, toxins, traumas and nutritional disturbances or inadequacies. Such interferences in the metabolic processes in individual cells result in reduced, slower or impaired function of the circulatory system and mental responses, giving rise to rise to impairments and diseases. Difficulties in working, nervous ailments, impairment of sense organs, greater need for sleep, fatigue, impaired memory, fear and loss of confidence are symptoms of old age. The quality of life is limited by the aging of the nervous system. For the behavioral scientist, aging has an important dual aspect, in which the cellular changes of the nervous system may determine behaviour capacities and this behaviour pattern may influence the rate and mode of aging of cells of the nervous system. Biological incapability gives rise to several psychological and social conflicts in life.

After adolescence, old age is the period in life when the crisis of adjustment is said to occur. Both these stages of life are considered

A comparison of Twos, Teens and Ties

Twos	*Teens*	*Ties*
Rebel against parental requests. Do's and Don'ts	Rebel against parental requests. Do's and Don'ts	Rebel against children's requests. Do's and Don'ts
Are "fearfully fascinated" with peers.	Are "fearfully fascinated" with peers.	Are "fearfully fascinated" with peers. (Difficult for them to accept as growing old with peers.)
Need constant reassurance of parental presence (i.e. "quietly available" parents)	Need constant reassurance of parental presence (i.e. "quietly available" parents)	Need constant reassurance of children's presence (i.e. "quietly available" children)
Issues of control: a) Toilet training b) The clenched teeth of 18-month-old who will not eat.	Issues of control: (a) Curfew setting (b) The defiant refusal of teenager to talk to their parents	Issues of control: (a) Food restriction (b) The defiant refusal of elderly to listen to their children
Will not share toys	Will not share personal corners of life.	Will not share responsibility and authority (can not accept the role reversal)
Struggle to dominate in play	Struggle to dominate in peer approval	Struggle to dominate with grown-up children
Put things into their mouths, from buttons to bugs	Put things into their mouths, from alcohol to drugs	Put things into their mouths, from alcohol to drugs

to be periods of storm and stress, caused by the several biological and psychological changes that take place, leading to depression.

Development, Separation and Individuation are the important tasks of childhood, adolescence and old age. Old age ("the trickier ties") brings a third shot at separation. The last time this struggled ensued was around age 13 ("troublesome teens") and before that around age 2 ("the terrible twos"), and every parent who survived remembers. The dynamics during old age is not any different.

In old age, a combination of biological, psychological and social factors such as deterioration of physical health, identity crisis, fear of losing financial independence, loss of power and social status, dilution of one's image or authority, inability to utilize one's time constructively or meaningfully, and the individuals capacity to fulfill the social, economic, physical, and emotional demands, may act as stressors. These stressors may result in old people adopting certain set of behaviours with which neither they themselves nor others around then are comfortable or happy. People in their old age often find it difficult to adjust themselves to the changes in their own selves as well as the rapid changes in the world around them, and are perceived as a burden on their families and societies.

Considering the rise in the median age of the elderly over the last few decades, and the increasing population of the elderly in India, both in proportion and in absolute numbers, it is important to understand the problems of adjustment that they face.

This paper is based on the findings of a study of the effect of old age, sex and socioeconomic status on adjustment problems conducted by the author in 2000. The study aimed to get an insight into the nature of problems of retired and non-working elderly men and women. The sample of elderly women in the study was 500, who included women who were retired and non-working, in the age groups of early old age (60-70 years) and advanced old age (over 70 years). The study tools comprised the Standardized Adjustment Inventory developed by P. V. Ramamurthy and semi-structured interviews. The Standardized Adjustment Inventory covers eight areas of adjustment such as health, home and family, economics, personal betterment, personality, occupation, religion and leisure. This paper confines itself to the findings of the study on women's adjustment problems and their perceptions regarding old age.

Adjustment Problems of Elderly Women

The women who were working and had retired found it more difficult to adjust as compared with women who had been housewives all their lives. Though the problems of women in advanced old age (70 years and above) and those in early old age (60-70 years) were similar, they differed in terms of their intensity and frequency of occurrence. The major problems at advanced old age were associated more with deteriorating health, psychological and social isolation, when compared with the problems in early old age (60-70 years).

Overall, the major problems of adjustment common to both groups of elderly women were as follows:

Health problems

The health problems reported by both groups of women were: Muscular pain, swelling, rheumatism, skin problems, deterioration of hearing and vision, general weakness, and inability to function normally, and sleep disturbances, problems of teeth, gums, throat, gastric problems, sensitivity to climate change, frequent bouts of cold and cough, headaches. Tension and nervousness and lack of concentration were also mentioned as health problems.

Economic problems

Both groups of women reported depletion of savings, inability to reduce/curtail expenditure, lack of independent source of income, difficulty in meeting recreational needs, lack of freedom to use money, as adjustment problems related to finances.

Home and family related problems

Most of the women felt that they were playing a leading role in the family earlier but now with their children assuming this role, they feel sidelined. Their problems were related mainly to their children, the attitude and behaviours of their family members, and the lack of freedom and choice to act on their wishes. Their major complaints against their children were: "children are careless", "they are away from us", "they are not too close to us", "they are not looking after us well". Lack of stability and unhappiness of their children were also problems, "children are not settled", "they have an unhappy family life", "they are not happy in their life". Women also complained about the constant "fault finding of family members", about being "irritated frequently by the behaviour of the family", and feeling "discriminated against by the family". Having too many dependents at home, inability to carry out their religious pursuits, lack of freedom to enjoy at home, inability to attend social functions of their choice and entertain guests, were also problems reported by women.

Psycho-social and personal problems

In this category, problems related to personal betterment, personality, occupation, religion and leisure are grouped. With advancing age, elderly women lack the courage and self confidence, they are unable to break or give up certain habits, find it difficult to control temptation, to adjust to modern life, and are unable to exercise their choice or realize their wishes. They have poor memory and worry about their future, the future state of their physical and mental health. They often fear about their state at advanced old age. Becoming short tempered, developing high sensitivity, being hurt easily, becoming highly suggestible, feeling lonely, isolated, identity crisis, are problems of elderly women. They are also worried about their inability to judge other's intentions. They often feel as though they are the object of ridicule by others.

Thus the major problems perceived by elderly women were:

Isolation: due to missing companionship, poor interpersonal relationship, reduction in social activities or functioning, loneliness, and lack of direction in life.

Rejection: when children leave them on their own or even if they are staying together, they feel they have failed to find a place of respect in the family. Very often they feel neglected, ignored, rejected, especially when they are not involved in important or routine decisions and they are viewed as interfering in these matters. They perceive that they are compelled to live a life as is given.

Misery: physical impairment, diseases or other conditions make them diminish their physical strength, making them less energetic and less mobile and more dependent on other family members. Dependence on others for everyday matters, for every small thing, makes them feel miserable. What adds to their misery is their financial dependency, especially when they have to remind their children to buy them medicines, buy gifts for others on their behalf, or ask their children for money when they wish to spend on recreation, etc.

Feeling of deprivation and worthlessness: Many a times elderly women have to compromise on several issues, which gives rise to feelings of self deprecation and worthlessness. For example, having to eat food which is difficult to chew or for which they have never developed the taste (eating *roti*, *pani puri*, noodles for dinner); having to wear maintenance free or inexpensive clothes (wearing synthetic clothes, which they have never worn earlier, even though they are more comfortable in cotton clothes).

Elderly women feel neglected or ignored also by their grandchildren. They wish to talk to their grandchildren, share their ideas and spend time with them, but feel rejected by their grandchildren who do not seem to like their ideas, advice and suggestions.

For many elderly women, their place of residence is not permanent. They may have to move to the homes of their various children as per the latter's convenience. For example, when their grandchildren have exams, during daughter's or daughter-in-law's pregnancy, or when their children are traveling, or want to go out on trips. In the absence of their children, they are asked to take care of their grandchildren. When there is some social function at home, like a party or a get-together, they are kept away at a friend's or relative's house, assuming they may not enjoy the function.

The feeling of deprivation becomes more acute due to their financial dependence on others, not having the resources to spend on their wishes. This intensifies with their increasing fear of the future. There is a constant fear that their savings will be exhausted and they anticipate the uncertainty of their health.

Not finding meaning or any purpose in their existence leads to feelings of worthlessness in them.

Coping with Problems

To help the elderly overcome their feelings of dependence, isolation, rejection and worthlessness, the elderly women have a few suggestions to meet their financial, health and psycho-social needs. According to these women, elderly people should be offered employment, even post retirement, as per their abilities so that they can spend their time constructively. This will not only ensure they are gainfully occupied, but also help them regain their self-respect, become self-sufficient, and lead a meaningful life.

The responsibility of maintaining good physical and mental health should be taken by the elderly themselves. They have to understand their own needs and accordingly they must try to plan their activities. For example, if they are mobile, they should go for morning and evening walks, they should try to find space for themselves and rather than asking others or allowing others to plan their life.

Finally, elderly people must learn to accept the realities of life and their own strengths and weaknesses in the given contexts. Instead of surrendering themselves to their situations, they should understand and adapt themselves to the new situation. Being demanding may be counter productive. Instead they should try to be adaptive. The elderly must also learn to accept others unconditionally to receive the same kind of acceptance from others.

References

Binstock, R., and Shanas, E. (1976). *Handbook of Aging and the Social Sciences*. New York: Van Nostrand Reinhold Company.

Birren, J. (2000). *The Psychology of Aging. National Institute of Health* (3rd edition). Englewood Cliffs, New Jersey: Prentice Hall Inc.

Oza, D. (2000). *The effect of old age, sex and socioeconomic status on the adjustment problems*. Unpublished project at Centre for Advanced Study in Education (CASE), The M. S. University of Baroda, Vadodara.

SECTION - II
Gender and Depression

5

Gender Differences in Depression: Findings from a Controlled Study

Tushar Agravat

Introduction

Major depression is the leading cause of disability and ranks fourth among the ten leading causes of the global burden of diseases. If projections are correct, within the next 20 years it will have risen to second place. According to WHO Report 2001, an estimated 450 million people alive today suffer from mental and behavioral disorder or from psychological problems. Between the suffering and the prospect of care stand the barriers of stigma, prejudice, shame and exclusion. About 10 to 20 million people attempt suicide every year. One million of them including many who are young do kill themselves. Major depression in both women and men is a debilitating disorder that disrupts relationships and daily lives and affects nearly 10 per cent of the general populations. Though depression is a treatable disease, about 80 per cent of episodes of depression go undiagnosed and untreated.

Gender and Depression: A Review of Literature

There is growing interest in the relationship between gender and depression. This interest arises from the consistent finding that women are 2-3 times more likely than men to experience a depressive episode. Considerable debate and research has focused on whether this difference has an intrinsic origin, such as biological vulnerability, or whether it can be attributed to indirect effects such as specific gender roles. Few studies have examined whether psychosocial factors, that operate to maintain depressive symptoms, have differential impact on depression in men and women. Theoretical formulation of gender differences suggest that women receive more learned helplessness training than men because of prior victimization experiences, restricted opportunities, and assigned social roles of passivity. Consequently, women are less equipped to manage negative life events and thus are more prone to feeling of hopelessness and depression.

Here are a number of possible explanations for the sex differences in the case of depression:

- Biological: Genetic transmission predisposes women to depression; female endocrine physiology predisposes women to depression.
- Social: Women are exposed to more stressful events. Women have a disadvantage of lower social status in many cultures as they are more vulnerable to the effect of poor social support.
- Cognitive: women develop a cognitive scheme similar to learned helplessness model.
- Women are more likely to have a ruminative response style.

Almost all studies report a female preponderance over males in depressive illness. The female to male ratio varies from 2:1 to 4:1.

Socio-demographic characteristics

The incidence of depression is approximately twice as high in women as compared with men. The causes of this difference have been attributed to other factors such as childbirth, hormonal factor and varying stress (Shah and Parker, 2000).

Scott (1988) reported that chronicity of depression is more frequent in females. The same was also found in several other studies (Kornstein et al., 2000; Angst, 1992; Bracke, 1998; Stefansson et al., 1994).

Winokur and colleagues (1993) reported that woman with unipolar major depression were more likely to experience multiple episodes during 5 years in the NIMH collaborative study.

The nature of modern urbanization may have deleterious consequences for mental health through the influence of increased stressors and adverse life events, such as overcrowded and polluted environments, poverty and dependence on cash economy, high level of violence and reduced social support (Desjarlais et al., 1995).

A one stage study of 330 high school students aged 15-17 years found prevalence of depressive syndrome in 22 per cent, with sexual abuse being reported by 13 per cent boys and 6.7 per cent girls, and physical abuse by 16 per cent boys and 3 per cent girls, in the depressed group. (Mishra et al., 2000)

In studies by Scott (1988), Bebbington (1991) it was concluded that being married and having to take care of young children appears to reduce the risk of depression for men. Paykel (1991) and Bertakis (2001) concluded that separated; divorced or widowed women were almost five times as likely to be diagnosed as depressed compared to controls.

Patel (2001) stated more prevalence of depression in the low socioeconomic status. Urbanized areas face more noise, pollution, contamination, frictions, more challenges and more depression.

In a study of 733 school-going adolescents, prevalence of depressive syndrome was 37 per cent, physical abuse 10 per cent, sexual abuse 6 per cent, and emotional abuse 26 per cent. All three kinds of abuses were found to be significantly related to depression (Mishra et al., unpublished dissertation)

Clinical manifestations

Shah and Parker (2000) found no statistically significant differences in the symptom profile in male and female patients.

Silverstein (1999) found that female subjects exhibited a higher prevalence of somatic depression but not of pure depression as compared to their male counterparts. Somatic depression was associated with high prevalence of anxiety disorder and among female subjects with bodyache and onset of depression during early adolescence (Frank, Carpenter and Kupfer, 1988; Young et al., 1990).

Salokangas and colleagues (2002) in their study of 330 patients found that Beck Depression Inventory scores were slightly higher in females than males.

Bhatia and Bhatia (1999) observed that women experience depression twice as often as men. The diagnostic criteria for depression are the same for both sexes, but women with depression more frequently experience guilt, anxiety, increased appetite, sleep, weight gain and comorbid eating disorder. Women may achieve higher plasma concentration of antidepressants and the may require lower doses of medication.

Kockler and Houn (2002) observed that women suffer more frequently from Major depression than men. The somatic and the atypical subtype of depression seem to be more prevalent in women. Women had more appetite disturbance and joylessness.

Derasari and Shah (1988) found higher frequency of somatic symptoms in Indian sample as compared to US sample.

Bracke (1998) in reviewing outcome studies of major depression found high rates of relapse and chronicity in women. The social role theories also imply that chronicity should be greater for women. (Usall, 2001; Stefansson et al.,1994).

Prince et al. (2001) reported that EURO – D (depression scale) scores tended to increase with age, women scored higher than men and widowed and separated subjects scored higher than others.

Stressful life events

Stress response is important for survival and adaptation. The stress response that involves both emotional and physiological changes is an adaptive response that motivates our behavior.

Some people may have the ability to shut down quickly their emotional, behavioral and hormonal responses to stressful situation, while others may have prolonged responses. Over time, their prolonged responses could affect physiology and brain function, for example, increased release of cortisol over a long time could affect glucose regulation, bone density, immune function, and function of specific brain cells. These individuals could become vulnerable to developing physical and mental diseases. Evidence suggests that overactivity of corticotrophin releasing factor, a brain neurochemical, may play a role in some people who become excessively anxious for depressed. For example above 50 per cent of depressed patients have over activity of stress hormone response, which is regulated by corticotrophin releasing factor.

Halbreich and Lumley (1993) showed that age has a differential effect on the increase of cortisol plasma, and dysregulation of noradrenaline levels in males/females.

Kendler and associates (2001) observed that women consistently reported higher rate of housing problems, loss of confidence, crises and problems in getting along with individuals in their proximal network and illness of individuals within distal network. Men reported higher rate of job loss, legal problems, and robbery and work problem. Men were more sensitive to the depressogenic effects of divorce or separation and work problem.

Wilhelm and associates (1998) found no gender differences in frequency of life events or in anticipated impact of pleasant and unpleasant events, whereas female rated the actual impact of unpleasant events higher.

Depressive episode in childhood and adolescence, predict more episodes and longer duration of depression in adult life and provide strong link between adverse experiences in childhood and adult depression (Kendler, 1993; Parker, 1997; Bifulco, 1998).

A review of epidemiological findings suggests that marriage may have detrimental effect in females, possibly due to gender specific demands posed by marriage and the resulting limited number of roles available to females (Bebbington et al., 1996, 1998).

Severity of depression was not found to be associated with significantly higher life events, which shows that the life events are associated with occurring of depression and not its severity. (Satija, Advani and Nathawat, 1998)

Another study found that elderly depressed patients experienced significantly higher number of stressful life events as compared to those in the control group. The stressful life events were significantly more in females, those with low per capita income and those who perceived crisis in family (Agarwal and Jhingan, 2002).

Singhal et al (1991) concluded that chronic depression tends to report more life stressors during the course of illness.

Gada (1987) used Presumptive Life Event Scale (Singh 1983). He observed that depressed patients had significantly more number of life threatening events and total life events than controls, during the previous one-year of illness.

Risk factors

Several studies found parental separation, divorce (resulting in lack of child care) and effect of physical and sexual abuse in childhood as possible risk factor for depression in adult life (Kendler et al 1993, Bifulco 1998, Weiss 1999, Wilhelm 2001). Adverse experiences in childhood have been shown to increase the risk of depression through several pathways, including biological mechanism (disregulated Hypothalamo-pituitary-adrenal axis), personal vulnerability (low self esteem, helplessness, external locus of control, poor coping style), adverse environmental factors (lack of social support, low social status, ongoing difficulties like single parenthood or unplanned pregnancy) and depressive episode in teenage years.

According to some studies, early traumatic experiences might be partly responsible for female preponderance in depression (Rodgers et al., 1994; Veijola, 1998, Bifulco, 1998). Since females are at greater risk of certain events (sexual abuse, childhood neglect, etc.)

Separated, divorced and widowed women were almost five times as likely to be diagnosed as depressed as those who were never married (Bertakis, 2001).

Tilwani and Vankar (1998) concluded that there are no gender differences regarding most socio-demographic and clinical characteristics and illness variables like duration and severity in major depressive disorder.

Study Objectives

Considering the inconclusive finding of previous studies on gender differences in the outcome of depression, the present study aimed to examine whether gender is the main effect or its interaction with type of treatment received, life events, social supports and dysfunctional attitude to predict major depression. The objectives of this study were to determine the gender differences in major depression with respect to following:

- Demographic characteristics
- Clinical manifestations
- Stressful life events
- Risk factors

Materials and Methods

One hundred patients (50 men, 50 women) meeting criteria for DSM-IV diagnosis of major depression (American Psychiatric Association, 1994) were interviewed at the Department of Psychiatry, B. J. Medical College and Civil Hospital Ahmedabad.

Instruments used for the present study included:

1.Hamilton Rating Scale for Depression: HAM-D Scale was developed in early 1960 to monitor the severity of major depression with focus on somatic symtomatology. For this study the 24-item version of this scale had been used. Items on the HAM-D are scored 0 to 2 or 0 to 4. The examiner, on the basis of the interview of patient and observations, completes the rating.

2.Presumptive stressful life events scale (PSLE)(Singh, 1983): Based on the Life Events Scale by Holmes and Rahe, its Indian adaptation (Presumptive stressful life events scale) was developed by Gurmeet Singh. PSLE scale consists of 51 common life events, each are experienced by people at some time or other in their life. The time period of each life event was recorded for lifetime and for the past one year. The scale items were further divided into desirable, undesirable and ambiguous and also into personal and impersonal categories. The scale is simple to administer to literate and illiterate subjects.

The PSLE scale was administered on a one to one basis with the patients, in the language that was convenient to them, i.e. Gujarati, (Vankar, 1991). The help of a reliable attendant was sought in some cases.

Statistical analysis was done for comparison of different factors and dimensions. Statistical analysis included the calculations of the range; the mean, the standard deviation and following tests were done as appropriate.

- 'X^2'test for comparison of categorical data
- 't' test for comparing difference between mean of continuous data.

The analysis was done by using the Statistical Package for Social Sciences (SPSS), version 9.

Results and Discussion

Socio-demographic characteristics

A total 100 patients (50 men and 50 women) having Major Depressive Disorder (MDD) were interviewed. Their ages ranged from 18 to 70 years. Most of the patients were married, were from rural area, and from nuclear families. The income of most of the patients was rupees 1000 or less. Most of the female patients were housewives and were the first born in their family. More than 50 per cent of patients had received primary education.

Urban life has been shown to be associated with increased life events and stressors in earlier studies in India, by Rao (1964), Chatterjee (1966), Sethi (1970) and Reddy (1998); and studies in the

Table 1: Background characteristics of the study participants and the duration of depression

Characteristics	*Male (per cent)*	*Female (per cent)*
Age		
<25Yrs	16	10
25 to 35Yrs	28	48
36 to 45Yrs	24	26
>45Yrs	32	16
Range	10-69	17-70
Mean(SD)	35.7(10.8)	39.6(13.1)
Residence		
Urban	82	84
Rural	18	16
Monthly income (in rupees		
Up to 1000	40	48
2000 to 3000	50	42
> 3000	10	10
Occupation		
Housewife	0	70
Unemployed	20	0
Employed	80	30

(Contd.)

(Contd. Table 1)

Characteristics	*Male (per cent)*	*Female (per cent)*
Education		
Uneducated	12	32
Primary	68	54
Secondary	10	10
Graduate and above	10	4
Marital status		
Single	16	16
Married	78	72
Divorced	2	2
Widowed	4	10
Family		
Nuclear	56	78
Joint	44	22
No. of patients interviewed	**50**	**50**

West by Desjarlais (1995), Hirschfeld (1982) and Tueting (1983). In the present study too, depression was found to be more common in urban areas in both males and females.

An earlier Indian study has linked poverty with depression (Patel et al., 2001). Ninety percent of the subjects of the present study with depression were from low socio-economic class. However, as the present study was conducted in the psychiatry department of a general hospital, where most patients coming to the hospital belong to the low socioeconomic class, this finding cannot be generalized.

Duration of depression and past history

Most of the patients had less than 1 year of symptoms of major depression (Table 2). This may be an indicator of increasing awareness about psychiatric disorders in general and depression in particular. However, there is also likelihood of selection bias.

Regarding history of depression, 30 per cent of the males and 20 per cent of the females had a past history of depressive episode. In both genders, 22 per cent patients had a positive family history. Many of the earlier studies suggest that chronicity and relapse in course of depression is more adverse in females (Scott, 1988; Kornstein, 2000; Bracke, 1998; Stefansson, 1994; Usall, 2001).

Table 2: Duration of depression and previous history

Duration of depression	*Male (per cent)*	*Female (per cent)*
Up to 1 yr Up to 2 yr > 3 yr	84 10 6	74 16 10
Past history of depression	30	20
Family history of depression	22	22
No. of patients interviewed	**50**	**50**

Clinical manifestations of depression and gender

There were significantly more severe clinical manifestations of depression in women: general somatic symptoms, early insomnia, and middle insomnia.

Table 3: Clinical manifestations of depression

Manifestations	*Range mean(sd)*	*Female*	*Male*	*p =*
Depressed Mood	Range Mean(sd)	2-4 2.64(0.52)	1-4 2.62(0.60)	0.4
Feeling of guilt	Range Median	0-1 0	0-2 0	
Suicide	Range Mean(sd)	1-4 2.72(0.83)	0-4 2.58(1.01)	0.22
Insomnia early	Range Mean(sd)	0-2 0.86(0.78)	0-2 1.06(0.68)	0.08
Insomnia middle	Range Mean(sd)	0-3 0.94(0.65)	0-2 0.58(0.58)	0.002
Insomnia late	Range Median	0-2 0	0-4 0	
Work and activities	Range Mean(sd)	1-4 2.5(0.79)	1-4 2.62(0.73)	0.2
Retardation	Range Median	0-2 0	0-2 0	
Agitation	Range Median	0-3 0	0-3 0	
Anxiety psychic	Range Mean(sd)	0-4 2.08(0.90)	0-3 1.96(0.73)	0.23

(Contd.)

(Contd. Table 3)

Manifestations	*Range mean(sd)*	*Female*	*Male*	*p =*
Anxiety somatic	Range Mean(sd)	0-4 1.68(1.07)	0-3 1.36(0.83)	0.04
Somatic:GIT	Range Mean(sd)	0-2 0.94(0.31)	0-2 0.84(0.51)	0.12
Somatic: general	Range Mean(sd)	0-1 0.96(0.20)	0-1 0.84(0.37)	0.02
Genital symptoms	Range Median	0-2 1	0-2 0	
Hypochodriasis	Range Median	0-2 0	0-3 0	
Loss of weight	Range Mean(sd)	0-2 0.76(0.66)	0-2 0.96(0.78)	0.08
Insight	Range Median	0-2 0	0-2 0	
Diurnal variation	Range Median	0-1 0	0-2 0	
Depersonalization and derealization	Range Median	0-1 0	0-1 0	
Paranoid symptoms	Range Median	0-2 0	0-1 0	
OC symptoms	Range Median	0-2 0	0-2 0	
Helplessness	Range Mean(sd)	0-3 1.46(0.28)	0-3 1.3(0.74)	0.13
Hopelessness	Range Mean(sd)	0-4 1.56(0.86)	0-3 1.3(0.76)	0.05
Worthlessness	Range Mean(sd)	0-2 1.32(0.68)	0-2 1.26(0.60)	0.3

Table 4: Severity of depression on Hamilton Rating scale

Symptom		*HAM-D Score*				
		0	*1*	*2*	*3*	*4*
Depressed Mood	Female Male		0 2	19 16	30 31	1 1
Feeling of guilt	Female Male	48 43	2 3	0 4		
Suicide	Female Male	0 1	6 10	4 8	29 30	6 6
Insomnia early	Female Male	19 23	19 25	12 2		

(Contd.)

(Contd. Table 4)

Symptom		*HAM-D Score*				
		0	*1*	*2*	*3*	*4*
Insomnia middle	Female	11	32	6	1	
	Male	23	25	2	0	
Insomnia late	Female	38	8	4	0	0
	Male	40	5	4	0	1
Work and activities	Female		3	25	16	6
	Male		1	23	20	6
Retardation	Female	27	20	3		
	Male	26	21	3		
Agitation	Female	46	3	0	1	
	Male	38	8	3	1	
Anxiety psychic	Female	3	7	25	13	2
	Male	3	5	33	9	0
Anxiety somatic	Female	8	14	15	12	1
	Male	6	25	14	5	0
Somatic: GIT	Female	4	45	1		
	Male	11	36	3		
Somatic: general	Female	2	48			
	Male	8	42			
Genital symptoms	Female	23	19	8		
	Male	30	12	8		
Hypochodriasis	Female	48	1	1	0	
	Male	45	2	1	2	
Loss of weight	Female	18	26	6		
	Male	16	20	14		
Insight	Female	33	15	2		
	Male	38	10	2		
Diurnal variation	Female	42	8	0		
	Male	37	10	3		
Depersonalization and derealization	Female	49	1			
	Male	49	10			
Paranoid symptoms	Female	48	1	1		
	Male	49	1	0		
Obsessive and compulsive symptoms	Female	49	0	1		
	Male	46	2	2		
Helplessness	Female	6	16	27	1	
	Male	7	22	20	1	
Hopelessness	Female	5	18	22	4	1
	Male	6	26	15	3	0
Worthlessness	Female	6	22	22		
	Male	4	29	17		

On Hamilton Rating Scale for Depression (HRSD), there was no significant difference in males and females.

Figure 1: Gender differences in scores on Hamilton Rating Scale for Depression

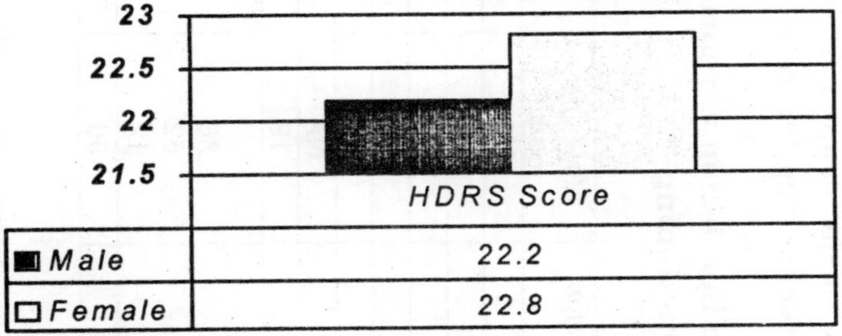

HRSD score	Male	Female
Range	12-32	13-35
Mean (SD)	22.2 (3.9)	22.8 (4.5)

In the present study, patients with depression presented with more somatic feature and insomnia. This has been found also in several other studies (Silverstein 1999; Kocklear 2002; Young 1990; Perugi 1991; Derasari 1988). This could be probably due to Indian patients having more anxiety combined with depression.

Biological factors and depression

Worsening of symptoms of depression in the premenstrual period was found in 8 per cent, while 2 per cent of women reported worsening of symptoms during peri- or postmenopausal period. Twelve per cent had onset of major depression during the post-partum period, while 10 per cent had postoperative onset.

Table 5 : Depression in relation to reproductive functioning

Onset and worsening of depression	*Male (per cent)*	*Female (per cent)*
Worsens Premenstrual	NA	8
Onset Post partum	NA	12
Onset Post abortion	NA	-
Onset post operative	8	10
Relation with pregnancy	NA	2
Peri post menopausal	NA	2
Functional limitation	18	24
Number of children 0 -1 2 to 3 >4	 36 52 12	 20 56 24
No. of patients interviewed	**50**	**50**

The female reproductive system, especially the hormonal changes during menstruation and pregnancy have a definite and complex relationship with mood disorders, the exact nature of which remains unknown even today. Studies by Sagud (2002), Kornstein (2001), Bebbington (1996), and Nazroo (1998) support this finding.

The Diagnostic and Statistical Manual of Mental Disorders-IV (DSM-IV) has postpartum onset in mood disorders as a course specifier. However, data supporting postpartum disorders, as a distinct clinical entity is yet not sufficiently strong.

A significant number of patients had a postoperative onset of depressive episode. The present study also found that women, who were housewives had more depression rates. A few earlier studies however suggest that depression is found to be more in professional and working women (Weissman and Mayers, 1974). This possibly only indicates the differential nature of stressors in working women.

Stressful life events

Ten most common life events in female patients were change in sleeping and eating habits, change in social activities, illness of family members, unfulfilled commitment, financial loss, sexual problems, self or family members unemployment, family conflicts and decreased number of family members.

The 10 most common life events in male patients were change in sleeping and eating habits, change in social activities, and illness of family members, financial loss, family conflicts, sexual problems, self or family members' unemployment, unfulfilled commitment, and property damage.

Table 6 : Life events in the past one year

Events	*Female (N)*	*Male (N)*
Change in sleeping habits	47	50
Change in eating habits	41	38
Change in social activities	41	45
Financial loss or problems	36	33
Son or daughter leaving home	35	24
Family conflict	31	20
Sexual problems	27	22
Self or family member unemployed	24	21
Unfulfilled commitments	21	30
Marital conflict	19	12
Illness of family member	13	6
Excessive alcohol or drug use by family member	12	10
Going on pleasure trip or pilgrimage	10	11
Change in working conditions or transfer	10	4
Death of a close family member	9	10

(Contd.)

(Contd. Table 6)

Events	*Female (N)*	*Male (N)*
Conflict a with in-laws (other than over dowry)	8	1
Reduction in the number of family functions	7	15
Wife begins or stops work	6	2
Change in residence	6	6
Gain of new family member	3	8
Large loan	3	5
Lack of son	3	5
Robbery or theft	3	4
Lack of child childlessness	3	0
Break-up with friend	2	0
Minor violation of law	2	2
Death of friend	2	0
Birth of daughter	1	3
Getting married or engaged	1	1
Major purchase or construction of house	1	3
Conflict over dowry (self or spouse)	1	0
Prophecy of astrologer or palmist, etc	1	4
Major personal illness or injury	1	5
Broken engagement or love affair	1	0
Death of spouse	1	0
Retirement	0	0
Begin or end of schooling.	0	1
Outstanding personal achievement	0	0
Change or expansion of business	0	1
Trouble with neighbor	0	11
Appearing for examination or interviews	0	0
Failure in examination	0	0
Death of a pet	0	1
Marriage of daughter or dependent sister	0	3
Pregnancy of wife (wanted or unwanted)	0	1
Trouble at work with colleagues, superiors or subordinates	0	1
Property or crops damaged	0	1
Detention in jail of self or close family member	0	1
Suspension or dismissal from job	0	1
Marital separation / divorce	0	0
Extramarital relations of spouse	0	0

Table 7 : Stressful life events (Past 1 year)

	Male	*Female*
Range	5-16	4-16
Mean (SD)	8.4(2.3)	8.8(2.8)

Table 8 : Significant Life Events Impact Score (Past 1 year)

	Male	*Female*
Range	159- 801	149-762
Mean (SD)	353.34 (119.50)	383.92 (135.62)

Men had higher mean life events score than women, but this was not statistically significant.

Table 9 : Severity of depression and life events

	Male	*Female*	*All*
1 year events	r=0.281 p=0.048	r=0.330 P=0.019	r=0.281 p=0.05
Impact score 1 year	r=0.305 p=0.031	r=0.335 p=0.017	r=0.290 p=0.03

As a whole, severity of depression as measured by HDRS score in this study was correlated with the number of life events in the last one year as well as with the impact score in one year. Thus as a whole, the number and impact of life events was significantly positively correlated with severity of depression.

In female patients, there was significant positive correlation between number of life events in one year and severity of depression as well as impact score during one year prior to onset of depression and Hamilton rating scores, i.e. higher the impact score of life events during one year in female patients, higher the HDRS score, i.e., more severe the depression.

In male patients, there was significant positive correlation between number of life events during one year and Hamilton rating scores, i.e. higher the number of life events during one year, higher the HDRS score, i.e. more severe the depression. Similarly in male patients, there was significant positive correlation between life event impact score during one year prior to onset of depression and Hamilton Rating scores, i.e. higher the impact score of life events during one year in male, higher the HDRS score, i.e. more severe the depression

Depression is caused by biological, psychological, social factors. Stressful life events, Psychological stress forms an inseparable part of life. Selye (1956) in his classic work postulated that any type of life change could act as a stressor, causing physiological arousal and enhanced susceptibility to illness. Individual subjective meaning of life events is important and it differs from person to person. In the present study, stressful life events occurring during the lifetime as well as during the last one-year has similar significance.

The present study revealed that if the total number of life events in the lifetime of a patient or the impact score in the last one year is increased, then Hamilton rating score is also increased meaning more severe depression. However, the study by Satija and colleagues (1998) in their study did not find severity of depression to be associated with significantly higher number of life events.

There was no difference between males and females in severity of Depression as measured by HDRS and this has been supported by previous studies also (Shah and Parkar 2000; Singhal, 1991; Tilwani and Vankar, 1998; Loewenthal, 1995).

Psychosocial risk factors for depression

Lack of a confiding relationship was found in 30 per cent of females and 18 per cent males. However this was statistically insignificant. Lack of a confiding relationship leads to increased risk for depression, especially in women.

Sixteen per cent women patients and only two per cent male patients had conflicts in their relationship with their spouses. Also, the spouses of 28 per cent of the female patients used substance in the present study. In India, alcohol use is commonly associated with physical abuse of spouse, conflicts in inter spousal relationship, loss of social status for the entire family and financial problems, with all these having a unique negative impact on women. Similarly unemployment of the spouse has a differential negative impact on women. In this study, 30 per cent of female patients reported that their spouse was unemployed.

Table 10: Risk factors for depression

Factor	*Male (per cent)*	*Female (per cent)*
Lack of confiding relationship	18	30
Conflict in relations with spouse	02	16
Spouse substance abuse	0	28
Housing problem*	40	62
Problem with in-law**	8	26
Unemployment spouse	0	30
No. of patients interviewed	**50**	**50**

Note: *X2= 4.84. df-1, p=0.02; **X2=5.74, df=1, p=0.016

Housing problems, problems with in-laws, were risk factors which were more in females than in males (Table 10).

Parental separation is a more common risk factor in females, while the risk factors death of parents, childhood abuse, and prolonged physical illness were almost equal by present in male and female patients (Table 11).

Table 11 :Risk factors

Particulars	*Male (per cent)*	*Female (per cent)*
Death of parents	14	20
Parental separation*	20	36
Childhood abuse	18	14
Prolonged physical illness	18	20
Early traumatic experience	4	6
No. of patients interviewed	**50**	**50**

*X^2=3.17, P=0.07

Parental separation in early childhood was more frequently found in females than in males, with 36 per cent of female patients and 20 per cent of male patients reporting parental separation during childhood. This seems to be a well replicated finding.

Other risk factors found equally important for development of depression in males and females were past history of childhood abuse, death of parents, prolonged physical illness. Previous studies support this finding, (Paykel 1991, Bertakis 2001).

Conclusion

This study explored the gender differences of depression with respect to other demographic characteristics, clinical manifestation, role of life events, and risk factors. It found that:

- Male and female patients with major depression did not differ as regards demographic characteristics, except that most women were homemakers and men were employed.
- Number of stressful life events experienced during 1 year prior to onset of Major Depressive Disorder (MDD) was similar.
- Early insomnia, middle insomnia and somatic symptoms general were more severely present in female patients.
- Higher the number of life events during the one year prior to the onset of MDD, more severe the depression- this was observed for both male and female patients.

References

Agrawal, N. and Jhingan, H.P. (2002). Life event and depression in elderly. *Indian Journal of Psychiatry 44*(1), 34 to 40.

Bebbington, P. E. (1996). The origins of sex differences in depressive disorder: bridging the gap. *International Review of Psychiatry*, 8, 295-332.

Bebbington, P. E. (1998). Sex and depression. *Psychological Medicine*, *28*, 1-8.

Benjetc, H. G. (2001). Gender difference in psychological well being of Mexican early adolescent. *Adolescence, 36*(141), 47-65

Bertakis KD, Helms LJ, Callahan EJ, Azari R, Leigh P, Robbins JA, Gender differences in the diagnosis of depression in primary care (Medline).

Bhatia, S. C. and Bhatia, S. K .(1999). Depression in woman, diagnostic and treatment consideration. *American Family Physician, 60*(1) 225-34, 239-40.

Bifulco, A., Brown, G. W., Moran, P., Ball, C., Campbell, C. (1998). Predicting depression in women: The role of past and present vulnerability, *Psycholo Med 28*(1): 38-50.

Bracke, P. (1998) Sex differences in the course of depression: evidence from a longitudinal study of a representative sample of the Belgian population. *Social Psychiatry and Psychiatric Epidemiology*, 33, 420-429.

Breslau, N., Schultz, L. and Peterson, E. (1995) Sex differences in depression: a role for preexisting anxiety. *Psychiatry Research*, 58, 1-12.

Burn,M. J. Cain, V. A Husaini, B. A. (2001): Depression, service utilization and treatment costs among Medicare elderly: Gender differences: Home Health Care Service 19(3):35-44.

Cadoret, R. J., Winokur, G., Langbehn, D., *et al* (1996) Depression spectrum disease, I: The role of gene-environment interaction. *American Journal of Psychiatry*, 153, 892-899.

Coryell, W, Endicott, J. Keller, M. Major depression in a non clinical smple, demographic and clinical risk factor for first onset, *Medline*

Dawson, D. A. and Grant, B. F. (1998) Family history of alcoholism and gender: their combined effects on DSM-IV alcohol dependence and major depression. *Journal of Studies on Alcohol*, 59, 97-106.

Desjarlais, R., Eisenberg, L., Good, B. and Kleinman, A. (1995). *World Mental Health: Problems and priorities in low-income countries*. New York: Oxford University Press.

Derasari, S., Shah,V.D. (1988) comparison of symptomatologic of depression between India and U.S.A. Indian Journal of psychiatry 30(2), 129 to 134

Egeland, J. A. and Hostetter, A.M. (1983) Amish Study, I: Affective disorders among the Amish, 1976-1980. *American Journal of Psychiatry*, 140, 56-61.

Frank, E., Carpenter, L. L. and Kupfer, D. J. (1988) Sex differences in recurrent depression: are there any that are significant? *American Journal of Psychiatry*, 145, 41-45.

Gada, M. (1987) Psychobiology of depression, *Indian Journal of Psychiatry*, 29(1), 15-31.

Gautam, S. and Kamal Preet. (1990). A study of impact of stressful life events in neurotic patients. *Indian Journal of Psychiatry, 32*, 356 – 361.

Gijsbers van Wijk, C. M., Huisman, H. and Kolk, A. M. (1999) Gender differences in physical symptoms and illness behavior: a health diary study. *Social Science and Medicine*, 49, 1061-1074.

Halbreich, U. and Lumley, L. A. (1993) The multiple interactional biological processes that might lead to depression and gender differences in its appearance. *Journal of Affective Disorders*, 29, 159-173.

Jenkins, R. (1985) Sex differences in minor psychiatric morbidity. *Psychological Medicine Monograph Supplement*, 7, 1-53.

Kendler, K. S. and Prescott, C. A. (1999). A population-based twin study of lifetime major depression in men and women. *Archives of General Psychiatry*, 56, 39-44.

Kendler, K. S., Davis, C. G. and Kessler, R. C. (1997). The familial aggregation of common psychiatric and substance use disorders in the National Comorbidity Survey: a family history study. *British Journal of Psychiatry*, 170, 541-548.

Kendler, K. S., Gardner, C. O. and Prescott, C. A. (1998) A population-based twin study of self-esteem and gender. *Psychological Medicine*, 28, 1403-1409.

Kendler, K. S., Kessler, R. C., Neale, M. C., *et al* (1993) The prediction of major depression in women: toward an integrated etiologic model. *American Journal of Psychiatry*, 150, 1139-1148.

Kessler, R. C., Kendler, K. S., Heath, A., *et al* (1992) Social support, depressed mood, and adjustment to stress: a genetic epidemiologic investigation. *Journal of Personality and Social Psychology*, 62, 257-272.

Kessler, R. C., McGonagle, K. A., Swartz, M., *et al* (1993) Sex and depression in the National Comorbidity Survey I: Lifetime prevalence, chronicity and recurrence. *Journal of Affective Disorders*, 29, 85-96.

Khan, A.A. Gardnerco, Prescohca, Kendlerks(2002) Gender difference in the symptoms of major depression in opposite sex dizygotic twin pairs,*Coll Antropol*, 26: 149-57

Kockler, M. Heun, R. (1977) Gender difference of depressive symptoms in depressed and nondepressed elderly person, *Archive Journal of Psychiatry*; 34:972-4

Kornstein, S.G. (2001) The evaluation and management of depression in women across the lifespan, *Journal of Clinical Psychiatry* 62 Suppli, 24: 11-7

Loewenthal, K., Goldblatt, V., Gorton, T., *et al* (1995) Gender and depression in Anglo-Jewry. *Psychological Medicine*, 25, 1051-1064.

Mavreas, V. G., Beis, A., Mouyias, A., *et al* (1986) Prevalence of psychiatric disorders in Athens: a community study. *Social Psychiatry*, 21, 172-181.

McGuffin, P., Katz, R., Watkins, S., *et al* (1996) A hospital-based twin register of the heritability of DSM-IV unipolar depression. *Archives of General Psychiatry*, 53, 129-136.

Mishra, A, Mehta, R.Y., Vankar G.K. (2000) Adolescence Depression; Are there gender difference. . Regional South East Asia Workshop on impact of gender based violence on the health of women. New Delhi, April 5-7,2000

Mukharjee, S.P., Chatarjee RN, Nandi DN (1981) life events and depression Indian journal of psychiatry 23(4) 333 – 337

Parker, G., Wilhelm, K. and Asghari, A. (1997) Early onset depression: the relevance of anxiety. *Social Psychiatry and Psychiatric Epidemiology*, 32, 30-37.

Perugi, G. Musetti, L. Simonini, E. Piagentini, F. Cassano, G.B. Akiskal, H.S. (1991) Gender mediated clinical features of depressive illness. The importance of temperamental difference, *British Journal of Psychiatry*; 158-438

Piccinelli, Marco., Wilkinson Greg (2000): Gender difference in depression, British Journal of Psychiatry, 177:486-492.

Ponnudurai, R. Somasundaram O. ,Balakrishnan S, Srinivasan N(1980) studies to evaluate the clinical profile of depressive patient. Indian Journal of Psychiatry, abstract – 35

Rao Shardamba (1967) sex distribution of mental disorder Indian Journal of Psychiatry :9, 264 – 271

Reddy, M.V., and Chandrashekhar, C. R. (1998). Prevalence of Mental and behavioral disorder in India. Indian Journal of psychiatry 40:149-157

Rodgers, B. (1994) Pathways between parental divorce and adult depression. *Journal of Child Psychology and Psychiatry*, *35*, 1289-1308.

Satija, Y. K., Advani, G. B., Nathavat, S. S. (1998) Influence of stressful life events and coping strategies in depression. Indian Journal of Psychiatry, *40*, 165 -171.

Selye, H. (1956). *The Stress of Life*. New York: McGrawHill.

Sethi, B.B., and Rudraprakash (1979) depression in industrial population Indian Journal of Psychiatry 21, 359 - 361.

Shah, and Parkar, S. (2000). Clinical profile of major depressive disorder and gender comparison, Indian Journal of Psychiatry, 42 (Supplements)

Silverstein, B. (2002) Gender difference in prevalence of somatic versus pure depression; a replication, *Journal of Affective Disorder* 68(2-3): 215-20

Silverstein, B. (1999) Gender Difference in the prevalence of clinical depression, the role played by depression associated with somatic symptoms, *American Journal of Psychiatry, 156,* 480-482; *The British Journal of Psychiatry, 174,* 339-345.

Singhal S., Kumar S, Agrawal A.K.(1991) A clinical study of clinical depression Indian journal of psychiatry 33, 261 - 265.

Spinhoven, P. and Kooiman, C. G. (1997) Defense style in depressed and anxious psychiatric outpatients: an explorative study. *Journal of Nervous and Mental Disease*, 185, 87-94.

Stallings, M. C., Cherny, S. S., Young, S. E., *et al* (1997) The familial aggregation of depressive symptoms, antisocial behavior, and alcohol abuse. *American Journal of Medical Genetics*, 74, 183-191.

Stefànsson, J. G., Lindal, E., Bjornsson, J. K., *et al* (1994) Period prevalence rates of specific mental disorders in an Icelandic cohort. *Social Psychiatry and Psychiatric Epidemiology*, 29, 119-125.

Tilwani, M. Vankar, G.K. (1998) Gender difference in depression, *Indian Journal of psychiatry*,Vol 40, Suppliment

Usall, I Rodie, J (2001) Gender differences in mood disorders. A literature review, *Actas Esp Psiquiatr*; 29(4), 269-274

Vázquez-Barquero, J. L., Diez-Manrique, J. F., Pena, C., *et al* (1987) A community mental health survey in Cantabria: a general description of morbidity. *Psychological Medicine*, 17, 227-242.

Veijola, J., Puukka, P., Letinen, V., *et al* (1998) Sex differences in the association between childhood experiences and adult depression. *Psychological Medicine*, 28, 21-27.

Venkoba Rao, A. (1976). Life changes and depressive disease Indian journal of psychiatry 18, 293-204.

Weiss, E. L., Longhurst, J. G. and Mazure, C. M. (1999) Childhood sexual abuse as a risk factor for depression in women: psychosocial and neurobiological correlates. *American Journal of Psychiatry*, 156, 816-828.

Wilhelm, K., Parker, G. and Hadzi-Pavlovic, D. (1997) Fifteen years on: evolving ideas in researching sex differences in depression. *Psychological Medicine*, 27, 875-883.

Young, M.A., Scheftner, W.A., Fawcett, J. *et al* (1990) Gender differences in the clinical features of unipolar major depressive disorder. *Journal of Nervous and Mental Disease*, 178, 200-203.

6

Depression in Middle Aged Women

Aruna Khasgiwala

Introduction

It is only since the last one decade that issues related to women's mental health have begun to be addressed by academics, practitioners, government and non-governmental organizations. Until then whatever health needs and priorities were identified for women, were related to their reproductive functioning i.e., obstetrics and gynecology and family planning. Women's mental health, a major problem area, remained unaddressed for many years. In fact, mental health of women poses as a challenge to public health, as a large number of women go unidentified and untreated.

There is sufficient research evidence from around the world to show that women suffer more severe mental health problems than men, and women outnumber men among the mentally ill. The rate of mental illness is found to be consistently higher for women than men. The ratio varies from 1:1 to as much as 3:1 or 4:1 (Women's Health Project, May 1994).

Studies in India also show that mental illness is more common among women (Verghese, 1973; Dube, 1970; Issac and Kapur, 1980); Shah, Goswami and Maniar, 1980). A study by Amita Dhanda (1995) found no class barrier for mental illness in women as compared to men. The study found that the male psychiatric ward admissions were mainly from the lower classes, while the female ward had patients from a cross section of economic classes. Some of the earlier studies have also shown that when subjected to extensive stress and emotional tension, women tend to become emotionally ill, while men tend to become physically ill.

Women's role stresses are greater in magnitude and complexity, but they suffer silently. While men cope with their stresses through substance dependency, turning to alcohol, drugs, etc., women do not surrender to these so-called relaxants. While some researchers explain women's vulnerability to psychiatric disturbances as biologically determined (Nandi, 1979), others explain it as being caused by social stressors and biological changes such as menopause (Verghese, 1973; Shah, 1980).

Depression in Women

Depression is a state of despondency characterized by feeling of inadequacy, lowered activity and pessimism about the future. It is an emotional state marked by sadness, loss of pleasure, quiet feeling, self dislike, punishment feeling, self criticalness, suicidal thoughts, loss of interest, agitation, indecisiveness, sleep disturbances, changes in appetite, tiredness, irritability, concentration difficulty, worthlessness and loss of interest in self.

Owing to its wide prevalence, depression is called the "common cold" of mental illnesses. About 340 million people around the world are estimated to suffer from depression, making it the fourth leading cause of Global Burden of Disease and a leading cause of disability worldwide. A WHO study (1996) where 25,000 adults were screened at 15 sites in 14 countries and found depression and anxiety disorders were present in 25 percent patients and commonest was depressive disorders. Depression reduces the quality of life of individuals and their families, is a risk factor for suicide and often worsens the outcome of other physical health problems.

Clinical depression is more common among women than men. A common explanation for the greater prevalence of depression in women is the hormonal changes occurring during different stages of their reproductive cycle. There is a strong relationship between women's reproductive process from menarche to menopause and mental health of women. Clinically these are identified as pre-menstrual syndrome, pre-natal depression, post-natal depression, post partum psychoses or menopausal syndrome.

Some studies found that peaking of depression is more in the immediate pre-menopausal years (McKinley, 1989; Cooke, 1984). A study by Mamta Sood and A.K. Sood (2003) on depression in pregnancy and post partum period revealed that there was significant co-relation between depression in pregnancy and early postpartum period and between depression in early and late postpartum period.

Depression has been found to be greater among women from low socio-economic background (Sethi, 1979), with low educational attainment and among women in urban areas (Chaudhary et al., 2004). Age is another factor that increases vulnerability to depression, due to deterioration in physical health. A hospital based study of males and females age 65 and above found that their physical health aggravated depression, sleep disturbances, mild cognitive impairment, agitation and retardation, irritability and hypochondriac symptoms most frequently present in elderly depressed (Acharya, 2004).

Many researches argue that women's multiple roles as both caregivers and family breadwinner in one-third of households worldwide are also to blame for women's ill mental health. Marital status has been found to be a strong predictor for depressive mood (White, 1986). Stressful life events such as death of husband or lack of male children have also been linked with depression in women. Case studies from India show that low education, low income and difficult relationships are critical determinants of mental ill health for women.

Depression in Middle Aged Women

Women in middle years experience a great deal of personal change and major life events. They have completed their tasks of child rearing and socialization. With children grown up, leaving home for higher education and employment, children getting married and starting their family life, they begin to experience the "empty nest" syndrome, making them feel lonely, isolated and helpless. women have a shift in attitude in middle age from positive to neutral or from neutral to negative in a few (McKinley, 1989).

Women in middle years experience menopause between the age 51 and 55 years. However, their life expectancy increases, by almost a third of their life span. Also, women live longer than men. So the number of widowed women is also greater with increasing age.

There are also a few other negative stressors like onset of major illness in self / spouse, care giving to older parents / in-laws, etc. By and large women carry out their daily tasks and responsibilities unless any symptoms of depression aggravate to the extent that it begins to affect their social functioning.

Rationale of the Study

Depression is experienced by all of us sometime in life. However, some groups may be more vulnerable to depression than the others. One such group is of Muslim women. Women from the Muslim community who experience low status, like other women, may become more vulnerable owing to their different life style and culture which keep them behind the doors, with limited access to resources like education and income. However, very little is known about the mental health status of Muslim women in India. Therefore it was thought worthwhile to undertake as small study on depression in middle aged Muslim women.

Methods and Materials

The present study aimed to assess the severity of depression in the middle aged Muslim women, age 40 years and above, of lower middle-socioeconomic status. The study was conducted in Vadodara city. In all 50 middle aged women were selected for the study, from the areas Sayajigunj (Bhatta) and Akota, which are inhabited by the target population. These women, who gave their consent to participate in the study were administered the Beck's Depression Inventory (BDI). The BDI is a 21-item self-report to measure the severity of depression symptomatically. Each group of items consists of four self-discipline statements. The 21-items measure:

(1) Sadness of an individual.

(2) Disappointment, failure guilt

(3) Feelings of withdrawal

(4) Sleeplessness

(5) Suicidal thoughts
(6) Indecisiveness
(7) Feelings of worthlessness etc.

Four options are provided as answers for each question: A= 0; B= 1; C= 2; D= 3. The following range of scores indicate severity of depression:

- below 8: no depression
- 8-10: borderline depression
- 13-15: mild depression
- 16-18: mild to moderate depression
- 20-29: moderate depression

Scores between 15-30 indicate that cognitive therapies were needed, while scores above 40 require medication.

Major Findings

- Majority of the respondents having depression were in the age group of 45-50 years (pre-menopausal age).
- 54 percent of respondents were found to have moderate level of depression, while 4 percent of them had severe depression, but none of them was taking any treatment.
- Two cases of severe depression were from the low and middle income group. They had very low educational attainment. These women were in the age group of 45-50 years.
- Women who were at borderline depression were from middle socio-economic strata with low level of education.
- Women having borderline depression experienced physical problems, while those with moderate depression experienced variations in mood, quiet and suicidal thoughts. Women who had severe depression reported both physical and psychological symptoms with the persistent feeling of rejection / isolation.
- While examining the causal factors, it was found that by and large all of these women experienced stressful life events, whether it was financial crisis, worries about their children not being settled and their inability to cope, their dependence on parents (i.e., on these women and their husbands), their inability to adjust with their children, childlessness, death and loss of an important family member.

- The other factors causing depression were: male dominance, which causes women's subjugation, discrimination and disparity (inequality) due to certain socio-cultural norms. The Joint Family System is another factor causing depression. This hampers the privacy of a couple and differences or conflicts occur between families living under the same roof. Greater number of children, reluctance to move out of the residential cluster and cultural differences are also the factors leading to depression.

Discussion and Conclusion

Depression in women may not be considered a severe mental health problem till it proves to be crippling and even fatal. Both, women who suffer and their family members are unaware of the signs and symptoms of depression and overlook these as normal phenomenon. Efforts should be made to sensitize family members and create awareness in the community about depression and its health consequences. Preventive steps are always desirable to check relapses and chronicity. Early detection and timely treatment are the mantras for preventive programmes.

Depression with its wide prevalence and potential to impair the quality of life of people, particularly that of women, needs to be addressed at the community level. Women do not seek clinical intervention, they need to be attended to in the community at their doorsteps. Therefore community based interventions need to be planned and implemented. There is a need for Crisis Intervention Centres in the community run by either NGOs or Government Hospitals/ Clinics. NGOs can take up sensitization and advocacy roles, can also provide supportive services, meaningful activities to such women to alleviate their suffering.

Depression can be addressed by short term or long term psychotherapy and counseling. Trained non-medical/ para-professionals can take up this role effectively. Medications will provide calmness and tranquility to women, but counseling provide the required emotional support and will enable them to think rationally while making decisions. Continuous effort in the direction of enhancing their self-esteem and aspirations will go a long way in helping women to come out of depression.

Exploring alternatives to make their life meaningfully occupied at middle age should also be facilitated through counseling. It is imperative that mental health professionals should promote a positive self concept, free women from the bondage of traditional role-stereotypes, and further their emotional and psychological well being. A paradigm shift of patriarchal construction of social relationship to an equal egalitarian construction of social relationship could be the only answer. It is necessary to evolve a feminist perspective and a feminist model of professional help that will challenge the subjugation of women, reject stereotyped roles. Women need to take charge of their lives, experience their existence, draw attention towards their powerlessness, lack of resources and create an agenda for social change.

The present study was conducted on women from one community and the findings cannot be generalized. However, whatever insights one gets out of these findings are that women's mental health issues must constitute an important part of the Mental Health Policy and programmes. The health needs of women need to be highlighted in the health education curriculum. Health service providers to be reoriented to place health in the context of women's unequal status and prioritization of funds should be on women's health issues.

References

Bettridge, B. (1987). The Self in Relation: Understanding Suicidal Behaviour in Women. *Canadian Women Studies Journal, Special issue on Women's Psychology, 8*(4)

Davar, B. (1999). *Mental Health in Indian Women*. New Delhi: Sage Publication.

Desjarlais, R., Eisenberg, L., Good, B. and Kleinman, A. (Eds.). (1995). *World Mental Health: Problems and Priorities in Low Income Countries*. New York: Oxford University Press.

Dhanda, A. (1995). *Minutes of the meeting on Women and Mental Health*. Organised on February 8, 1995 by Co-ordination Unit, Delhi.

Kaplan, H. and Saddock, B. (1991). *Synopsis of Psychiatry, Behavioural Sciences, Clinical Psychiatry*. Baltimore: Williams & Wilkins

Mane, P. and Gandevia, K. (1993). *Mental Health in India: Issues of Concerns*. Mumbai: Tata Institute of Social Sciences

Patel, V. (1999). The Epidemiology of Common Mental Disorders in South Asia. *National Institute of Mental Health and Neurosciences Journal 17*(4), pp. 307-27.

Scott, J. and Dickey, B. (2003). Global Burden of Depression: The Intersection of Culture and Medicine. *British Journal of Psychiatry, 183*, pp. 92-94.

Srinivasan, T. N. and Suresh, T. R. (1990). Non-specific symptoms and screening of non-psychotic morbidity in primary care. *Indian Journal of Psychiatry, 32*, 77-82.

Ustun, T. B., Ayuso-Mateos, J. L., Chatterji, S., Mathers, C. D., Murray, C. J. L. (2005). **Global Burden of Depressive Disorders in the Year 2000**. *British Journal of Psychiatry,* 184, pp. 386 – 92.

Women's Health Project, *Newsletter no.10*, May 1994.

SECTION - III
Social Realities and Mental Health of Women

7

Determinants of Stress in Older Women

Geeta Challa, K. Mayuri

Old age: *"Last of all that ends this strange eventful history, is second childishness, sans teeth, sans eyes, sans every thing."*

- William Shakespeare

Introduction

Human life is a long journey whereby a person crosses many stages: infancy, childhood, adolescence, adulthood and old age. These stages have different developmental tasks coupled with different developmental and degeneration processes, which are both physiological and psychological in nature. About one fourth of a person's life is spent in growing up and preparing for active participation in society, while one half of a person's life is spent in a variety of activities in an attempt to gain happiness, and the final quarter of life is spent in a progressive process of reduced activity leading to physical decline. Aging may be defined in broad terms as the totality of post-maturational changes that occur in an individual. Old age is an unavoidable and irreversible process of life. As aptly described by Shakespeare, this is the last stage of the journey of human life, in which a person is reduced to a state similar to infancy, marked by complete dependence on others.

The rapid growth in the number of older people worldwide is creating an unprecedented global demographic change. The number of elderly in India has risen from 12.1 million in 1901 to 76.6 million in 2001, due to the decline in the birth as well as death rates. With the increase in elderly population, the number of the elderly women is also likely to increase, as is the case in other countries of the world.

Stress and Old age

Selye (1974) has defined stress as "the state manifested by a specific syndrome which consists of all the nonspecifically-induced changes within a biologic system." Stressors or stressor events are those life events or changes in life circumstances that are of a significant magnitude to provoke a change in the family system (Boss, 1988). Stressors can be events that occur within the family or they can be external to the family. Stress is how a family responds to a stressor event.

Developmental milestones, like adolescence and old age create and increase stress. Old age is therefore termed as a developmental stressor event. Old women in particular are likely to experience greater stress than old men.

In 1990, the ratio of stress among aged women was 98 women per 100 men over the age of 65. Demographic predictors suggest that older women are more disadvantaged than older men in terms of both physical and mental health (Arber and Ginn, 1991). Old women are much more likely than old men to live alone and be poor (UN 1999). There are more than 20 million aged women in India. A good number among them do not have their spouse living. Most of them stay with their children, relatives and may not have any independent source of income (Jamuna, 1984).

The rapid growth in the number of older people worldwide, including India, due to the decline in birth as well as death is creating an unprecedented global demographic change. With the increase in the elderly population, the number of the elderly women is also increasing in India as in other countries of the world, which demands our attention.

In India, available studies on the psychological aspects of aged women have found them to be more unhappy than aged men

(Purohit and Sharma, 1972). The elderly face social-psychological problems such as economic dependency, and lack of care and health related problems which create difficulties in coping with aging. This has been found more among widows than among women who lived with their spouse (Sharma, 1990).

Widowhood is among the most stressful of all life events and requires more psychological and behavioural adjustments than any other life transition (Barrett, 1980; Schneweis, 1981; Gallagher and Peterson, 1984). The presence of spouse is said to be associated with positive emotions and absence of a spouse with negative emotion (Hong and Duff, 1997). A study by Chadha, Aggarwal and Mangala (1990) found that married older people were low on loneliness and high on life satisfaction as compared to their widow/widower counterparts. Widowhood results in many physical and psychological problems, likely to cause stress. While aged widowers have been found to have more difficulties in carrying out their daily activities (Chadha, 1997), aged widows tend to suffer more from health problems (Mann and Chakrabarti, 1990). Besides health problems Singh and Sharma (1987) have reported financial hardships and conflicting relationship with the daughter-in-law, as causes of psychological problems in aged women.

Gerontology in general, and stress and coping with stress among elderly women in particular, are topics that have been little explored in research in India. A review of research in psychosocial gerontology has underscored the need for studies on stress and interventions and education to reduce stress and popularising particularly good and useful stress coping procedures, as stress and coping are important areas the of research in Gerontology in India (Jamuna, 2001).

The present paper is based on a study of stress and coping among elderly men and women. The study aimed to develop a Stress Scale and examine the stress levels among elderly women; find out the determinants of stress among elderly women; and suggest effective methods for elderly women to cope with stress. The study is based on a stress model developed by Boss (1986), which is a revised form of Hill's ABCX model (1958). In Boss's model of stress, A- represents the stressor event (Aging), B – represents resources at personal, family and community level, C – is perception of the stressor event by family members and community, X – is stress resulting from the comprehensive effect of the ABC elements.

Materials and Methods

As the variables selected had already resulted in cause and effect relationships, Ex-post facto research design was adopted for the present study and the In-depth Interview method was used.

The study was conducted in the city of Hyderabad, Andhra Pradesh. The city was selected as the location of the study because of its cosmopolitan nature, as people from diverse backgrounds, varying in their socioeconomic status and level of education are found in this city.

The sample of elderly men and women was selected using the random sampling method. The criteria for selection were:

- The elderly respondent should be in the age group of 60-75 years.

Independent Variables	*Measuring Tools*
Personal variables Age, gender, education, religion, occupation, income, marital status, health status	General Information Schedule Developed for eliciting information regarding the variables.
Self Esteem	Self esteem scale, Rosenberg (1965)
Emotional intelligence	Emotional Intelligence inventory (shorter format) developed by Dr. L.Uma Devi and Dr. K. Mayuri
Family variables Family type, family size, family income, type of house	General Information Schedule
Process Variables Resources available at personal, family and community level.	A resource inventory for elderly developed by the investigator.
Attitudes of family members and members of the community towards the elderly	Inventory of attitudes towards elderly developed by the investigator.
Dependent variables Symptomatic Stress among the elderly	Symptomatic Stress Scale developed by the investigator
Sources of Stress among the elderly	Stress source scale developed by the investigator

- He/she should not be bed ridden.
- He/She should be living in a three-generation family.

In all, 120 elderly men and women aged 60-75, were interviewed. This paper is based on the findings of the 60 elderly women who were interviewed.

As the study aimed to assess levels of stress among the elderly, it looked into the relative role of personal, family, process variables as sources of stress as well as coping for the elderly. The personal variables were: age, gender, education, religion, occupation, income, marital status, health status, emotional intelligence and self esteem. The variables related to family were: family type, family size, family income and type of house, and the process variables were: resources available for elderly and attitudes of children, adults and community towards the elderly. The variables and their empirical measurements are as below:

Frequencies, percentages, F ratio for mean differences, correlation coefficient (r) to examine the relationship, and step down multiple regression were statistical measures and procedures used to find out the contributing factors for stress and coping among the elderly.

Results and Discussion

Background of the elderly women

Out of 60 elderly participants of the study, 67 per cent were in the 'young' old age of 60-65 years, about one-fifth of them were in the age group of 71-75 years and the remaining 13 per cent were between 66 and 70 years old. Seventy per cent of these women were widows, while the rest had their spouse living. Majority of these women had studied up to Intermediate level, and interestingly, none had any professional qualification. None of these women were previously engaged in any gainful employment or occupation, and they had been housewives throughout their lives. The individual monthly income for nearly two-thirds of these women (73 per cent), was below Rs. 1000 and none of them had income above Rs. 5000. As 70 per cent of these women were widows, and none of them had ever worked, the low level of individual income is not surprising. Moreover, for as many as 73 per cent of these women the monthly income of their family was less than Rs.10, 000 per month (Table 1).

Over half of the elderly women (56 per cent) were living in joint families, while 44 per cent were living in nuclear families. Fifty per cent of the elderly women were from families having 5-6 members and 20 per cent from 7-10 member families. Majority (77 per cent) of the respondents lived in independent houses and 23 per cent lived in apartments.

Regarding their health, 60 per cent of the elderly women perceived their health status as average, 37 per cent perceived themselves to be in good health and only 3 per cent perceived themselves as having poor health (Table 1).

Table 1: Background of the elderly women

Particulars	*N*	*Percentage*
Age (in years)		
60-65	40	66.67
66-70	8	13.34
71-75	12	20.00
Marital status		
Spouse living	18	30.00
Widowed	42	70.00
Education		
Up to class 10	4	6.67
Class 10 to Intermediate	38	63.33
Graduation	16	26.67
Post-Graduation	2	3.33
Professional course	0	0.00
Occupation		
Retired	0	0.00
Working in private sector	0	0.00
Business	0	0.00
Never worked	60	100
Monthly income		
Up to Rs.1000	44	73.33
Rs.1001 to Rs.2000	8	13.33
Rs.2001 to Rs.3000	6	10.00
Rs.3001 to Rs.5000	2	3.33
Rs.5001 and above	0	0.00
Family type		
Nuclear	26	43.33
Joint	34	56.67

(Contd)

(Contd. Table 1)

Particulars	*N*	*Percentage*
Family Size		
Up to 4 members	16	26.67
5 to 6 members	30	50.00
7 to 10 members	12	20.00
11 members and above	2	3.33
Monthly Family income		
Rs.2000 to Rs.5000	26	43.33
Rs.5001 to Rs.10000	18	30.00
Rs.10001 to Rs.20000	8	13.33
Rs.20001 and above	8	13.33
Type of house		
Independent House	46	76.67
Apartment	54	23.33
Health status		
Good	22	36.67
Average	36	60
Poor	2	3.33
Total elderly women interviewed	**60**	**100.00**

Symptomatic stress in elderly women

Symptomatic stress refers to the feeling of stress or strain felt by the elderly women and exhibited through physiological, psychological and behavioral symptoms.

As evident from Table 2, most of the elderly women who participated in the study were experiencing medium or low level of stress. The results also show that in these women stress is exhibited mostly by physiological and psychological symptoms and very rarely by behavioral symptoms. The physiological symptoms mostly exhibited by the women were: trembling of the body, fatigue, indigestion, acidity, high blood pressure, palpitations, cold hands and feet, perspiration and body pain. The psychological symptoms mostly seen in these women were restlessness, inability to express feelings, loss of memory, depression, feeling of dependency, dissatisfaction, and anxiety and feeling of being neglected. The behavioral symptoms shown by elderly women were, wanting to be alone, using high-pitched voice, nail biting, neglect of personal care and grooming. They also reported of insomnia and nightmares.

The level of overall symptomatic stress experienced by nearly two-thirds of these women was low. The low level of symptomatic stress may be attributed to their place of residence (i.e., living in an urban area), resources available to them, and also to the presence, in higher levels, of other personal factors such as emotional intelligence and self-esteem.

Table 2: Symptomatic stress levels among elderly women

Category	*Level*	*F*	*Percentage*
Physiological symptoms	Low Medium High	32 16 12	53.33 26.67 20.00
Psychological symptoms	Low Medium High	24 28 8	40.00 46.67 13.33
Behavioral symptoms	Low Medium High	48 12 0	80.00 20.00 0.00
Overall symptomatic stress	Low Medium High	36 22 2	60.00 36.67 3.33

Determinants of symptomatic stress in elderly women

As mentioned earlier, the present study made an attempt to find out the variables contributing to symptomatic stress in women. The variables that were considered for analysis were personal and family variables such as age, gender, education, occupation, religion, income, emotional intelligence, self esteem, family size, family type, family income, place of living and type of house. In addition to these, process variables i.e., resources available for elderly and attitudes of family members and members of community towards elderly were also considered for analysis.

Step down regression analysis was used to find out the stronger variables contributing towards the symptomatic stress experienced by elderly women. Table 3 presents the determinants of symptomatic stress among the elderly women.

Table 3: Determinants of symptomatic stress among elderly women (Step-down regression)

S. No.	Variable	Regression co-efficient (SE B)	Standard Error of B	't' value
1	Age	1.069**	0.239	4.481
2	Education	2.515	2.192	1.147
3	Religion	-15.749**	3.384	-4.654
4	Occupation			
5	Income	2.692*	1.432	2.069
6	Marital Status	1.441	2.360	0.611
7	Health Status	4.291*	2.042	2.102
8	Family Type	13.913**	3.119	4.461
9	Family Size	-3.794	2.472	-1.534
10	Family Income	0.393	1.375	0.286
11	Type of House	-11.799**	3.490	-3.381
12	Emotional Intelligence	0.137	0.134	1.028
13	Self-esteem	-1.086**	0.384	-2.832
14	Resources	-0.615**	0.214	-2.867
15	Attitudes of children	0.290	0.155	1.871
16	Attitudes of adults	-0.239	0.324	-0.736
17	Attitudes of members of community	-0.228	0.315	-0.727
18	Coping with stress	0.159	0.271	0.582

Note: **Multiple R = .853, R2 = .727, F = 7.160**
*** significant (p>0.05), **significant (p>0.01), NS = not significant**

The overall regression coefficient indicates the fact that eight variables listed in the above table are contributing significantly to the symptomatic stress among the elderly women (F= 7.160: P<0.01). The model explains that 73 percent of variance is caused by eight variables (out of 18 variables studied) namely age, religion, income,

health status, family type, type of house, self-esteem, and resources. Among the eight variables age (t= 4.481); religion (t= -4.654); income (t= 2.069); health status (t= 2.102); family type (t= 4.461); type of house (t= -3.381); self-esteem (t= -2.832); resources (t= -2.867) were closely related to symptomatic stress among the elderly women.

In other words, as age increases the stress also increases. Elderly women with very high and very low income exhibited high stress. Elderly women in joint families had more stress. It was also found that elderly women living in apartments, with high availability of resources, and who had good health status and high self-esteem, tended to exhibit low levels of symptomatic stress.

Conclusion

The present study found most of the elderly women participants to be experiencing medium to low level of stress. In these women, stress is exhibited mostly by physiological and psychological symptoms and very rarely by behavioral symptoms. The study also found that that age, religion, income, health status, family type, type of house, self esteem and resources availability affect the symptomatic stress among elderly women.

Aging affects the physical and mental activity, thoughts, emotions and feelings of the elderly women. These cause physical and mental health problems. In order to be able to cope with the process of aging old age should not be thought as a stressful period, but should be considered as a pleasant journey of one's life.

Any research study would be useful only when the findings and suggestions reach and are used by or for the people who need them. Hence on the basis of the findings of the present study, the investigator has developed guidelines for ageing gracefully. These guidelines are in the form a folder, and are intended for use by both the elderly and their caretakers.

A manual on effective ways and means of coping with stress has also been developed for the elderly. The manual provides suggestions and useful tips to the elderly for coping with stress.

The investigator of the study has also developed a software in Telugu named "JEEVANA SANDHYA" which provides information on the process of aging stress and coping among the elderly and facilities available for the elderly from government and non government organizations. This material will be a small contribution to the existing material on Gerontology and will be helpful for the elderly in society.

References

Arber, S., and Ginn, J. (1991). *Gender and later life: A sociological analysis of resources and constraints.* New Delhi: Sage Publications.

Boss P. (1987). Family stress: Perception and context. In M. Sussman and S. Stenetz (Eds.), *Handbook on marriage and the family* (pp. 32-38). New York: Plenum.

Boss, P. (1988). *Family stress management.* California: Sage Publications.

Boss, P. G. (1986). Family stress. In M. Sussman & S. Steinmetz (Eds.), *Handbook on marriage and the family* (pp. 695—723). New York: Plenum.

Chadha N. K., Aggarwal, V., and Mangala, A. P. (1990). Social network and ageing. *Spectra of Anthropological Progress 12*, 15-32.

Chadha, N.K. (1991). Self-Concept and Life Satisfaction among Aged. *Indian Journal of Gerontology, 5*(1) 47-54.

Hill, R. (1958). Generic features of families under stress. *Social Casework, 49*, 139-150.

Hong, L. and Duff, R. (1997). Relative importance of spouses, children, and friends in the life satisfaction of retirement community residents. Journal of Clinical Geropsychology, Vol. 3, No. 4, pp. 275–82.

Jamuna, D. (2001). A review of trends and perspectives of research in psychosocial gerontology. *Journal of Family Issues, 22*(7)

Purohit, C.K. and Sharma, R. (1972). A study of aged 60 years and above. Social Profile. Indian Journal of Gerontology, Volume 4 (3&4).

Ramamurti, P.V. and Jamuna, D. (1984). Psychological Research on Agedin India. *Journal of the Anthropological Society of India.*

Rosenberg, M. (1965). *Society and the adolescent self-image.* Princeton, NJ: Princeton University Press.

Selye, H. (1974). *Stress without Distress.* New York: Lippencott.

8

Mental Illness: A Risk Factor for Domestic Violence in Women?

Khyati Mehtaliya, G.K. Vankar

Introduction

Around the world at least one woman in every three has been beaten, coerced into sex, or otherwise abused in her lifetime. Most often the abuser is a member of her own family. Globally, violence within the home is universal across culture, religion, class, and ethnicity.

Violence against women encompasses physical, sexual and psychological violence, occurring in the family and in the general community, including battering, sexual abuse of children, dowry-related violence, rape, female genital mutilation, and other traditional practices harmful to women, non-spousal violence and violence related to exploitation, sexual harassment and intimidation at work, in educational institutions and else where trafficking in women, forced prostitution, and violence perpetrated or condoned by the state.

Domestic violence or wife/intimate partner abuse is one of the most common forms of violence against women. According to the WHO (2000), around the world between 10-50 per cent of the women report having been physically abused by an intimate partner in their life time. Large percentages of women are subjected to emotional and psychological violence, which many women consider as an even worse form of violence.

Prevalence of Domestic Violence in India

In India, both government statistics, including crime statistics, from various sources (Crime Statistics, Demographic and Household surveys) as well as community based studies have shown high prevalence of domestic violence (NCRB 2005; ORC-Macro and IIPS, 2000; CWDS, 2002).

Table 1: Studies on Domestic Violence (DV) in India

Authors	*Year*	*Place*	*Population*	*Physical violence(%)*
Jejeebhoy*	1998	Tamil Nadu	859 currently married	37
Jejeebhoy *	1998	Uttar Pradesh	983 currently married	45
Martin, et al.	1999	Uttar Pradesh 5 districts.	6695 married men reporting DV	30
ICRW	1999	6 states	9938 ever married	40
Sanchetna	2000	Ahmedabad	400	42.6
Mahajan*	1990	Jullunder, Punjab	Married Scheduled caste Higher caste	75
Rao and Bloch	1993	Karnataka	Married Rural	22
Visaria	1993-97	Rural Kheda, Gujarat	346 married	23
International Clinical Epidemiologists Network (INCLEN)	1997	Bhopal, Chennai Lucknow Nagpur Trivendrum Vellore	Nearly 10,000	40

(Contd.)

(Contd. Table 1)

Authors	*Year*	*Place*	*Population*	*Physical violence(%)*
Kumar, Gupta & Abraham#	2001	Rajasthan rural	486 married men reporting DV	37.4
Anandhi and Jeyaranjan#	2001	Tamil Nadu rural	872 Dalit men 382 Non-Dalit men	45 43
Dagar#	2001	Amritsar, Bhatinda Punjab	SC men Non SC Hindu men Non SC Sikh men	69.6 27.9 21.3

Sources: * WHO-SEARO, 2000; #ICRW (2002)

The following table summarizes the findings from several community based studies conducted in India to assess the prevalence of domestic violence. As can be seen from the table, between 22-75 per cent of the women in the population studied reported having experienced domestic violence.

Why does Domestic Violence Occur?

While several theories exist to explain the dynamics of domestic violence, Lori Heise's Ecological Model provides a holistic analysis of the various factors at play that contribute to a person's violent behaviour. The ecological model, as illustrated in the Figure 1 , shows that violent behaviour grows out of a complex interplay of in individual, relational, communal and societal dynamics. It asserts that violence does not occur as a result of one factor in one of the fcur spheres of influence, but is rather more complex with multiple factors within different spheres influencing a person's attitudes, behavior and choices.

Figure 1: Ecological Framework of Domestic Violence

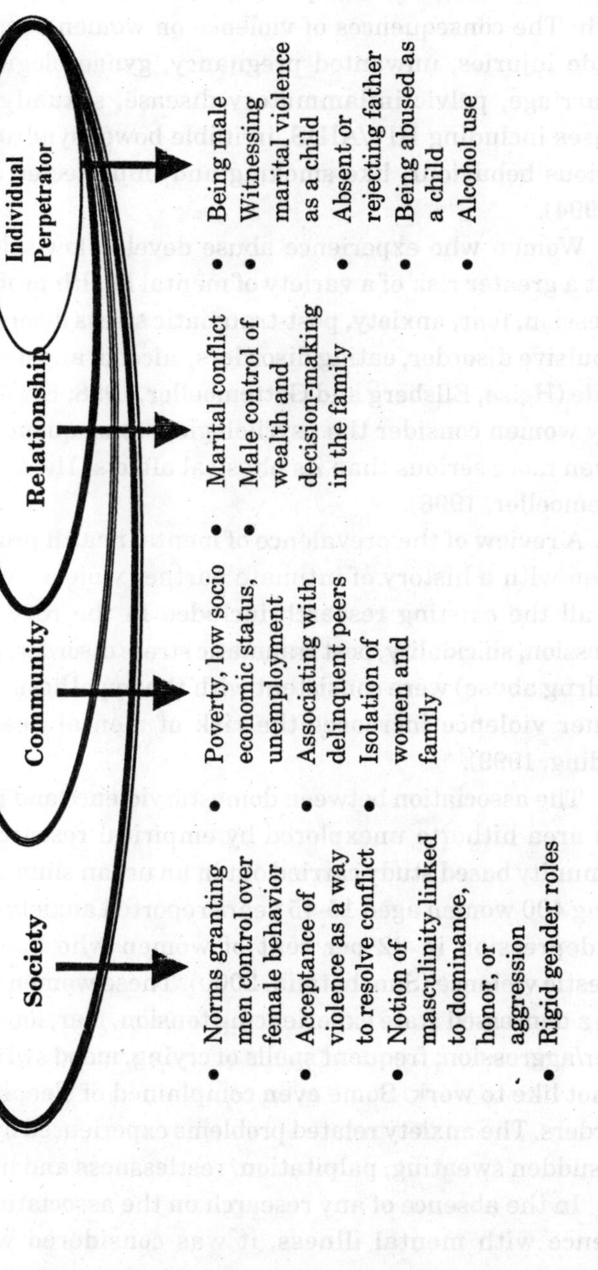

Source: Reproduced from from Heise et al, 1998.

Domestic Violence and Women's Health

Violence not only affects all aspects of women's health including their survival but is also a risk factor for their ill health. It can have adverse consequences on their physical and mental health. The consequences of violence on women's physical health include injuries, unwanted pregnancy, gynaecological problems, miscarriage, pelvic inflammatory disease, sexually transmitted diseases including HIV/AIDS, irritable bowel syndrome, and self-injurious behaviour, like smoking and unprotected sex (Heise et al., 1994).

Women who experience abuse develop low-self esteem and are at a greater risk of a variety of mental health problems such as depression, fear, anxiety, post-traumatic stress disorder, obsessive compulsive disorder, eating disorders, alcohol and drug abuse, and suicide (Heise, Ellsberg and Gottemoeller, 1998; Heise et al., 1994). Many women consider the psychological consequences of abuse to be even more serious than its physical affects (Heise, Ellsberg and Gottemoeller, 1998).

A review of the prevalence of mental health problems among women with a history of intimate partner violence was concluded that all the existing research included in the review (studies of depression, suicidality, post traumatic stress disorder, alcohol abuse, and drug abuse) were consistent with the hypothesis that intimate partner violence increases the risk of mental health problems (Golding, 1999).

The association between domestic violence and mental health is an area hitherto unexplored by empirical research in India. A community based study carried out in an urban slum of Ahmedabad among 400 women aged 15-45 years reported anxiety in 68 per cent and depression in 82 per cent of women who had experienced domestic violence (Sanchetana, 2000). These women were found to be in a depressed state experiencing tension, fear, loneliness, shock, anger/aggression, frequent spells of crying, mood swings and hence did not like to work. Some even complained of sleeping and eating disorders. The anxiety related problems experienced by women were like sudden sweating, palpitation, restlessness and uneasiness.

In the absence of any research on the association of domestic violence with mental illness, it was considered worthwhile to undertake a hospital based study on the subject. This paper is based on the study of domestic violence among women psychiatric patients visiting a government hospital.

Study Objectives

The study aimed to find out

- the frequency of domestic violence among female psychiatric patients,
- the demographic as well as domestic violence related factors
- To find out association of domestic violence with mental illness

Material and Methods

One Hundred consecutive women psychiatric patients attending the psychiatry department of a general hospital were evaluated for physical, psychological and sexual abuse. The inclusion criteria were: A woman of any age, who was ever married, who was diagnosed with a psychiatric disorder, and was in a position to be interviewed. Women patients who needed emergency care, those who were not cooperative or those who, in the investigator's opinion, were not in a position to give an interview were excluded.

Women patients were interviewed using a semi-structured Proforma, which was pre-tested. Information collected included their socio-demographic characteristics, experience of physical, psychological and sexual violence and frequency of such experiences and their effects. Women's perceptions about the causes of trauma and consequences of domestic violence were also assessed.

Computer aided data analysis was carried out using the Statistical Package for Social Sciences, Version 11, and appropriate statistical tests were applied. Categorical data was compared using chi square test and quantitative data was compared using't' test. As the study examined not only the frequency of domestic violence but also the subjective experiences of women, women's narration were recorded verbatim. In the analysis of the qualitative data, the recurring themes were identified by content analysis.

Results and Discussion

As mentioned earlier, 100 consecutive women psychiatric patients visiting a government general hospital were interviewed in the present study. Among these women were 91 Hindus and 9 Muslims. Their age ranged from 18-63 years with their mean age being 36.5 (SD 10.2) years. Of these women, 80 were married, 9 were divorced or separated, and 11 were widowed. Sixty-eight women lived in nuclear families.

Frequency of Domestic Violence

The study found that out of 100, as many as 88 women had suffered from at least one type of abuse, and over a third (38 women) had suffered from all three kinds of abuse, i.e., physical, sexual as well as psychological. For the majority of women, experience of abuse was not a one time experience but had occurred several times (Table 2).

Table 2: Type and frequency of abuse experienced by women

Type of abuse	*Physical*	*Psychological*	*Sexual*
Prevalence	69	73	53
Abuse by husband	61	51	52
Abuse by others	29	56	11
Frequency:			
Once/ twice	16	7	7
Many	53	66	46

Other than physical, psychological and sexual abuse, as can be seen from Table 3, 25 per cent of the women patients were controlled by their husbands as well as in-laws in various ways and 16 per cent were not even allowed to seek help from other well-wishers.

Table 3: Abuse by way of controlling behaviours

Type of controlling behaviour	*Husband %*	*Other perpetrator %*
Not allowing to go to parents	26	20
Not allowing to meet friends	22	16
Constantly monitoring with whom interacts	25	23
Keeping away from help	16	16

Figure 2 : Experience of domestic violence by women psychiatric patients in the last one year and in their lifetime

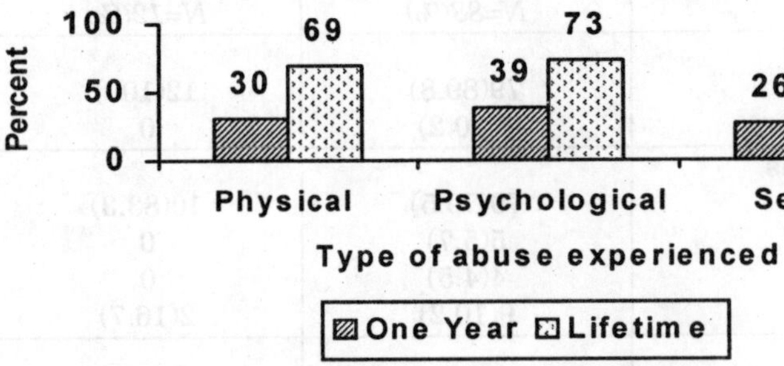

Almost one-fifth of patients had physical abuse; one-fifth had sexual abuse and a quarter from psychological abuse during lifetime. Twice the number of patients reported physical abuse by husband as compared to the number of patients reporting abuse by other perpetrators, whereas more number of patients reported psychological abuse by other perpetrators (mainly in-laws, especially mother-in-law) as compared to that by husband. Around half of the patients reported sexual abuse by husband. It is also worth noting that 11 women reported having experienced sexual abuse by someone other than the husband.

Domestic violence and socio-demographic characteristics of women psychiatric patients

Table 4: Background characteristics of women who had experienced domestic violence

Background characteristic	*Domestic violence Present N=88(%)*	*Domestic violence Absent N=12(%)*
Age		
Range	18-63	20-60
Mean (sd)	36.1(10.2)	39.6(9.6)
14-24	12	1
25-35	35	3
36-50	32	7
50+	9	1

(Contd.)

(Contd . Table 4)

Background characteristic	*Domestic violence Present N=88(%)*	*Domestic violence Absent N=12(%)*
Religion		
Hindu	79(89.8)	12(100)
Muslim	9(10.2)	0
Marital Status		
Married	70(79.5)	10(83.3)
Divorced	5(5.7)	0
Separated	4(4.5)	0
Widowed	9(10.2)	2(16.7)
Family		
Nuclear	58(66.7)	10(83.3)
Joint	30(33.3)	2(16.7)
Education		
Illiterate	23(26.1)	4(33.3)
Primary	33(37.5)	5(41.7)
Secondary &Above	32(36.3)	3(24.9)
Domicile		
Urban	70(79.5)	11(91.7)
Rural	18(20.5)	1(8.3)
Caste		
SC/ST	28(31.8)	7(58.3)
SEBC	25(28.4)	3(24.9)
Muslim	9(10.2)	0
Sindhi	14(15.9)	1(8.3)
Others	12(13.6)	1(8.3)
Family assets		
Pucca house	57(64.8)	10(83.3)
Vehicle	42(47.7)	10(83.3)
TV	64(72.7)	9(75)
Fridge	21(23.9)	2(16.8)
Phone	15(17)	0
Computer	1(1.1)	0
Tractor	1(1.1)	0
Land	8(9.1)	1(8.3)

Table 4 shows the socio-demographic characteristics of women psychiatric patients having experienced domestic violence and those who had not experienced domestic violence. The age ranges of both the groups were similar and the means were comparable. About 10 per cent of the women psychiatric patients among those who had experienced domestic violence were divorced or separated, whereas none of the women in the group without any experience of domestic violence was divorced or separated.

Table 5: Background characteristics of the husbands of women psychiatric patients

Characteristic of the husband	*Domestic violence Present N=88 (%)*	*Domestic violence Absent N=12 (%)*
Age of husband		
Range	23-65	23-53
Mean(sd)	40.4(10.1)	44.1(7.8)
14-24	2	1
25-35	27	0
36-50	38	9
50+	13	1
Education of husband		
Illiterate	11(12.5)	1(8.3)
Primary	30(34.1)	2(16.7)
Secondary & above	47(53.3)	9(74.9)
Working	80	9
Unemployed/ Retired	8	2

More number of women who had not experienced domestic violence were living in nuclear families as compared to those who had experienced domestic violence (83 per cent vs. 67 per cent respectively), but this difference was not statistically significant. Moreover, it was also found that a higher number of spouses of women with no experience of domestic violence had higher education (secondary schooling or above) as compared to the spouses of women who had experienced domestic violence (74 per cent vs. 53 per cent respectively) but this difference was also not statistically significant. Also there was no statistically significant difference between the socio-demographic characteristics of patients and spouses of the women who experienced domestic violence and those had not.

Effects of Domestic Violence as Reported by Women

A significant proportion of the women patients exposed do domestic violence reported psychological distress. The most common symptoms were persistent depression and anxiety, and sleep

Figure 3 : Self-reported psychological effects of domestic violence in women psychiatric patients

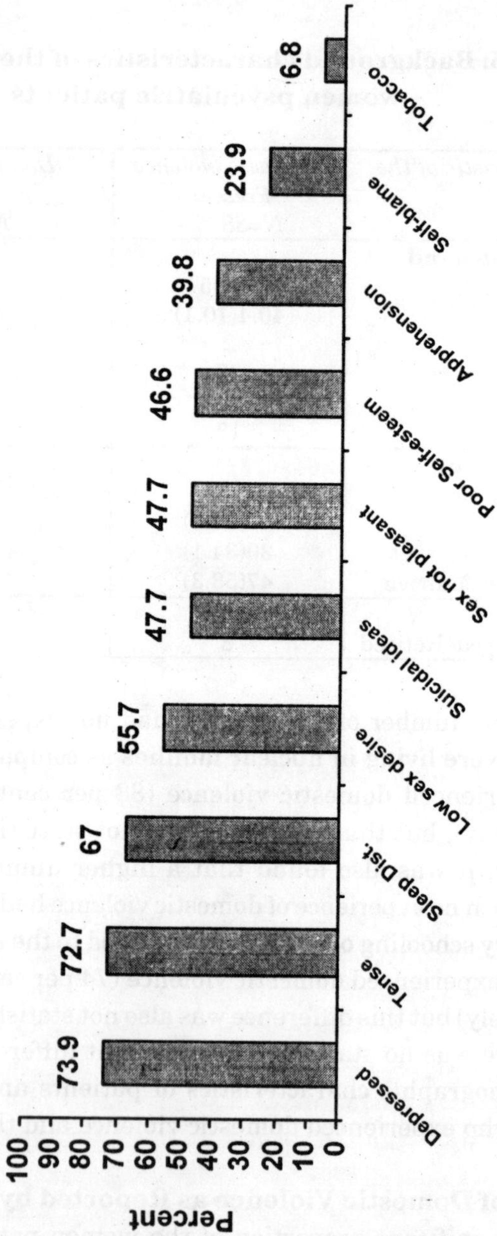

disturbance. Low sexual desire and lack of pleasure in sex were present in 56 per cent and 48 per cent patients. Domestic violence they experienced was belittling resulting in poor self-esteem.

One in four subjects in this study blamed themselves for the domestic violence they experienced. About half of the subjects reported suicidal ideation. Substance use, particularly use of tobacco, was reported by 7 per cent patients as an effect of domestic violence.

Reasons for Domestic Violence as Perceived by Women

Out of the 87 women patients who had experienced physical or psychological abuse or both, 52 per cent felt that their husbands became violent with them because they answered back or disobeyed their husbands. The second most common reason for being subjected to domestic violence was 'not doing chores' (44 per cent), followed by 'not making food properly or in time' (39 per cent). Moreover over one-third (36 per cent) of the women who had experienced violence were beaten or scolded/criticized for refusing to have sex with their husband. There was only one woman in among them who had isolated sexual abuse. None of these reasons was given by her or anybody for sexual abuse. Sexual abuse in context of intimate partner violence was related to mismatch of sexual desires.

Table 6: Reasons for domestic violence

Reason	*N=87 (%)*
Answering back / disobey	51.7
Do not do chores	43.7
Do not make food in time/ properly	39.1
Refuse to have sex	35.6
You do not take care of parents/relatives	28.7
Talk to people whom he does not like	27.6
Expressing contrary opinion	24.1
Has extra-marital relation	23.8
Ask about money	23.8
Go without asking permission	19.5
You do not take care of children	18.4

Response to Domestic Violence as Reported by Women

Table 7 shows how the patients responded to abuse. Not surprisingly, three-fourths of the women i.e. 76 per cent, tolerated silently most of the time; 41 per cent talked to their parental family about this, while 25 per cent talked to the in-laws, whereas 33 per cent did not talk about this to anybody. There were 17 per cent of women patients who hit back the perpetrator. Only three women lodged a complaint with the police.

Table 7: Response to domestic violence by women patients

What women did when they experienced abuse	*N=88 (%)*
Tolerated silently	76.1
Talked to parental family	40.9
Gave in to what the husband asked	35.2
Did not talk about it with anyone	33.3
Talked to friends	31.8
Left for parents	31.8
Ran away/locked herself in a room	30.7
Shouted for help	25
Talked to in laws	25
Had physical symptoms	22.7
Hit back	17
Complained to police	3.4

Reasons for Tolerating Violence as Reported by Women

Table 8 shows the reasons given by the patients for tolerating the abuse. Nearly two-thirds (60 per cent) stuck to the traditional helplessness of women believing that it was a woman's lot to tolerate. They too tolerated silently. About 44 per cent tolerated the violence for the sake of their children. Lack of social support for any retaliatory action to be taken by then and the hope that one day the husband would change were the reasons given by one third of the women each for tolerating violence. About 30 per cent of the women held the view that it was not good to separate from a violent spouse.

Table 8: Reasons for tolerating violence from spouse as reported by women patients

Why do you tolerate this?	*N=88 (%)*
Woman has to tolerate	60.2
For sake of children	44.3
No one else would support me	35.2
Hope that he will change	32.9
To separate is not ok	29.5
He will leave me/ divorce me	17
I do not have my income	17
I love him a lot	17

Perceived Freedom to Act one's Will and Confiding Relationship with Others

Women in the index group reported that they had time for themselves less often compared to the control group. DV survivor women especially lacked more frequently a person in whom they can confide their personal problems or to whom they can go for support when they felt low.

Table 9: Perceived freedom and confiding relationship enjoyed by women patients

Particulars	*DV + N=88(%)*	*DV – N=12(%)*	*P value*
Doing at will			
Visiting parents	70(79.5)	11(91.6)	0.45
Going to doctor for treatment	70(79.5)	12(100)	0.11
Spending money at will	54(61.4)	12(100)	0.072
Having time for self	52(59.1)	11(91.6)	0.0296
Having someone whom one can			
Tell good news	67(76.1)	12(100)	0.659
Tell personal problems	52(59.1)	12(100)	0.0036
Go for support if feeling low	49(55.7)	11(91.6)	0.0248
Care for during illness	54(61.4)	10(83.3)	0.202

Why their Spouse is Abusive: Women's perception

According to majority of the women who experienced physical abuse (75 per cent), their husbands are abusive, because it is part of their nature of personality ("His nature is like that, he gets angry easily). Over one-third of the women who experienced physical abuse blamed their spouses abusive behaviour on male dominance in society ("I am a man, I can do anything, you are a woman, you have to tolerate). A similar percentage of women explained the abusive behaviour of their husbands as a result of witnessing others being beaten. Forty-two per cent of the women blamed their husbands abusive behaviour on their alcohol dependence and nearly half of the women who experienced physical violence thought that their husbands had turned violent as they had seen poverty in their childhood.

Table 10: Women's perception about the reasons for their husbands being abusive

Reasons	*Physical abuse N=61(%)*	*No physical abuse N=39(%)*	*P value*
Personality	46(75.4)	16(41.0)	0.0005
Male-dominated society	22(36.1)	5(12.8)	0.0106
Dowry	8(13.1)	0	0.0251
Possessiveness	11(18.0)	1(2.6)	0.025
Witnessed others being beaten	19(31.1)	5(12.8)	0.036
Alcohol use	26(42.6)	9(23.1)	0.045
Was himself beaten	5(8.2)	0	0.153
Low self-esteem	9(14.8)	2(5.1)	0.194
Financial strain	13(21.3)	5(12.8)	0.281
Poverty in childhood	30(49.2)	23(59)	0.338
All are beating	12(19.7)	5(12.8)	0.373
Low income	18(29.5)	13(33.3)	0.68
Depression	14(23.0)	8(20.5)	0.774
Quarrels in marriage	8(13.1)	1(2.6)	0.086
Less education	17(27.9)	12(30.8)	0.81

When the characteristics of the spouses described by the women who had experienced physical abuse and that described by those who had not experienced physical abuse were compared, it was found that the characteristics husbands personality, male dominance in society, dowry, possessiveness, witnessing other being beaten, and alcohol use were significantly associated with domestic violence.

Diagnosis and Duration of Psychiatric Disorder in the Women Patients

Table 11 shows that diagnosis of psychiatric disorder in women patients who had expericned domestic violence and those that had not. It was found that both the groups had similar frequencies of different psychiatric diagnosis and there was no statistically significant difference between frequencies of any particular diagnosis between the two groups.

Table 11: Diagnosis of psychiatric disorder in women patients

Group	*Diagnosis*	*Domestic violence present N=88(%)*	*Domestic violence absent N=12(%)*
I	Major Depression	38(42.6)	6(50)
	Depression + Somatoform	10(11.2)	0
II	Schizophrenia and related disorders	14(15.7)	2(16.7)
	Bipolar Disorder	6(6.7)	0
III	Anxiety Disorder	6(6.7)	0
	OCD	1(1.1)	1(8.3)
	Somatoform Disorder	11(12.4)	2(16.7)
	Adjustment Disorder	1(1.1)	1(8.3)
	Dissociative disorder	1(1.1)	0

A comparison of the three broad diagnostic groups viz. mood sorders, psychotic disorders and nonmood nonpsychotic disorders not suggest increased domestic violence with a specific diagnosis(=0.23, df=2, p=0.23)

Table 12: Duration of psychiatric disorder and domestic violence

Duration of illness	*DV Present N=88(%)*	*DV Absent N=12(%)*
</= 6 months	15(18)	3(25)
6-12 months	12(13.5)	5(41.6)
1-2 years	13(14.6)	1(8.3)
2-5 years	19(21.3)	0
5-10 years	17(19.1)	2(16.7)
>10 years	12(13.6)	1(8.3)

Chronic illness (duration of illness 2 years or longer) comparec to shorter illness was associated with more frequent domesti violence (54% vs. 25%, X^2=3.69, df=1, p=0.05).

The present study can claim to be the first of its kind to stud domestic violence among women psychiatry patients of diagnosti categories in a general hospital setting. The study has explored th relationship of domestic violence and psychiatric disorder relate characteristics like diagnosis and duration of illness.

Having described the findings of the study, the question arises do women with mental illnesses suffer from domestic violence mor frequently?

In the present study, a vast majority of female psychiatri patients (88 per cent) suffered from at least one type of abuse an one third (38 per cent) suffered from all the three kinds of abus i.e. physical, sexual as well as psychological. Physical abuse i intimate relationships is often accompanied by psychological abus and in one-third to over one half of cases by sexual abuse in a revie of intimate partner violence studies (Krug et al., 2002).

For the majority of women experiences of abuse were n one or two time experiences, they were occurring several time This figure is higher compared to those cited in studies by Visar (1999) and Sanchetana (2000) studies done in rural and slu populations of Gujarat respectively.

Is mental illness a risk factor for domestic violence? Tl question cannot be conclusively answered by this study, thou definitely women with psychiatric disorders have reported domestic violence more frequently compared to women in community based studies from Gujarat (Visaria, 1999; Sanchetana, 2000). The stigma related to psychiatric disorders, burden of care to caregivers caused by the psychiatric disorders, and manifestations of psychiatric disorders leading to interpersonal friction may be contributing to this. High expressed emotions may also be generated by the faulty perception of caregivers that the abnormal behaviors are intentional and not manifestations of psychiatric disorder.

Is Domestic Violence an important issue in mental health? About 33 per cent of women patients who had experienced domestic violence reported that their mental illness had contributed to domestic violence in some way. Over half (55 per cent) of women patients who had experienced domestic violence believed that domestic violence had caused or increased the severity of mental illness, whereas almost half (49 per cent) believed that if domestic violence would not have occurred, they would not have had mental illness.

Is mental illness a cause or effect of domestic violence? This study cannot conclusively answer whether domestic violence is a cause or effect of psychiatric disorder. Though domestic violence is a very important issue to be addressed in the treatment of psychiatric disorders.

The present study showed that none of the demographic characteristic was associated with increased domestic violence. Domestic violence cuts across all barriers and clinicians need to consider possibility of domestic violence in all women seeking their treatment.

A wide range of studies from both industrialized and developing countries have produced a remarkably consistent list of events that are said to trigger partner violence (39–44). These include not obeying the man; arguing back; not having food ready on time; not caring adequately for the children or home; questioning the man about money or girlfriends; going somewhere without the man's permission; refusing the man sex; the man suspecting the woman of infidelity (Krug et al. 2002). In many developing countries, women often agree with the idea that men have the right to discipline their wives, if necessary by force.

A woman's response to abuse is often limited by the alternatives at her disposal. Qualitative studies of women in the U.S. and Africa, Latin America, Asia and Europe show that various factors can keep women in abusive relationships. These commonly include: fear of retribution, a lack of alternative means of economic support, concern for the children, emotional dependence, a lack of support from family and friends, and an abiding hope that the man will change (Krug et al. 2002). In developing countries, women also cite the stigmatization associated with being unmarried as an additional barrier to leaving abusive relationships.

The duration of illness as well as type of psychiatric disorder was not associated with rate of abuse in the present study. Thus it seems that presence of psychiatric disorders rather than its type or duration is associated with abuse. Sexual abuse during lifetime was reported by as many as 53 per cent of women, and sexual abuse during the last one year was reported by 36 per cent women. The only study of sexual coercion in female severe mental disorder patients in India found this in 30 per cent of women (Chandra, 2003).

The most important reasons cited by women why their men are abusive were that it was his nature only, alcohol abuse, possessiveness. Alcohol abuse and dependence ranked only second important factor. Several studies have associated alcohol abuse and domestic violence. However, nature of the relationship between alcohol use and violence and whether it is truly causal is debatable. Many researchers believe that alcohol operates as a situational factor, increasing the likelihood of violence by reducing inhibitions, clouding judgement and impairing an individual's ability to interpret cues. Excessive drinking may also increase partner violence by providing more reasons for arguments between couples. Others argue that the link between violence and alcohol is culturally dependent, and exists only in settings where the collective expectation is that drinking causes or excuses certain behaviors. Despite conflicting opinions about the causal role played by alcohol abuse, the evidence is that women who live with heavy drinkers run a far greater risk of physical partner violence, and that men who have been drinking inflict more serious violence at the time of the assault.

Dowry as the reason for domestic violence was cited infrequently. This may be because women in this study mostly belonged to the lower socioeconomic strata. Dowry is more often a middle class or upper caste feature. Visaria (1999) has also observed that only three women in her study of 346 women from rural Gujarat reported dowry related harassment.

Violence in the family of origin has emerged as an especially powerful risk factor for partner aggression by men. Rates of abuse are higher among women whose husbands had either themselves been beaten as children or had witnessed their mothers being beaten .Although men who physically abuse their wives frequently have violence in their background, not all boys who witness or suffer abuse grow up to become abusive themselves.

Implications of the Present Study

In light of the above, should healthcare professionals in primary care routinely screen patients for domestic violence? To answer this question Ramsay and colleagues (2002) conducted a systematic review of published papers on domestic violence to assess the evidence for the acceptability and effectiveness of screening women for **domestic violence** in healthcare settings. In four surveys, 43-85 per cent of women respondents found screening in healthcare settings acceptable. Two surveys of health professionals' views found that two-thirds of physicians and almost half of emergency department nurses were not in favor of screening. In nine studies of screening compared with no screening, most detected a greater proportion of abused women identified by healthcare professionals. Six studies of interventions used weak study designs and gave inconsistent results. Other than increased referral to outside agencies, little evidence exists for changes in important outcomes such as decreased exposure to **violence.** No studies measured quality of life, mental health outcomes, or potential harm to women from screening programmes. Hence they concluded that although **domestic violence is** a common problem with major health consequences for women, implementation of screening programmes in healthcare settings cannot be justified. Evidence of the benefit of specific interventions and lack of harm from screening is needed.

However given competence of mental health professionals, screening psychiatric patients for domestic violence may enhance therapeutic relationship, may provide opportunity to intervene and improve overall social functioning of the patient, and hence asking about domestic violence should be an integral part of social history of patient.

References

Centre for Women's Development Studies (CWDS). (2002). *Crimes against women: Bondage and beyond: Revelations of data*. New Delhi: CWDS.

Chandra, P.S., Carey, M. P., Carey, K. B., Shalinianant, A., and Thomas, T. (2003) Sexual coercion and abuse among women with a severe mental illness in India: an exploratory investigation. *Comprehensive Psychiatry, 44*, 205-12

Daga, A. S., Jejeebhoy, S. and Rajgopal, S. (1999). Domestic Violence: What Hospital Records Tell Us. *Lawyers Collective, 16*(3), 14-16.

Department of Health. (2000). *Domestic violence: a resource manual for health care professionals*. London: Department of Health. Accessed on 11 March 2003, from www.doh.gov.uk/pdfs/domestic.pdf

Domestic violence in India - A summary report of three studies (pp. 9-17). Washington DC: International Centre for Research on Women (ICRW).

Evaluation Project/PERFORM, Carolina Population Center. (1997). *Uttar Pradesh Male Reproductive Health Survey, 1995-96*. Chapel Hill: University of North Carolina.

Family Violence Prevention Fund. (1997). *Best practices: innovative domestic violence programs in health care settings*. San Francisco: Family Violence Prevention Fund.

Golding, J. M. (1999). Intimate partner violence as a risk factor for mental disorders: A meta-analysis. *Journal of Family Violence, 14*(2), 99-132.

Heise, L. L., Pitanguy, J., and Germain, A. (1994). *Violence against Women: The Hidden Health Burden. World Bank Discussion Papers, no. 255*. Washington, D.C.:World Bank.

Heise, L., Ellsberg, M., & Gottemoeller, M. (1998). Ending violence among women. *Population Reports, Series L, No. 11*. Baltimore: Population Information Programme, Johns Hopkins University School of Public Health.

International Centre for Research in Women (ICRW). (2002). *Domestic Violence in India. Exploring strategies, promoting dialogue. Men, Masculinities, and Domestic Violence in India. Summary Report of 4 studies*. Washington D. C.: ICRW.

International Institute for Population Sciences (IIPS) and ORC Macro. (2000). *National Family Health Survey (NFHS-2), 1998–99: India*. Mumbai: IIPS.

Krug, G., Dahlberg, L., Mercy, J., Zwi, A., Lozano Generve, R. (Eds.). (2002). World Report on Violence and Health. Geneva: World Health Organization. Accessed from www5.who.int/violence_injury_prevention/main.cfm?p = 0000000117

Mahajan, A. (1990). Instigators of wife battering. In S. Sood (Ed.), *Violence against Women*. Jaipur: Arihant Publishers.

Mirlees-Black, C. (1999). *Domestic violence: findings from a new British crime survey self completion questionnaire*. Home Office research Study 191. London: Home Office.

National Crime Records Bureau (NCRB). (n.d.). *Crime in India 2005*. New Delhi: Ministry of Home Affairs. Available at http://ncrb.nic.in

ORC Macro and IIPS. (2000). *National Family Health Survey (NFHS-2). India (1998-99)*. Mumbai: ORC Macro and IIPS.

Ramsey, J., Richardson, J., Carter, Y.H., Davidson, L., and Feder, G. (2002). Should health professionals screen women for domestic violence? Systematic review. *BMJ, 325:314*.

Rao, V. (1996). Wife-Beating in Rural South India: A qualitative and econometric analysis. *Social Science Medicine 00(0),* 1-12.

Sanchetna Community Health and Research. (2000). *Angst – theirs and ours. Domestic violence: an epidemic on the upsurge*. Ahmedabad: Sanchetana.

Visaria, L. (1999). Violence against women in India: Evidence from rural Gujarat. In

Wolfe, D. A., and Korsch, B. (1994). Witnessing domestic violence during childhood and adolescence: implication for pediatric practice. *Pediatrics, 94*, 594-599

World Health Organization, South East Asia Regional Office (WHO-SEARO). (2000). *Prevalence of violence against women (adolescent childbearing). Chapter 6. Women of South-East Asia: a health profile*. New Delhi:WHO/SEARO.

World Health Organization. (1997). *Violence against women: a health priority issue*. Geneva: WHO (FRH/WHD/97.8.).

9

Is There Light at the Other End of the Tunnel? Travails of Widows from Rural Gujarat whose children have out-migrated

Indira Mallya and Parul Dave

Introduction

"Mental Health is the successful performance of mental function, resulting in productive activities, fulfilling relationships with other people, and the ability to adapt to change and to cope with adversity; from early childhood until late life. Mental health is the spring board of thinking and communication skills, learning, emotional growth, resilience, and self esteem". This definition was given by the World Bank (at the seminar on Mental Health and the Global Development Agenda: What Role for the World Bank, November, 2003, at Washington D.C.) Mental Health also refers to a positive state. It is the capacity of the individual, the group and the environment to interact with one another in ways that promote subjective well-being, the optimal development and use of mental abilities (cognitive, affective and relational), the achievement of individual and collective goals consistent with justice and the attainment and preservation of conditions of fundamental equality" (WHO, 1981).

In 1964, the World Health Organization depicted health as a state of complete physical, mental and social well -being and not merely the absence of disease.

Today, the scope of mental health includes the aim of developing the mental health of "normal persons" and not just of the mentally ill, as was the case, earlier. Positive mental health consists of protection and development at all levels of human society to secure, affectionate and satisfying human relationships, and in the reduction of hostile tensions in persons and groups (Govindaswamy cited in Murthy, 1993). Mental health concepts may be used with adults to deal with their selves and their environment.

Widows in Indian families

In Indian culture, the elderly have been integrated into the family which includes the joint, extended and nuclear family structures and the local community according to the norms of society. However, a woman in the family, especially if she is a widow, is surrounded by the culture that seldom allows her to exercise her freedom (Thara Bhai, 2004).

There are an estimated 33 million widows in India (Girish, 2004). Apart from having to face economic problems constantly, widows in India, even those in educated, middle class families, continue to be placed under immense psychological and social pressures. Martha Alter Chen's extensive survey of widows across seven states of India reveals that even today widows are accused of being 'responsible' for their husband's death. They are pressurized to observe restrictive codes of dress and behaviour. They are excluded from religious and social life. They are physically and sexually abused. And they are done out of their property. Chen concludes that in theory, 51 per cent of widows have rights to a share in their husband's land. However, these rights are often violated in practice by brothers-in-law.

The incidence of widowhood rises sharply with age, 64 per cent among women aged 60 and above, and 80 per cent among women aged 70. An Indian woman who survives to old age is therefore almost certain to become a widow. In contrast, only 2.5 per cent of Indian men are widowers, and even in the older age groups only a small minority of men is widowed. The main reasons for this are the much higher rate of remarriage for widowers, and the fact that male mortality rates are higher than female mortality rates. Deprivations that cause mortality rates for widows have been estimated to be a shocking 85 per cent higher amongst widows than among married women (Chakravarti cited in Chen, 1999). It is thus possible to imagine the emotional turmoil and the state of mental health of an average widow in an Indian family who is subjected to unwarranted social pressures, forced isolation and cultural restrictions.

These issues need to be addressed before they get translated into suicides or deaths of despair or unfortunate circumstances among the widows.

Stage of development and mental health

Developmental theories on the elderly demonstrate that at this stage of life the elderly are given to reminiscing about and reviewing their life events and defining old age. Usually, feelings, satisfactions and constraints felt by them maybe used to gauge their sense of wellbeing (Mallya, 2003). By and large, successful aging consists in somehow adjusting to physical and social setbacks. Though they cannot be as active as they once were, they have an inner struggle of this period that holds potential for growth and even wisdom. Erikson calls this struggle **ego integrity vs. despair.**

As older people face the prospect of death, they engage in life review. They look back and wonder whether their lives were worthwhile. In this process, they confront the ultimate despair i.e., the feeling that life was not what it should have been, but now time has run out and there is no chance to try alternate life styles.

As the older person faces despair, he or she is trying to find a sense of ego integrity that includes "the acceptance of one's one and only life cycle as something that had to be and that, by necessity, permitted no substitutions (Erikson, 1963; Crain, 1985). Gaur and Kaur (2001), reiterate that life satisfaction is related to successful aging by meeting the developmental challenges presented to individuals in a "satisfying manner." Among the aged this reflects psychological, physical, social and financial adjustments (Mallya et al., 2005).

The present article deals with the review of life events of six widows through oral histories. The respondents were a part of a larger, case study by Mallya (2003), which included elderly parents whose children have migrated to other countries. Life review was one of the study objectives, from which select findings are presented in this paper. The widowed women gave an account of major events during their life course that included births, marriages, deaths, major trauma and life satisfactions. They also expressed feelings about life events and the future, and, their concept of old age.

Methods and Materials

Five villages in Kheda, Anand district of Gujarat, India, namely, Alindra, Dharmaj, Karamsad, Mehlav and Sojitra formed the **population** selected on the criterion of heavy international out-migration, and availability of adequate communication systems with the outside world. The **primary sample** was selected for the in-depth case study comprising a unit of 10 women and 9 men from the five villages, using the snowballing technique. They were aged between 55 years and 85 years, having at least one daughter or a son who had migrated to another country.

The in-depth interviews of the sample were tape recorded with their prior permission. The women, especially the widows found it difficult to recall their past life. It needed a lot of cajoling and subsequent visits to get information out of them. Sometimes, a relative would help jog their memory.

The interviews were transcribed and cross case analysis and triangulation were used to validate the results and quantifying data by age, sex and marital status, when necessary.

Results and Discussion

Life course events

Widowed women gave were asked to recall, as part of the life review, important events during their life course.

Labors of early life: The widowed women were quite reticent when asked to recall their past, as in Lataben's words "memory diminishes" and therefore it is not easy to delve way back into childhood. Besides, their past was too uninteresting to be recounted and there had been no major hiccups. For most of the women, life really began when they arrived as new brides in a joint family they were married into. On the whole, they unfolded their roles of a traditional housewife, long-suffering daughter-in-law and self-sacrificing parent. Vignette No.1 captures a glimpse of their experiences.

Laxmiben, I had to grind grains, pound masala, tolerate fumes from the stove, milk the buffaloes, care for younger brothers and sisters in-law...it went on and on, the poverty..."Kirtiben added, 'not to forget the "lippan" i.e. plastering cow dung on the floor ... which did not allow me to go out marketing or for dropping children off to school". **Vignette 1.** The arduous tasks of Daughters-in-law of Yore

Other incidents: The incidents recalled were about their deliveries, fetal deaths and miscarriages, trauma of accidental deaths of young relatives, support provided by maternal family and birth of grand children. For example, Leelaben had been very happy at the birth of a grandson in an "all daughters family" and had distributed sweets called "pendas", which are given at the birth of boys, "chokrine babo aavyo etle khushino prasang kehvaay ney? To khushina penda vehechyaa hataa...paanch kilo" (when the daughter gives birth to a boy, is it not a happy occasion? So five kilos of pandas (of happiness) were distributed). Whereas Sarlaben had distributed pendas at the birth of a daughter because "sons belong to their wives "bairana thaay ane maabaapni laagni na thaay".

Some women recalled how the major decisions were made by the husband or the son such as selling a house or getting registered for a pilgrimage... the women were passive observers.

Some sadness in later life

Serving the mothers-in-law and husbands (in that order) seemed to preoccupy the women's married lives. They thought of it as their duty and would go to great lengths and physical strain to care, nurse and look after them personally; despite the former being bedridden. Jeeviben recalled how her husband had his brother's ashes brought over from abroad, for his mother's sake, as she had wanted the funeral to be held in India.

Leelaben juggled home and work as a nurse along with nursing her ailing and bedridden husband for three long years. She called this period as the worst crisis "evi bimari koyi dushmanne pan na aape"! (even an enemy should not be inflicted with such a disease!). She had sponged fed and cared for her husband, daily, before leaving for her job, till the day he died. She sighed deeply and admitted to feeling relaxed now, "pan have free thayaa thodak, I can spare some time for myself now".

Dared to be different

Jeeviben loved sports and even participated in village games right upto the age of 60 plus years and had won many prizes till a few years back. She had recently celebrated her own shraddh (death rituals) in advance, along with that of her deceased husband's, in order to avoid future expenses for her sons. She had even given away two "tola" of gold to each of her four daughters.

Feelings

It is very important to look at feelings and concerns after the life review by older persons, as it helps in gauging their sense of wellbeing and satisfaction, in perspective. The respondents displayed mixed reactions to feelings regarding their life course events. The situations included feelings about their present life, children's

Table 1: Life Satisfactions and Concerns of Widows (N= 5)

Satisfactions	*Concerns*
• No regrets as fulfilled all responsibilities	• The first son migrated at the cost of his studies
• All five children are living happy lives	• Repayment of huge loans
• Happy as children have migrated for a good purpose	
• Sent son abroad to Africa/USA for a secure foothold on foreign soil, so that others can follow	
• Looking after sick husband and mother-in-law right up to their deaths	

migration and fulfilling children's responsibilities in life. Table 1 indicates the women's feelings of satisfactions and concerns in life.

It shows that the satisfactions and concerns of women centered on their children and family members serving whom was considered supremely important. However, settling their children abroad was foremost on their list. They were most happy about the son taking over the mantle of their father. All women were emphatically proud of having fulfilled their duties and obligations and were happy with their lot in life.

Their concern was mainly for the son's welfare as well as repayment of huge loans they had incurred.

The women did not express any feelings of loneliness possibly because living in a close rural community, they had neighbours to interact with, as and when the need arose. Prakash (2003), who interviewed 40 women and 35 men, urban parents of Non Resident Indian children, found that two thirds of the sample felt lonely, especially the women. However, none of her sample said that they were unhappy or dissatisfied with life. This could be because the urban neighbourhoods do not have a strong social support network as in a rural setting.

Future expectations

As far as future expectations of helpful persons were concerned, the women expected mainly the family to help. The son was mentioned first, followed by the daughter-in-law, grandson, self (pension), neighbours (for day to day problems), daughter (in emergency) and paid help (in emergency.

Concept of old age

The respondent's concept of old age was consonant with the concept of old age in the last two stages of the Ashrama Dharma theory, in which the individual is expected to pass on the wisdom and experiences gained over the years to the next generation, give up worldly pursuits and attachments and devote herself or himself to spiritual matters and spend the remaining years of life awaiting death.

They also saw it as the last stage of development at 60 years, which was troublesome, characterized by deteriorated health and mobility. One just waited for death and the abode of God!

Alternatively, old age was seen as a stage of engrossing self in religious activities, as all worldly responsibilities had been completed; thus leading a peaceful and satisfied life.

Mehta and Mallya (2000) in a sample of elderly persons from a low income neighbourhood, found that the concept of old age was associated with life milestones such as marriages of children and birth of grandchildren, along with physical changes caused by deterioration of health.

On the whole, the elderly women in the present study had come to terms with the situations in their lives, and, despite their struggles in the past they did not show any despair. Therefore if Erikson is to be quoted they had achieved a sense of **tranquility** and it may be said, **ego integrity** as well; which is obvious in their philosophical wisdom about life and its truths, in their narratives, (Mallya et al., 2005). Their life history narratives were replete with idioms, religious quotes and sayings which had been passed down over the years by the family. Thus, it appeared that they did not bear anyone any grudges but took things in their stride.

Conclusion and Recommendation

In conclusion, it appears that the widows from the rural setting appeared to "adjust" to their environment by expressing many satisfactions and by not expressing any despair about their life situation. They seemed to accept what life had to give them in a stoic manner. Though this attitude augers well for an existence of sound mental health among the women, one need to keep in mind that they hardly venture out of their immediate environment and, appear helpless when it comes to solving their problems, such as settling financial debts.

It is thus imperative to offer them avenues of self-expression, wider social interactions and exposure to a wider world, which will empower them to meet their needs and problems independently.

The Government of India Policy on Older Persons of 1999 does mention some sops for widows, but only in passing. What are needed are aggressive interventions by NGOs and stakeholders of rural communities for concrete actions to empower the rural widows before they are engulfed in the turmoil of the fast emerging "modern" life in the rural areas. Such empowerment will help the women live a life of fruitful adjustment and happier lives.

References

Chen, M. A. (Ed.) (1999). *Widows in India: Social Neglect and Public Action*. New Delhi: Sage.

Crain, W.C. (1985). *Theories of development: Concepts and applications* (2nd ed.). New Jersey: Prentice - Hall Inc.

Erikson, E.H. (1963). *Childhood and society* (2nd ed.). New York: W.W. Norton.

Gaur, R., & Kaur, K. (2001). Life satisfactions among institutionalized and non- institutionalized elderly. *Indian Journal of Gerontology, 15*(3-4), 323-361.

Girish, U. (2004). *India's Outcast Widows Have New Havens*. Retrieved on February 22, 2005 from http://www.womensenews.org/article.cfm/dyn/aid/1794/context/archive.

Mallya, I. (2003). *Implications of international migration of children on older persons: A case study in rural Gujarat*. Doctoral Dissertation, Department of Human Development and Family Studies, The M.S.University of Baroda, Vadodara, India

Mallya, I. P., Dave, P., & Sharma, D. (2005). Journey Through Life: Reminiscences of older people from rural Gujarat, India. *Indian Journal of Gerontology, 19*(1), 61-68.

Mehta, B., & Mallya, I. (2001). Self appraisal of elderly in slums of Vadodara city. *Helpage India- Research and Development Journal, 7*(2), 22-32.

Ministry of Social Justice and Empowerment, Government of India (2000). *National policy on older persons, 1999*. New Delhi: Author.

Murthy, S. (1993). Evolution of the concept of mental health: From mental illness to mental health. In P. Mane and K. Gandevia (Eds.), *Mental Health in India: Issues and concerns*. Bombay: Tata Institute of Social Sciences.

Prakash, I. J. (2003). Impact of out migration of the young on older people. *Help Age India - Research and Development Journal, 9*(1), 34-39.

Thara Bhai, L. (2004). *Widows in India*. New Delhi: Vedams eBooks.

WHO (1981). *Social dimensions of mental health: A report*. Geneva: Author.

10

Traumatic Widowhood and Major Depression: A Study of Widows affected by Communal Violence

M.S. Saiyad, Arun Kumar, Chetan Patel, Rahul Shidhaye, Seema Garg, Nilesh Bhaiya, G.K. Vankar

"Bereavement is a darkness impenetrable to the imagination of the unbereaved."
- Iris Murdoch

Introduction

Loss of spouse through death may result in profound consequences for the surviving spouse (Dohrenwend and Dohrenwend, 1984). After spending several years with someone, sharing smiles and stories, tears and troubles, growing together and making adjustments to each other, as a unit, it is reasonable to say that once a spouse dies, the life of the one left behind will never be the same.

Spousal bereavement is unique in that the loss is usually unpreventable and always irreversible, may involve the shattering of the long term attachment bonds, often necessitates the assumption of new roles, frequently leads to financial hardships, and may leave the survivor without his or her major support

(Osterweis et al., 1984). Thus it is important to identify the factors that may influence the surviving spouse's vulnerability to the potential adverse consequences of widowhood.

Following factors are known to predict the outcome of bereavement (Stroebe and Schut, 2001):

- situational factors related to the death, such as whether the death was sudden or anticipated;
- personal factors such as gender and characteristics prior to the death such as emotional stability, religious beliefs and practices and self- esteem; and
- interpersonal factors such as the availability of social and emotional support from family and friends.

These factors may act to increase risk of adverse consequences following bereavement (e.g., sudden death, or lack of social and emotional support) or may play a protective role in better outcome after bereavement in the survivors (e.g., availability and use of social and emotional support from family, friends and community) (Hansson and Stroebe, 2003).

Violent circumstances surrounding the death such as suicide, homicide, or accidents result in worse bereavement, as indicated by greater severity of depressive symptoms (Range and Niss, 1990; Farberow et al., 1992) and symptoms of Post Traumatic Stress Disorder (PTSD) (Zisook et al., 1998). In a study of traumatic grief as a risk factor for mental and physical morbidity, 75 per cent of bereaved individuals had depression after 2 months which gradually declined to 36 per cent at 13 months and 33 per cent at 25 months (Prigerson et al. 1997). Perceptions of the death as more violent (than peaceful) were associated with major depressive disorder at the baseline but not at follow-up. The perception of being unprepared for the death may be indicative of possible difficulties in acknowledging and accepting the impending loss, and may also be an indicator of potential complications of bereavement (Barry et al., 2002).

Bereavement is associated with elevated risk of suicidality (Szanto et al., 2001), which itself proves to be risk factor of completed suicide (Shaffer et al., 1988). Pathologic grief reactions or complicated grief is also associated with traumatic bereavement. Risk factors for this include traumatic circumstances of death, multiple deaths and personal vulnerabilities (Parkes, 1998). Complicated Grief symptoms include those of separation distress and traumatic distress. Symptoms of separation distress were found to be significantly higher for those bereaved by deaths from violent acts relative to those bereaved by accidental deaths (Prigerson et al., 2002).

Sex, age, and family income are significantly related to outcome of spousal bereavement, with women and the lower age and lower income groups tending towards poorer outcomes of widowhood (Zisook et al., 1987). A high percentage of bereaved individuals report a subjective sense of decline in health. An increase in the number of bereaved patients with illness, more visits to general practitioners and an increase in physical symptoms unrelated to major illnesses have been noted. Striking physical features include sighing, indigestion, chest pain, palpitations, headaches and psychosomatic medical diseases (Khin and Sunderland, 2000). Depression associated with widowhood has a strong effect on physician utilization, with higher numbers of physician visits than by those who were not depressed (McHorney and Mor, 1988).

There is sufficient evidence that loss of spouse is a major stressful event in an individual's life and spousal bereavement increases the risk for psychiatric illness in the surviving spouse. Spousal bereavement due to violence results in worse bereavement and increases the severity of depressive symptoms. In light of this evidence, the present study was undertaken.

Study Objectives

The present study aimed to find out: the prevalence of major depression among riot affected widows; the demographic characteristics, and manifestations of major depression; and the correlates of major depression in riot affected widows and other associated psychiatric co-morbidities.

Methods and Materials

The study was conducted in the months of February and March 2004, two years after the communal violence that broke out in Gujarat, during February-March, 2002. In all 110 widows from four districts of Gujarat, namely Ahmedabad, Vadodara, Kheda, and Mehsana, were interviewed. These widows had lost their husbands in the communal violence and at the time of the study, were under the rehabilitation program run by SEWA – Self-employed Women's Association. SEWA is an internationally known NGO having 5,30,000 members active in 11 districts of Gujarat. SEWA's mission is to provide sustainable livelihood to women in the informal sector, including employment, insurance, health care, child care so that women will have income security, food security, and social security. It is an organization of women, for women, and its institutes are owned, managed, and used by its members.

The study instruments comprised semi-structured interview guide and the following tools to measure major depression, PTSD, complicated grief, emotional impact of traumatic events, and psychological distress, and disability in doing daily work.

- **The Brief Patient Health Questionnaire** (Spitzer et al., 1999). It consists of 9 items (corresponding to nine criteria for Major depression as per DSM IV) for the reference period of the previous two weeks to be rated on a 4-point scale (0 = Not At All, 1= Frequently, 2 = More than half of the days, 3 =Almost Daily). Major depression was diagnosed when person rated at least five symptoms as two or more with sadness of mood or lack of pleasure as essential criteria. Women who have these essential criteria present, plus two to three responses rated as 2 or 3, were considered as having other depressive disorder.
- **PTSD Symptom Scale** (Foa et al., 1997). This 17 item-screening instrument measures three symptom clusters of PTSD: re-experiencing of trauma (4 items), avoidance (7 items) and hyper arousal (6 items). A self-report instrument in Gujarati language was used. The respondents recorded frequency/ severity of manifestation, and the items were rated on 4 point scale:(0 = not at all or only once,1 = once a week or less/ once in a while, 2 = 2-4 times a week/ half of the time, 3 = 5 or more time a week/ almost always). Though the original instrument considers any severity of symptoms, the researchers of this study wanted to disregard the clinically less significant minor manifestations. Only those symptoms with moderate severity were considered as present. For diagnosis of PTSD the presence of one of the four re-

experiencing symptoms, plus three of the seven avoidance symptoms, plus two of the six hyper-arousal symptoms was considered.

- **Inventory of complicated grief** (Prigerson et al., 1999). This is an instrument comprising a constellation of symptoms including preoccupation with the deceased, yearning, disbelief and inability to accept death, bitterness or anger about the death, and avoidance of reminders of the loss. This is also called traumatic grief (Prigerson et al., 1999). Traumatic or complicated grief is associated with impairment and poor outcomes (Prigerson et al., 1997). It includes **criteria** for separation distress, for traumatic distress, for duration and functional impairment.
- **Impact of Events Scale (IES)-Revised** (Weiss and Marmar, 1997). This is a 22-item scale that assesses the emotional impact of a traumatic event on a person by looking at intrusive thoughts, emotional numbing, and avoidance. Respondents answer items related to the frequency of each symptom experienced from 1= not at all to 4 =often.
- **Self-Reporting Questionnaire** (Harding, et al., 1980). This is one of the most widely used measures of psychological distress in communities. It has twenty questions with option of 'yes' or 'no'. A score of 4 or more indicates psychological distress.
- **Disability Assessment Score** (WHO, 2000). This is a self reported questionnaire used to assess the health during the last one month as well assess difficulties in doing daily work.

In the semi-structured interviews various factors related to trauma were explored such as death of a family member, injury to family members, assault on family members, injury to self, assault on self, damage to house, damage to property, damage to workplace, separation from family members and watching mutilated dead bodies, and living in relief camps.

These instruments were administered to the 110 women by a consultant psychiatrist and six resident doctors of the Department of Psychiatry, Civil Hospital Ahmedabad conducted this study. The residents were trained in the administration of the study instruments and conducting the interviews.

The Statistical Package for Social Sciences (SPSSx 11.5 version) was used to analyze data. Women who had major depression and those who did not have major depression were compared in terms of their demographic characteristics. They were also compared regarding psychological distress as measured by the Self-Reporting Questionnaire (SRQ), impact of the event and posttraumatic stress on Impact of Events (IES) and PTSD scale scores, and disability caused by the symptoms as measured by Disability Assessment Scores (DAS). These subjects were also screened with Inventory of Complicated Grief to look for presence of complicated grief in them. Women with major depression and those with other psychiatric disorder present were compared with 'normal' women, i.e., those who had neither, as regards trauma related events.

Results and Discussion

Out of the 110 women who participated in the study, 79(71.8 per cent) were Muslim, while the rest were Hindus. The age of these women ranged between 20 and 65 years, with their mean age being 34.2 years. Nearly three-fourths of them (71.8 per cent) belonged to low-income group (having monthly income less than Rupees 1000). Twenty six women (23.6 per cent) had lived in relief camps after the communal violence. Seventy seven women belonged to Ahmedabad, 14 to Kheda, 7 belonged to Vadodara and 12 came from Mehsana.

Prevalence of psychiatric disorders in riot affected widows

Of the 110 women interviewed, major depression was present in 68 (61.8 per cent) women. Of these 29 (42.6 per cent) had comorbid PTSD, and complicated grief was present in 23 (33.8 per cent) subjects. Table 1 provides the break up of the types of psychiatric disorders prevalent in these women.

The rate of MDD obtained in the present study (61.8 per cent) is much higher than those reported in other studies among women in the community, where it was reported to be around 10 to 25 per cent (Eaton, et al., 1989), and in bereaved individuals after 25 months of death of spouse (Prigerson et al., 1997), where the rate of MDD was found to be 33 per cent

Table 1: Prevalence of psychiatric disorders in communal riot affected widows (N=110)

Type of disorder	*N (%)*
No Psychiatric disorder	37 (33.6)
Major depression Major depression + PTSD Major depression + Complicated Grief Major depression + Complicated Grief + PTSD	30 (27.2) 15 (13.6) 09 (8.2) 14 (12.7)
Total Subjects with Major Depression	68 (61.8)
Major Depression Subjects with comorbid PTSD	29 (42.6)
Major Depression Subjects with comorbid Complicated Grief	23 (33.8)
PTSD	04 (3.6)
Panic disorder + agoraphobia	01 (0.9)

Table 2: Background characteristics of widowed women, by presence of major depressive disorder and other psychiatric disorders

Demographic Characteristics	*MDD Present n=68*	*Other Psychiatric Disorder Present n=05*	*Normal n=37*	*Test for Difference*[a]
	n (% of subjects)	*n (% of subjects)*	*n (% of subjects)*	
Age: Mean Years	34.4 years	32 years	34.1 years	ns
Religion:				ns
Muslim (%Subjects)	76.4	40	67.5	
Hindu (%Subjects)	23.6	60	32.5	
Monthly income< Rupees 1000	70.5	100	70.2	ns
Residence (District):				ns
Ahmedabad	48 (62.3)	01(0.01)	28 (36.3)	
Mehsana	10 (83.3)	01(8.3)	1 (8.3)	
Baroda	4 (57.1)	0 (0.0)	3 (42.9)	
Kheda	6 (42.9)	3 (21.4)	5 (35.7)	
Experience of living in relief Camp (% who said yes)*	29.4	60	8.1	**X^2=5.17, dF=1, p=0.02**

Note: [a] F test for means; Chi-sq test for categorical measures were used; ns= not significant

* = significant

Table 2 shows background characteristics of the study participants by presence of major depressive disorder and other psychiatric disorders.

As can be seen from the table, the mean age of women with MDD were found to be 34.4 years, whereas the subjects having other psychiatric disorder had a mean age of 32 years.

Prevalence rate of MDD in Muslim women (76.4%) was found to be higher than that in Hindu women (23.6%), but was not found to be significant. Women from Mehsana had higher rates of MDD as compared to those from other districts, but there was no specific demographic characteristic present in women from Mehsana that increases risk of MDD in them.

About 71 per cent of MDD women were from low income families with a monthly income of less than Rs. 1,000. Low income groups are reported to experience poorer outcome from the state of bereavement (Zisook et al., 1987), however in the present study, no significant difference in this regard was found between women with major depression and those who were not depressed.

Manifestations of major depression in riot affected widows

As shown in Table 3, most of the women with major depressive disorder (n=68), reported diminished interest in activities, sadness

Table 3: Manifestations of major depression in women

Type of manifestation	*Percent women with MDD (n=68)*
Diminished interest in activities	94.1
Depressed Mood	98.5
Sleep disturbances	92.6
Fatigability or loss of energy	98.5
Appetite Disturbances	89.7
Feeling of Worthlessness, excessive or	73.5
inappropriate guilt	80.9
Difficulty in concentration	60.3
Pychomotor activity retardation or agitation	67.6
Recurrent thoughts of death and suicidal ideations	

of mood, sleep and appetite disturbances and fatigability. Suicidal ideations were reported by nearly seven out of ten subjects at the time of interview, while 60 per cent of subjects reported disturbances in psychomotor activity.

Manifestations of complicated grief

As shown in Table 4, depressed patients having complicated grief experienced most of the symptoms of complicated grief. Disbelief regarding death at time of interview was seen in six out of ten subjects with complicated grief. Identification with the deceased in form of similar physical symptoms or adopting similar behaviors was not uncommon; it was present in 30.4 per cent of the women.

Table 4: Manifestations of complicated grief in riot affected widows having major depression

Type of manifestation	*Percent women having complicated grief (n=23)*
Separation Distress	
Preoccupied with thoughts of death	95.7
Drawn to places and things related to husband	91.3
Longing and yearning	95.7
Feeling Lonely	95.7
Trauma Distress	
Avoids reminders of death	91.3
No meaning or purpose for future	95.7
Numb and detached	91.8
Stunned, dazed, shocked	95.7
Disbelief	60.9
Emptiness, meaninglessness	100
Cannot imagine fulfilled life	95.7
Feeling part of oneself has died	87.0
Changed worldview	91.3
Similar symptoms or behaviors as spouse	30.4
Bitter over death	73.9

Table 5: Factors related to trauma experienced by riot affected widows having major depressive disorder and other psychiatric disorders

Trauma related factor	*MDD Present n=68*	*Other Psychiatric Disorder Present n=05*	*Normal n=37*	*Test for difference* [a]
	n (%)	*n (%)*	*n (%)*	
Death of other family member	9 (13.2)	0	6 (16.2)	Not Significant
Injury to a family member	8 (11.7)	0	6 (16.2)	Not Significant
Injury to self	6 (8.8)	0	2 (5.4)	Not Significant
Assault on self	2 (2.9)	0	2 (5.4)	Not Significant
Damage to home	12(17.6)	0	6 (16.2)	Not Significant
Damage to property	12(17.6)	0	6 (16.2)	Not Significant
Damage to workplace	9 (13.2)	1 (20)	4 (10.8)	Not Significant
Separation from family	12(17.6)	0	2 (5.4)	Not Significant
Watching mutilated dead bodies	8 (11.7)	0	6 (16.2)	Not Significant
Experience of living in a relief camp	20(29.4)	3(60)	3 (8.1)	X^2=5.17, dF=1, p=0.02

Note: [a] Chi-square test for categorical measures were used.

Trauma related experiences

As shown in Table 5, of all trauma related experiences, separation from the family during riots, damage to workplace, and their stay at relief camps were reported more frequently. Women having major depression had lived in relief camps more often compared to normal women (29.4 per cent vs. 8.1 per cent, p=0.0004). Thus living in a relief camp was found to be a significant contributory factor for MDD.

Correlates of major depression and comorbidities

As shown in Table 6, on all measures, women with major depression had higher scores than those who had no psychiatric disorder. Psychological distress measured by Mean SRQ score was found to be more in women with major depression (15.7 vs. 7.6) when compared with normal women having no psychiatric disorders. Similarly, women with major depression also had higher scores on measures of traumatic stress, i.e. IES and PTSD scores as well as measures on disability i.e. DAS scores than those observed for other psychiatric disorders.

Table 6: Correlates of major depression in riot affected widows (n=110)

	Disorders	*SRQ score Mean (sd)*	*IES score Mean (sd)*	*PTSD score Mean (sd)*	*DAS score Mean (sd)*
A	Major depression	15.7(3.6)	40(18.1)	25.6(13.5)	36.1(9.1)
B	Other psychiatric disorders	14(2.4)	28.8(11.5)	24.4(9.7)	31.2(4.9)
C	No psychiatric disorder	7.6(4.5)	21.0(12.9)	11.6(8.8)	20.4(7.0)

Bereavement has physiological as well as emotional effects. It also affects physical health and there are endocrine changes as in other situations that evoke depression and stress (Parkes, 1998). Traumatic or complicated grief symptoms have been related significantly with higher risks of health impairments and disabilities than the bereaved individuals without traumatic grief. (Chen et al.,

1999). In the present study, women with major depression and complicated grief had higher mean SRQ score (16) as well as mean DAS score (37.4) than all other subjects.

PTSD is an important comorbidity associated with traumatic bereavement. Studies have found PTSD symptoms to be associated with death from accidents and as well as death related with natural disasters (Glaser et al., 1978) as well as man made disasters like wars(Green et al., 1990). In the study by Davis and Breslau (1994), 23 per cent of the subjects exposed to traumatic events developed PTSD which varied by the type of stressor. In terms of individual characteristics, women and men seem to be about equal risk for developing symptoms following disasters, but may present with different complaints. Women tend to report more PTSD, anxiety and depression symptoms than men (Gleser et al., 1981). In a study by Silverman and associates (2000), PTSD was present in 25 per cent of widowed subjects after 4 months of bereavement.

In the present study women with major depression had high rate of PTSD (42.6%) following traumatic bereavement. These women had had high mean PTSD score than normal women (25.6 vs. 11.5). The impact of traumatic event measured by mean IES score was also found to be more in women with major depression (40) than in those diagnosed with other disorders (28.8) and in women who were normal (21.1).

Traumatic bereavement is also associated with development of complicated grief. It occurs in 10 to 20 per cent of bereaved individuals and its symptoms are separation and traumatic distress (Shear et al., 2001). A study has found the presence of symptoms of complicated grief in around 20 per cent of the study subjects during second year of bereavement, and complicated grief symptoms as well as depressive symptoms decreased with time after death of spouse (Prigerson et al., 1997). Complicated grief also correlates with poor social functioning, lower mental health scores and lower energy scores (Silverman et al., 2000).

In the present study, the rate of complicated grief in women with major depression was 33.8 per cent, while the overall rate of complicated grief was found to be 21 per cent. Complicated grief subjects have been reported to have more symptoms of separation distress than traumatic distress, if bereavement was traumatic and violent (Prigerson et al., 2002). In the present study too, women with complicated grief reported more separation distress symptoms than traumatic one.

Conclusion

The present study has found major depression to be present in 61.8 per cent of riot-affected widows two years after the riots. The rate of major depression was found to be higher in Muslim women than in Hindu women, but was not statistically significant. Also, high rate of comorbidities in the form of PTSD was found in women who had traumatic bereavement and suicidal ideations were also more prominent in them. Complicated grief was present in 33.8 per cent of women with major depression (out of 68 subjects with MDD, 23 of them developed Complicated Grief). Psychological distress, impact of traumatic events (most importantly separation from the family, damage to the workplace, and being forced to live in relief camps) and disability, i.e. poor health and difficulty in doing daily work were present more frequently among women with major depression and women having complicated grief, than in women having no psychiatric disorder. Further, thus social as well as psychological support is required in order to overcome complicated grief. Assistance in seeking livelihoods to such women, as the study indicates, could be an important intervention for the riot affected.

The present research is a pioneering effort, as it is the first of its kind in India, to study the prevalence of major depression and traumatic widowhood among the riot affected, and the presence of PTSD, complicated grief, psychological distress, impact of traumatic events, and disability. However, as the study was conducted two years after the riots, there is a possibility of recall bias in the accurate reporting of symptoms over this period by the study subjects. This study has been conducted among riot-affected widows, comparison with normally bereaved women would shed more light on the nature of depression associated with traumatic bereavement. Also, gender differences in this regard could not be studied as the subjects were only women. Further research in this direction would help in gaining a deeper insight into this topic.

References

Barry, L., Kasl, S. and Prigerson, H. (2002). Psychiatric disorders among bereaved persons: The role of perceived circumstances of death and preparedness for death. *American Journal of Geriatric Psychiatry, 10*(4), 447-457.

Chen, J. H., Bierhals, A.J., Prigerson, H. G., et al.(1999). Gender differences in the effects of bereavement related psychological distress on health outcomes. *Psychological Medicine, 29*, 367-380.

Davis, G. C., and Breslau, N. (1994, June). Post traumatic Stress Disorder in victims of civilian trauma and criminal violence. *Psychiatric Clinics of North America, 17*(2), 289-299.

Dohrenwend, B. S. and Dohrenwend, B. P. (1984). *Stressful Life Events and their contexts*. New Brunswick, New Jersey: Rutgers University Press.

Eaton, W. W., Kramer, M., Anthony, J.C., Dryman, A., Shapiro, S., and Locke, B. Z. (1989). The incidence of specific DIS/DSM-III mental disorders: Data from the NIMH Epidemiologic Catchment Area Program. *Acta Psychiatr Scand, 79*, 163.

Farberow, N.L., Gallagher-Thompson, D., Gilewski, M., et al. (1992). Changes in grief and mental health of bereaved spouses of older suicides. *Journal of Gerontology, 47*, 357-366.

Foa, E. B., Cashman, L., Jaycox, L., Perry, K. (1997). The validation of a self-report measure of posttraumatic stress disorder: The Posttraumatic Diagnostic Scale. *Psychological Assessment, 9*, 445-451.

Gleser, G.C., Green, B.L., and Wingert, C. N. (1978). Quantifying interview data on psychic impairment of disaster survivors. *Journal Nerv Ment Dis, 166*, 209-216.

Gleser, G. C., Green, B. L., and Wingert, C. N. (1981). *Prolonged psychosocial effects of disaster: A study of Buffalo Creek*. New York: Academic Press.

Green, B.L., Grace, M.C., Lindy, J.D., Gleser, G.C. (1990). War stressors and symptoms persistence in posttraumatic stress disorder. *Journal of Anxiety Disorders, 4*, 31-39.

Hansson, R. and Stroebe, M. (2003). Grief, older adulthood. In T. P. Gullotta and M. Bloom (Eds.), *Encyclopedia of primary prevention and health promotion* (pp. 515-521). New York: Plenum.

Khin, N. A., and Sunderland, T. (2000). Bereavement in older Adults: Biological, Functional and Psychological Consequences. *Psychiatric Times*, volume XVII, Issue 1.

McHorney, C. A., and Mor, V. (1988). Predictors of bereavement depression and its health services consequences. *Med Care, 26*(9), 882-893.

Osterweis, M., Soloman, F., and Green, M. (1984). *Bereavement reactions, consequences and care.* Washington, DC: National Academy of Sciences.

Parkes, C.M. (1998). Coping with loss: Bereavement in adult life. *British Medical Journal, 316*, 856-859.

Prigerson, H. G., Bierhals, A. J., Kasl, S. V., Reynolds, C. F. III, Shear, M. K., Day, N., Beery L. C., Newsom, J.T., and Jacobs, S. (1997). Traumatic grief as a risk factor for mental and physical morbidity. *American Journal of Psychiatry, 154*, 616-623.

Prigerson, H. G., and Latham, A.E. (in press). *Suicidality and Bereavement: Complicated Grief as Psychiatric Disorder presenting Greatest Risk for Suicidality*

Prigerson, H. G., Maciejewski, P. K., Reynolds, C. F. III, Bierhals, A. J., Newsom, J. T., Fasiczka, A., Frank, E., Doman, J., and Miller, M. (1995). Inventory of Complicated Grief: A scale to measure maladaptive symptoms of loss. *Psychiatry Research, 59*, 65-79

Prigerson, H. G., Shear, M. K., Jacobs, S. C., Reynolds, C. R. III, Maciejewski, P.K., Davidson, J. R., Rosenheck, R., Pilkonis, P. A., Wortman, C. B., Williams, J. B., Widiger, T.A., Frank, E., Kupfer, D. J., and Zisook, S. (1999). Consensus criteria for traumatic grief: A preliminary empirical test. *British Journal of Psychiatry, 174*, 67-73

Prigerson, H., Ahmed, I., Silverman, G. K., Saxena, A. K., Maciejewski, P. K., Jacobs, S. C., Kasl, S.V., Aqeel, N., and Hamirani, M. (2002). Rates and risks of complicated grief among psychiatric clinic patients in Karachi, Pakistan. *Death Studies, 26*, 781-92.

Range, L. M., and Niss, N. M. (1990). Long term bereavement from suicide, homicide, accidents, and natural deaths. *Death Studies, 14*, 423-433.

Shaffer, D., Garland, A., Gould, M., Fisher, P., and Trautman, P. (1988). Preventing teenage suicide: A critical review. *Journal of American Academy of Child Adolescent Psychiatry, 27*, 675-687.

Shear, M. K., Zuckoff, A., and Frank, E. (2001). The Syndrome of Traumatic Grief .*CNS Spectrums, 6*(4), 339-346.

Silverman, G. K., Jacobs, S. C., Kasl, S. V., Shear, M. K., Maciejewski, P. K., Noaghuil, F. S., and Prigerson, H. G. (2000). Quality of life impairments associated with diagnostic criteria for traumatic grief. *Psychological Medicine, 30*, 857-862.

Spitzer, R. L., Kroenke, K., and Williams, J. B. W. (1999). Validation and utility of a self-report version of PRIME-MD: The PHQ primary care study. *The Journal of the American Medical Association, 282, 1737-1744.*

Statistical Package for Social Sciences (SPSS) (2002): SPSS for Windows, Release 11.5.0(6 September 2002).

Stroebe, M.S., and Schut, H. (2001). Models of coping with bereavement: a review. In M.S. Stroebe, R. O. Hansson, W. Stroebe and H. Schut (Eds.), *Handbook of bereavement: consequences, coping, and care* (pp. 375-403). Washington, DC: American Psychological Association.

Szanto, K., Prigerson, H. G., and Reynolds, C. F. (2001). Suicide in the elderly. *Clinical Neuroscience Research, I*, 366-376.

Weiss, D. and Marmar, C. (1997). The Impact of Event Scale-Revised. International Journal. In J. Wilson and T. Keane (Eds.), *Assessing Psychological Trauma and PTSD* (pp 399-411). New York: Guildford.

Harding, T.W., de Arango, M.V., Baltazar, J., Clement, C.E., Ibrahim, H.H., Ladrido-Ignacio, L., Murthy, R.S., Wig, N.N. (1980). Mental disorders in primary health care: a study of their frequency and diagnosis in four developing countries. *Psychological Medicine, 10*, 231–241.

Zisook, S., Chentsova-Dutton, Y., Shuchter, S. R. (1998). PTSD following bereavement. *Annals of Clinical Psychiatry, 10*, 157-163.

Zisook, S., Shuchter, S. R., Lyons, L. E. (1987). Predictors of psychological reactions during the early stages of widowhood. *Psychiatric Clinics of North America, 10*(3), 355-367.

SECTION - IV
Some Aspects of Physical and Mental Health in Aging Women

SECTION A

Some Aspects of Physical and Mental Health in Ageing Women

11

Effects of Nutrients on Mental Health

N. Somashekara, Sandeep H. Shah, C. N. Ramchand

Introduction

Mental health is fundamental to health and human functioning. Appropriate treatment can alleviate, if not cure the symptoms and associated disability of the mental illness. Today, integrative neuroscience and molecular genetics point to some of the most exciting basic research opportunities in medical science. Molecular and genetics tools are being used to identify the genes and proteins that might be involved in the origin of mental illness. Genes and gene products promise to provide novel targets for therapeutic applications. A plethora of new pharmacological agents for mental disorders affords new treatment opportunities for a variety of conditions.

Nutrigenomics is defined as interaction of dietary components like vitamins, minerals, fatty acids, and phytochemicals with genes. The Nutrigenomics approach has been used for the last few years for certain genetic diseases. Nutrients alter the phenotypic expression of a given genotype, particularly during fetal and postnatal development. Many hormones act as nutritional signals and their receptors play a key role in mediating the effects of nutrition on numerous genes involved in differentiation, growth and metabolism. The preliminary results involving the gene-diet interactions for cardiovascular diseases and cancer are promising.

The relationship between nutrition and mental illness is a relatively new area of research. Most of the existing studies focus on the use of dietary supplements in individuals with mental disorders, but there is a lack of consistent data on the impact of nutrition, diet and eating habits on mental health. The long-term goal of nutrigenomics is to help to understand how we can use nutrition to prevent many of the same diseases for which pharmacogenomics is attempting to identify cures. Nutrigenomics is a potential goldmine for the discovery of genes that are important as dietary targets. It should also have an important role in elucidating nutrient signaling pathways that might contribute to certain diet-related diseases, such as cancer or metabolic syndrome.

Mental illness

The term mental illness covers a wide range of mental disorders including severe psychotic illness (such as schizophrenia) and chronic non-psychotic illness (depression and anxiety). Mental illness is characterized by the alteration in thinking, in mood or behavior (or combination thereof) associated with significant distress and impaired functioning over an extended period of time. The symptoms of mental illness vary from mild to severe, depending on the type of mental illness, the individual, the family and the socioeconomic environment (Kessler and Ahangang, 1999). Mental health is as important as physical health for daily living. In fact, the two are intertwined. Individuals with mental illness can develop physical symptoms and illness, such as weight loss and blood biochemical imbalance, associated with eating disorders or state of disease. Mental illness takes many forms such as mood disorders, schizophrenia, anxiety disorders, personality disorders, eating disorders and suicidal behavior (Health Canada, 2002).

Research indicates that some people may have genetic predisposition to developing mental illnesses such as anxiety disorders, depression and psychotic disorders. Anxiety is characterized by extreme distress, panic, worry, high blood pressure, increased heart beat, upset stomach, tremors, muscle tension, restlessness, and sleeplessness. Depression affects mood

(Queensland Transcultural Mental Health Centre). Depression is an illness that affects the thoughts, feelings, behaviour, and overall health. One feels sad and down for long periods of time. Depression can even have physical effects on the body (McKeough). Mood disorders take a monumental toll on human lives in the form of suffering, lost productivity and suicide. Moreover, when unrecognized, they can result in undesirable health problems. Worldwide, mood disorders rank among the top 10 causes of disability (Mental Health, Report from Surgeon General). They are classified into mild and major depression. Mild depression is characterized by sadness and unwillingness to do anything. Major depression is characterized by the extreme sadness or despair, a loss of interest in doing things, sleeping problems, loss of appetite, weight loss, lack of energy, suicidal feelings, sense of guilt, hopelessness and feelings of worthlessness (Queensland Transcultural Mental Health Centre). Depression may be unipolar (general feelings of sadness / feeling low, negative view of self, the world and the future, lethargy, poor sleep and loss of appetite) or bipolar (characterized by the mood swings) (McKeough).

Depression can affect the immune system and can exacerbate existing medical conditions. Heart disease, diabetes and cancers are linked to depression. Depression may have adverse effects on blood clotting, blood pressure, blood vessel and heart rhythms.

The way we respond to situations (with thoughts of hopelessness, anxiety, anger, etc) affects the chemicals that are released within our body. All emotional responses have chemical consequences. Depression is associated with certain neurotransmitters (e.g. Serotonin, or adrenalin and to a lesser extent dopamine). Serotonin, a neurotransmitter has a major role in the depression cycle. When a person is depressed their serotonin level becomes low which leads to several changes in the body. Serotonin is involved in the many aspects of mood, personality and behavior (e.g. anxiety, depression, impulsiveness and addiction) (McKeough).

In psychotic disorders, the person loses touch with reality or is unable to distinguish between reality and fantasy. Two of the most common psychotic disorders are schizophrenia and manic-depressive illness. Schizophrenia affects about 1 percent of population, yet its severity and persistence reverberate throughout the mental health systems. Schizophrenia is marked by profound alterations in cognition (Mental Health, Report from Surgeon General). The symptoms of schizophrenia include feeling confused and depressed, withdrawal from family, friends, reduced social contact, hearing voices of people, who are not present or that no one else can hear, believing that people want to cause them harm, believing oneself to be some one famous or powerful, feeling and thoughts not matching, e.g. laughing at a sad thought for no apparent reason, and inability to perform everyday tasks, e.g. neglecting personal hygiene or diet (Queensland Transcultural Mental Health Centre). Symptoms frequently include hearing internal voices or experiencing other sensations not connected to an obvious source (Hallucinations) and assigning unusual significance or meaning to normal events or holding false personal beliefs (Delusions) (Mental Health, Report from Surgeon General). Although the causes of schizophrenia are not fully known, research points to the prominent role of genetic factors and to the impact of adverse environmental influences during the early stage of brain development (Tsuang et al., 1991).

Manic-depressive illness affects person's mood. A person may have extreme mood swings of highs and lows. Symptoms of low mood consist of feelings of failure or unworthiness, suicidal feelings, sleeping problems and poor appetite. Symptoms of high mood consist of irritability, jumbled speech due to rapid speaking, impulsiveness and belief in being someone important or having great powers. (Queensland Transcultural Mental Health Centre)

Women experience depression about twice as often as men. Many hormonal factors may contribute to increased rate of depression in women, particularly factors such as, menstrual cycle changes, pregnancy, miscarriage, postpartum period, pre-menopause and menopause (Kohen, 2004). To a lesser extent other factors such as, responsibilities both at work and home, caring for children and for aging parents also contribute to the depression in women. The female hormone, estrogen influences the depression in women. At McMaster University, Meir Steiner and his colleagues have been studying the role that estrogen and other reproductive hormones may play in gender differences in depression. Women are two to three times more likely than men to experience a major depressive episode during their lifetime. The underlying cause of the gender difference in depression and other mood disorders is not entirely clear, but the differences, which begin rather dramatically at puberty and become less marked after menopause, strongly suggest a link to fluctuating estrogen and progesterone levels. Although hormones fluctuate in both men and women, the fluctuations are much more pronounced in women, particularly around their menstrual cycles, during the weeks immediately after pregnancy (postpartum), and in the period leading up to menopause (perimenopause). These fluctuations cause disturbances along the hypothalamic-pituitary-adrenal axis, a part of the neuroendocrine system that is believed to play a primary role in the body's reaction to stress. Because hormonal fluctuations occur in all women, yet not all women experience clinical depression, it's likely that women who develop hormone-related depression and mood disorders have a genetic predisposition to them. Further research is needed, to identify the specific genetic markers that might lead to a better understanding of how the balance between estrogen, progesterone, testosterone, and other reproductive hormones affects brain function and increases women's susceptibility to depression (Medical Science News).

Causes of mental illness

Research suggests that mental illnesses are the results of a complex interaction of genetic, biological, personality and environmental factors. However, the brain is the final common pathway for the control of behavior, cognition, mood and anxiety. Most mental illnesses are found to be more common in close family members of person with mental illness, suggesting a genetic basis to the disorders. In some instances there is research evidence suggesting that genetic factor affecting the brain chemistry contribute to the onset and progression of mental illness. However there is also increasing evidence that long term changes in brain function can occur in response to factors in the environment such as stimulation, experiences of traumatic or chronic stress, or various kind of deprivation. Age and sex affects the rates of mental illness. Environmental factors such as family situation, work place pressures and socioeconomic status of the individual can precipitate the onset or reoccurrence of mental illness. Lifestyle choices (Substance abuse) and leaned pattern of thoughts and behavior can influence the onset, course and outcome of mental illness. Mental illness contributes to or result from or share a common pathway with physical illness such as cancer, heart diseases and chronic obstructive pulmonary disease (COPD) (Schwartz, 1999).

Neurological research has identified over fifty (50) neurotransmitters in the brain. Research also tells us that several neurotransmitters such as dopamine, serotonin, norepinephrine, and GABA (Gamma Aminobutyric Acid) are related to mental health problems. Too much or too little of these neurotransmitters are now felt to produce psychiatric conditions such as schizophrenia, depression, bi-polar disorder, obsessive-compulsive disorder, and ADHD (Attention Deficit Hyperactivity Disorder). High levels of Dopamine in the brain often cause us to lose our contact with reality. As though living in a science-fiction movie, we begin to develop unusual, if not bizarre ideas about what is happening to us. With our paranoia, we may experience delusions (false beliefs) of persecution or may think we have super powers (delusions of grandiosity) and can predict the future or read minds. High levels of dopamine are found in schizophrenia, drug intoxication, and other psychotic conditions where the ability to distinguish the inner world from the real world is impaired. Serotonin, first isolated in 1933, is the neurotransmitter that has been identified in multiple psychiatric disorders including depression, obsessive-compulsive disorder, anorexia, bulimia, body dysmorphic disorder, social anxiety, phobias, etc. Low serotonin levels are believed to be the cause of many cases of mild to severe depression, which can lead to symptoms such as anxiety, apathy, fear, feelings of worthlessness, insomnia and fatigue (University of Bristol). Low levels of norepinephrine are associated with a loss of alertness, poor memory, and depression. Norepinephrine appears to be the neurotransmitter of "arousal" and for that reason, lower-than-normal levels of this neurotransmitter produce below-average levels of arousal and interest, a symptom found in several psychiatric conditions including depression and ADHD. It is for this reason that medications for depression and ADHD often target both dopamine and norepinephrine in an attempt to restore both to normal level. Gamma-Aminobutyric Acid (GABA) is a neurotransmitter, which involved in level excitability. Low levels of GABA are associated with Bipolar Disorder, Mania (Carver, 2002).

Genetics and Mental Illness

Its long been known that certain diseases tend to run in families, and in fact, most of our understanding of mental illness comes from family, adoption, and twin studies. Now, researchers have discovered a gene that can double the risk of depression, another that can increase the risk of schizophrenia, and others that may play a role in heightening the risk of bipolar disorder (Griffin Kellicker).

The Genetics of Depression

One of the questions scientists have been trying to answer is why some people become depressed in reaction to life stresses while others do not. A study led by Avshalom Caspi, M.D. of Kings College London, sheds some light on this question. In their study, Caspi and colleagues followed 847 New Zealanders over five years and charted their reaction to different life stressors. Stressors included things like loss of job, death of a loved one, broken relationships, or prolonged illness. What they found was that participants with a short version of a particular gene were more likely to become depressed when faced with stressful life events than those who had the long version of the same gene. Specifically, 43% of people with the short form of the gene developed depression, in contrast to 17% of those with the long form. The findings suggest a genetic vulnerability to depression when certain environmental stressors activate the gene (Caspi et al., 2003).

The Genetics of Schizophrenia

The family link to schizophrenia is well established, but paring down the risk to one specific gene has proven difficult. For example, we each inherit two copies of the COMT (catecho-O-methyltransferase) gene, one from each parent. There are two COMT types possible: the *val* type (short for the amino acid valine) and the *met* type (short for the amino acid methionine). Research suggests that the *val* type may increase the susceptibility to schizophrenia by reducing dopamine activity (Griffin Kellicker).

A study performed by Michael Egan M.D. and colleagues tested the working memory of 181 schizophrenic patients, 219 of their well siblings and 75 controls. The researchers found that individuals who had two copies of the *val* type gene performed worse than those with only one copy, and those with the *met* type gene performed best of all. What this suggests is that the *val* type COMT gene may increase an individuals susceptibility to schizophrenia (Egan et al., 2001).

The Genetics of Bipolar Disorder

Bipolar disorder, also sometimes called manic-depressive illness, is a disease that causes extreme shifts of mood from depression to mania to a mixed state. While family and twin studies have shown that bipolar disease can be inherited, they have not yet pinpointed a particular gene. In fact, evidence suggests that bipolar disorder is affected by the presence and interaction of many genes (Griffin Kellicker). In one study, Alessandro Rotondo M.D. and colleagues studied 111 individuals with bipolar disorder, 49 of whom also had panic disorder, and 127 individuals with no history of psychiatric disorders. When the DNA from all the participants was compared, the researchers found that those with bipolar disorder had a significantly higher frequency of the COMT (Catechol O-Methyltransferase) and short 5-HTT (serotonin transporter gene) genes. These findings suggest that genes may increase an individual's vulnerability to bipolar disorder (Rotondo, 2002).

Nutrigenomics

The interaction of genetics and environment, nature and nurture is the foundation for all health and diseases. Nutrition is an environmental factor of major importance. Major advances have occurred over the past 25 years in the field of both genetics and nutrition. Methodological advances in molecular biology and genetics have facilitated the study of diseases at DNA level, and the study of nutrients at the molecular level. This has led to the studies on evolutionary aspects of diet and the role of nutrients in the gene expression called nutrigenomics. Nutrigenomics could provide a framework for the development of novel food, which will be genotype dependent for the promotion of health and prevention of chronic diseases (Simonopoulos and Ordovas, 2004). Diet represents one of the key environmental factors to which genes are exposed, from the conception throughout the life. Nutrients governs the concentration of different proteins in deferent organs by functioning as regulators of gene expression and translation, nuclear RNA processing, mRNA stability (IFT Expert Report).

Strategies for disease prevention can have a major impact on people' health. However, major gaps exist in our knowledge with regards to nutritional adequacy, nutrient and gene interaction, and effective strategies for implementation of dietary recommendations. Extensive review carried out in the field of gene-diet interactions, reinforcing the concept that, genetic variability at the classical candidate genes determines a small, but statistically significant, fraction of individual variability in response to dietary modification (Ordovas, 2002).

The interface between the nutritional environment and cellular/genetic processes is being referred to as nutritional genomics or "nutrigenomics". Nutrigenomics seeks to provide a genetic understanding for how common dietary chemicals (nutrients) affects the balance between health and disease by altering the expression and/or structure of an individual's genetic makeup. Common dietary chemicals act on the human genome, either directly or indirectly, to alter gene expression or structure. Some diet-regulated genes (and their normal, common variants) are likely to play a role in the onset, incidence, progression, and/or severity of chronic diseases (Kaput and Rodriguez, 2004).

The emerging field of nutrigenomics explores how nutrients in the food interact with the genes that contribute to chronic diseases. The goal of nutrigenomics is to understand the individual nutrient genotype to design dietary intervention that restore health or prevent disease (Ruskin, 2004). Scientists are finding biologically active components of the food can alter the gene expression. For example, a deficiency of folic acid may lead to break in DNA that mimic radiation damage. Other nutrients are involved in molecular processes related to DNA structure, gene expression and metabolism, which contribute to the development of chronic illness (Potera, 2004).

Nutrigenomics, proteomics and metabolomics are the three new disciplines that will contribute to the rapid development of functional food with known bioactive or nutrient component for a disease (Clydesdale, 2004). Nutrigenomics is defined as interaction of dietary components with genes. The dietary components of interest can be essential nutrients like vitamins, minerals and fatty acids and other bioactive substances like phytochemicals or metabolite of food components like retinoic acid, eicosanoids (IFT Expert Report). The nutrigenomics approach resembles pharmacogenomics, which looks at the relationship between SNPs in genes and patients. The nutrigenomics and pharmcogenomics are closely linked, as without nutrigenomics, pharmocogenomics data cannot be interpreted correctly, because diet may affect the expression of gene involved in drug metabolism (Potera, 2004).

Nutrition profoundly alters the phenotypic expression of a given genotype, particularly during fetal and postnatal development. Many hormones act as nutritional signals and their receptors play a key role in mediating the effects of nutrition on numerous genes involved in differentiation, growth and metabolism (Dauncey et al., 2001).The research has shown that nutrient affects gene expression and formation of various proteins. Thus, the amount and even the form of nutrient present during gene expression can affect the synthesis of protein, resulting in less of protein being produced, production of less than optimally functional form or no protein at all (Clydesdale, 2004). Nutrients serve as substrates, cofactors or co enzymes for metabolic processes that are familiar from traditional research and epidemiological observation. The premise, that food consumed during the first weeks and months of life may have permanent effects on metabolism is not new. Studies on humans and animals showed permanent effects of early diet on adult metabolism, cognitive formation and body composition through activation or suppression of gene expression or turning genes "on" or "off"(Barker et al., 1993).

The concept of "personalized" medicine is now being extended to the field of nutrition. It is now accepted that, nutrients (i.e., macronutrients, micronutrients and antinutrients) alter molecular processes such as DNA structure, gene expression, and metabolism, and these in turn may alter disease initiation, development, or progression (Kaput and Rodriguez, 2004).

Table 3: Gene expression processes leading to protein formation and selected nutrient regulators in the process

Gene Expression Sequence	*Nutrient Regulator*	*Reference*
Gene transcription	Fatty acids, glucose, cholesterol, amino acids, zinc, bioactive components	Berger et al., 2002; Brown et al., 2003; Carluccio et al., 2003; Chowanadisai et al., 2004 ; Lizuka et al., 2004 ; Jousse et al., 2004; Koo et al., 2001 ; Stoeckman and Towle, 2002 ; Uyeda et al., 2002
mRNA processing	Methionine, choline, vitamins B-6,& B12, fatty acids	Mater et al., 1999; Niculescu and Zeisel, 2002
mRNA stability	Amino acids, vitamin D, calcium	Fafournoux et al., 2000; Slattery et al., 2004
mRNA translation	Glucose, fatty acids, minerals, amino acids, choline, conjgated linoleic acid (CLA)	Brown et al., 2004; Campos et al., 2001; Doering and Danner, 2000; Fafournoux et al., 2000 ; Hasty et al., 2000 ; Liu et al., 2000 ; Niculescu et al., 2004 ; Redonnet et al., 2002 ; Slattery et al., 2002
Post-translational modification	Minerals and vitamin cofactors	Bailey and Gregory, 1999; Campbell et al., 1999; Escher and Wahli, 2000
Protein transport to functional location	Vitamins, mineral	Kelleher and Lonnerdal, 2002

Source: *Expert Report –Institute of Food Technologists.*

Table 4: Examples of nutrient involvement in gene expression and potential phenotypic results

Nutrient Deficiency	*Phenotypic Expression*	*Reference*
Folate	Elevated homocysteine (cardiovascular disease), neural tube defects, central nervous system dysfunction	Clarke, 2001; Kolling et al., 2004; Regland et al., 1997; Shields et al., 1999 ; Susser et al., 1998 ; Verhoef et al., 1997 ; Yoo et al., 2000 (also, Kunugi et al., 1998 and Virgos et al., 1999 for contrasting views)
Fatty acids	Cognitive function (depression), obesity, inflammation	Covault et al., 2004; Escher and Wahli, 2000; Saugstad, 2001; Takahashi et al., 2002; Vlassara et al., 2002
Vitamin D	Osteoporosis	Chen et al., 2002; Sowers et al., 1999

Source: *Expert Report –Institute of Food Technologists*

Dietary chemicals can affect gene expression directly or indirectly. At the cellular level, nutrients may: *1*) Act as ligands for transcription factor receptors *2*) Be metabolized by primary or secondary metabolic pathways, thereby altering concentrations of substrates or intermediates; or *3*) Positively or negatively affect signal pathways (Kaput and Rodriguez, 2004).

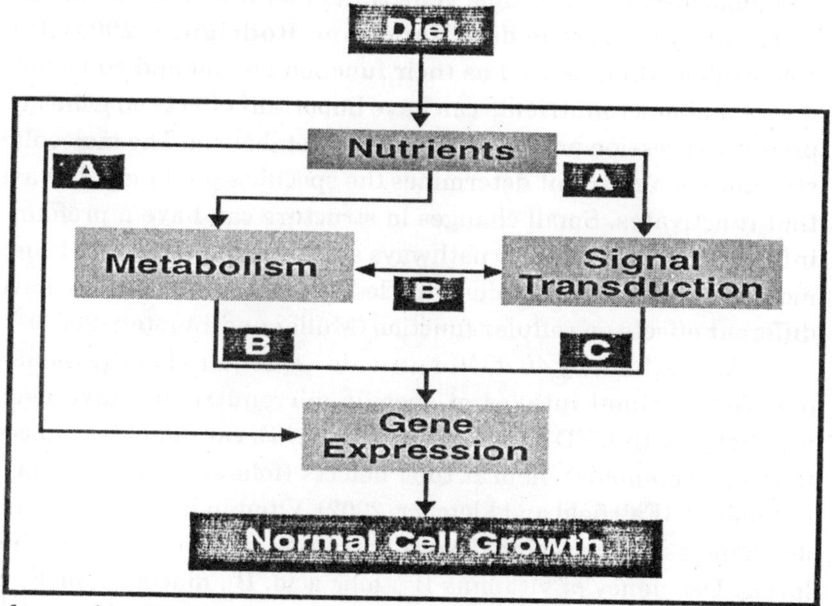

the next frontier in the post genomic era, Physiological Genomics 16:166-177 (2004)

Some dietary chemicals are ligands for nuclear receptors. Many, but not all genes involved in fatty acid metabolism are regulated by one of the three members of the peroxisome proliferator-activated receptor family ($PPAR_\alpha$, $PPAR_\beta$, $PPAR_\gamma$) (Auwerx, 1992). The surprising finding (at the time) was that the fatty acids, palmitic (16:0), oleic (18:1 n9), linoleic (18:2 n6), and arachidonic (20:4 n6) acid, and the eicosanoids, 15-deoxy-$\Delta^{12,14}$ prostaglandin J_2 and 8-(*S*) hydroxyeicosatraenoic acid, are ligands for PPARs (Kliewer et al., 2001). Metabolic conversion of dietary chemicals also serves as a control mechanism for gene expression. Dietary chemicals also can directly affect signal transduction pathways.Green tea contains the polyphenol, 11-epigallocatechin-

3-gallate (EGCG). EGCG inhibits tyrosine phosphorylation of Her-2/neu receptor and epidermal growth factor receptor, which, in turn, reduces signaling via the phosphatidylinositol 3-kinase (PI-3) Akt kinase NF-B pathway. Activation of the NF-B pathway is associated with some virulent forms of breast cancer. PKU (Phenylketonuria) and galactosemia are single gene traits and thus easy to identify and treat by changes in diet (**Kaput and Rodriguez, 2004**). It is now evident that, as well as their function as fuel and co-factors, micro- and macronutrients can have important effects on gene and protein expression and, accordingly, on metabolism. The molecular structure of a nutrient determines the specific signaling pathways that it activates. Small changes in structure can have a profound influence on which sensor pathways are activated. This fine-tuned molecular specificity explains why closely related nutrients can have different effects on cellular function (Müller and Kersten, 2003).

Approximately 40 micronutrients are required in the human diet. Sub optimal intakes of specific micronutrients have been associated with CVD (B vitamins, vitamin E, carotenoids), cancer (folate, carotenoids), neural tube defects (folate), and bone mass (vitamin D) (Fairfield and Fletcher, 2002). Vitamin B_6, B_{12}, and folate deficiencies are associated with increased serum homocysteine levels. Deficiency of vitamins B_{12}, folic acid, B_6, niacin, C, or E, or iron or zinc appears to mimic radiation in damaging DNA by causing single- and double-strand breaks, oxidative lesions, or both. Unbalanced intake of any of the three major macronutrients, such as, fat, carbohydrates, or protein, contributes to the initiation, development, progression, and/or severity of chronic diseases. Intake of saturated fatty acids (SFA) is correlated with increased levels of low-density lipoprotein (LDL) cholesterol, the principal target of intervention for coronary disease risk reduction (Krauss, 2001). In addition to CVDs, SFA may contribute to obesity and diabetes because these diseases are also characterized by dyslipidemias. Large numbers of human and laboratory animal experiments support the associations predicted from epidemiological studies. The hunt for a single macronutrient or micronutrient that will prevent chronic diseases is destined to fail. It is more likely that dietary imbalances, from micronutrient deficiencies to over consumption of macronutrients or dietary supplements, are the modifiers of metabolism and potentiators of chronic disease. Although the complexity of food and genotypic variations appears daunting, molecular and genetic technologies may provide the means for identifying causative genes (or their variants) and the nutrients that regulate them (Kaput and Rodriguez, 2004).

There has been a growing recognition that micronutrients and macronutrient can be potent dietary signals that influence the metabolic programming of cells and have an important role in the control of homeostasis. Nutrition researchers have increasingly started to recognize that genetic predisposition can be an important contributor to the main causes of mortality that are linked to diet, such as cardiovascular disease, diabetes type II and cancers. Furthermore, nutrigenomics aims to identify the genes that influence the risk of diet-related diseases on a genome-wide scale, and to understand the mechanisms that underlie these genetic predispositions (Müller and Kersten, 2003).

Nutrient sensors

Transcription factors are the main agents through which nutrients influence gene expression. The nuclear hormone receptor superfamily of transcription factors, with 48 members in the human genome, is the most important group of nutrient sensors. Numerous receptors in this superfamily bind nutrients and their metabolites. These include retinoic acid (Retinoic acid receptor (RAR) and retinoid X receptor (RXR)), fatty acids (Peroxisome proliferatoractivated receptors (PPARs) and liver X receptor (LXR)), vitamin D (vitamin D receptor VDR)), oxysterols (LXR), bile salts (Farnesoid X receptor (FXR), also known as bile salt receptor) or other hydrophobic food ingredients (constitutively active receptor (CAR) and pregnane X receptor (PXR)) (Müller and Kersten, 2003).

In metabolically active organs, such as the liver, intestine and adipose tissue, these transcription factors act as nutrient sensors by changing the level of DNA transcription of specific genes in response to nutrient changes (Francis, 2002). Nuclear hormone receptors have important roles in the regulation of numerous processes, including nutrient metabolism, embryonic development, cell proliferation and differentiation. So, it is easy to envision how nutrients, by activating these receptors, are able to influence a wide array of cellular functions (Müller and Kersten, 2003).

Transcription-factor pathways mediating nutrient–gene interactions

Nutrient	*Compound*	*Transcription factor*
Macronutrients		
Fats	Fatty acids	PPARs, SREBPs, LXR, HNF4, ChREBP
	Cholesterol	SREBPs, LXRs, FXR
Carbohydrates		
	Glucose	USFs, SREBPs, ChREBP
Proteins		
	Amino acids	C/EBPs
Micronutrients		
Vitamins		
	Vitamin A	RAR, RXR
	Vitamin D	VDR
	Vitamin E	PXR
Minerals		
	Calcium	Calcineurin/NF-ATs
	Iron	IRP1, IRP2
	Zinc	MTF1
Other food components		
	Flavonoids	ER, NF?B, AP1
	Xenobiotics	CAR, PXR

AP1, activating protein1; CAR, constitutively active receptor; C/EBP, CAAT/enhancer binding protein; ChREBP, carbohydrate responsive element binding protein; ER, oestrogen receptor; FXR, farnesoid X receptor; HNF, hepatocyte nuclear factor; IRP, iron regulatory protein; LXR, liver X receptor; MTF1, metalresponsive transcription factors; NF?B, nuclear factor ?B; NF-AT, nuclear factor of activated T cells; PPAR, peroxisome proliferator-activated receptor; PXR, pregnane X receptor; RAR, retinoic acid receptor; RXR, retinoid X receptor; SREBP, sterol-responsive-element binding protein; USF, upstream stimulatory factor; VDR, vitamin D receptor.

Source: *Michael Müller and Sander Kersten, Nutrigenomics: goals and strategies: Nature Reviews | Genetics Volume 4 | April 2003 | 315)*

Mental Illness and Diet

Nutrients play a critical role in mental health. They are the building blocks of the nervous system. Correct testing and understanding of deficiencies and overloads can pinpoint the causes of many severe mental symptoms, thus opening the door to hope and recovery. The medical and scientific communities agree on the tremendous influence of neurotransmitters on behavior disorders, ADHD, depression, and schizophrenia. Most persons with these disorders were born with a predisposition for these problems due to genetically aberrant levels of specific neurotransmitters. Our mental health is dependent upon having the proper amounts of these critical brain chemicals. The most common chemical imbalances we encounter include Over-methylation (too many added methyl groups) results in excessive levels of the neurotransmitters dopamine, norepinephrine and serotonin. Over-methylated persons have a physical tendency to be very depressed in folates (a form of folic acid), niacin and vitamin B-12, and biochemical treatment focuses on supplementation of these nutrients. Seasonal depressions are under-methylated, which is associated with low serotonin levels and Pyrrole Disorder, which results in a dramatic deficiency of zinc, vitamin B-6 and arachidonic acid (an omega-6 fatty acid). Certain pyrroles called kryptopyrroles (literally, "hidden pyrroles") bind with B-6, then zinc to deplete the body's supply. Common symptoms include explosive temper, mood swings, poor short-term memory and frequent infections (*Walsh, 2002*). Serotonin, a neurotransmitter, was found to be related to body temperature and the onset of sleep. Research also identified Serotonin as related to depression and later to a variety of mental health conditions such as anorexia and obsessive-compulsive disorder. High levels of Dopamine are found in Schizophrenia, drug intoxication, and other psychotic conditions, where the ability to distinguish the inner world from the real world is impaired (Walsh, undated). The brain is 20% fat (by dry weight) and these fatty substances fulfill very important functions. The myelin sheaths that surround our brain cells contain essential fatty acids that are directly involved in nerve receptor formation and nerve transmission. A 1998 Symposium at the National Institute of Mental Health presented strong evidence of the important roles for omega-3 oils (especially EPA and DHA[10]) and omega-6 oils (especially

AA and DGLA[11]) in "ADHD," depression and "schizophrenia." A recent Harvard study showed EPA and DHA supplements to be more effective than psychiatric medications in combating "bipolar depression."(Walsh, 2002). Although a multitude pharmaceutical agents are available for the treatment of mood disorders anxiety and insomnia, many patients have difficulty in tolerating side effects, do not respond adequately, or eventually lose their response (*Brown and Gerbarg, 2001*).

Diagnosis	*Neurotransmitter*	*Medication*
Stress-Produced Depression	Low Serotonin	Selective Serotonin Reuptake Inhibitor (SSRI)
Agitated/Anxious Depression	Low Serotonin Elevated Norepinephrine	SSRI and Antianxiety Medication or Serotonin Norepinephrine Reuptake Inhibitor (SNRI)
Major Depression with Psychosis (Severe depression with hallucinations/paranoia)	Elevated Dopamine Low Serotonin	Antipsychotic medication SSRI
Bipolar Disorder, Mania	Low GABA	Anticonvulsant or Lithium
Bipolar Disorder, Depressed	Low GABA Low Serotonin	Anticonvulsant or Lithium SSRI

Source: *Handout written by Joseph M. Carver, Ph.D., a Clinical Psychologist, Private practice in Southern Ohio. Revised: January 2002*

Diet has an effect on mood and cognitive function (Rogers, 2001). There is some evidence that deficiency or supplementation of nutrients can affect not only mood, but also behavioral patterns. A number of studies have shown that acute tryptophan depletion produces depressive symptoms and results in worsening of mood (Neumeister et al., 1998). Folic acid deficiency may also correlate with depression, and it has particular effects on mood, cognitive as well as social functioning (Reynolds, 2002). Recently, it has been reported that, low dietary folate is associated with elevated depressive symptoms (Tolmunen, 2003).

In general, a low-fat diet may have negative effects on mood. And altered dietary fat intake can lead to acute behavioral effects such as drowsiness, independent of energy consumption .A high intake of proteins also seems to increase alertness. Increased dietary serine and lysine may be linked to the pathogenesis of major depressive disorder. Apart from specific nutrients or vitamins, certain foods may have an effect on mental wellbeing. Warm milk, for instance, has been traditionally used as self-medication for insomnia. Individuals drinking regular coffee with caffeine have reported to have decreased total sleep time and sleep quality, and increased sleep latency. It has been reported that people with a high consumption of fish appear to have a lower prevalence of major depressive disorder. Recently, it has been also reported that increased fish intake in people without depressive symptoms had no substantial effect on mood (Hakkarainen, 2004). The balance of protein and carbohydrate consumed in a meal can influence brain serotonin (5-hydoxytryptamine) neurotransmission by altering the availability of tryptophan for uptake into the brain. Tryptophan is the precursor amino acid of serotonin and, paradoxically, high carbohydrate intake tends to increase brain uptake of tryptophan. Serotonin is involved in the modulation of various aspects of mood and behaviour, including depression, aggression, impulsivity, sleep and appetite (Rogers, 2001).

The brain is a chemical factory that produces serotonin, dopamine, norepinephrine and other brain chemicals 24 hours a day. The only raw materials for their syntheses are nutrients, namely, amino acids, vitamins, minerals, etc. If the brain receives improper amounts of these nutrient building blocks, we can expect serious problems with our neurotransmitters. For example, some depression patients have a genetic pyrrole disorder that renders them grossly depleted in vitamin B-6. A pyrrole is a basic chemical structure that is used in the formation of heme, which makes blood red. Pyrroles bind with B-6 and then with zinc, thus depleting these nutrients. These individuals cannot efficiently create serotonin (a neurotransmitter) since B-6 is an important factor in the last step of its synthesis (*Walsh, 2002*). Serotonin levels can be controlled through the diet. A diet deficient in omega-3 fatty acids may lower brain levels of serotonin and cause depression. Complex carbohydrates raise the level of tryptophan in the brain resulting in a calming effect. Vitamin C is also required for the conversion of tryptophan into serotonin (University of Bristol).

Serotonin levels can be controlled through the diet. A diet deficient in omega-3 fatty acids may lower brain levels of serotonin and cause depression. Complex carbohydrates raise the level of tryptophan in the brain resulting in a calming effect. Vitamin C is also required for the conversion of tryptophan into serotonin

Many of these persons appear to benefit from Prozac, Paxil, Zoloft or other serotonin-enhancing medications. However, as with all mind-altering drugs, side effects occur and the true cause of the mental difficulties remains uncorrected. Similar and more healthful benefits can be achieved by simply giving these patients sufficient amounts of B-6 along with supporting nutrients. Most neurotransmitter problems appear to be genetic in nature and involve abnormal absorption, metabolism or storage of key nutrients. As neuroscience advances, biochemical treatments to correct brain chemistry become well defined. Nutrient therapy can be very potent and does not involve side effects, since no molecules foreign to the body are needed. This therapeutic approach may eventually eliminate the need for most psychiatric medications (Walsh, 2002).

Conclusion

Mental illness is amongst the most common health problems. One in six adults will experience some form of mental ill health at some point in their life. Mental illnesses are characterized by alterations in thinking; mood or behavior (or some combination thereof) associated with significant distress and impaired functioning over an extended period of time. These disorders can affect persons of any age, race, sex, and religion or income. There are different types of mental disorders like depression, anxiety, schizophrenia etc, which are caused by the chemical imbalance in the brain. Mental disorders have no single cause but several factors such as genetical, biochemical, environmental or nutritional factors. The mental disorders are predominant in women, as it has shown direct relationship with the female hormones such as estrogen. Many hormonal factors may contribute to the increased rate of depression in women-particularly such factors as menstrual cycle changes, pregnancy, miscarriage, postpartum period, pre-menopause, and menopause. Mental disorders can be treated thereby drugs, by proper care and proper diet. The quality of food we take has a profound effect on mental function. There are several studies have been conducted about the role of diet in the prevention of mental disorders. Most of the studies shown that nutrients in the diet profoundly alter the phenotypic expression of given genotype. Previous research results indicate that the nutrition may have a role in expression of certain gene, there by regulating mental disorders along with few other chronic diseases. Nutritional treatment is considered as an alternative treatment or used along with the drug treatment. Fatty acids are crucial for the mental function, proper growth and development. Body cannot produce the two fatty acid families, omega 3 fatty acids and omega 6 fatty acids on its own and therefore must receive through the diet and supplementation. The association between vitamins and depression has been explained by their ability to decrease the serum total homocystein levels and by their connection with monoamine metabolism in the central nervous system Inadequate energy intake leads to the mental health problems such as concentration, decision, irritability, depression and social withdrawal. EPA and DHA found to play a key role in brain gene expression. EPA is directly related to the mental health and depression. Present research interest is to study the interaction between nutrients and the genes of risk of mental illness and other chronic diseases. The food and gene interaction may be direct or indirect. Many hormones act as a nutritional signals and their receptors play a key role in mediating effects of nutrition on numerous gene involved in the mental disorders. The term Nutritional genomics has been used to describe work at the interface of plant biochemistry, genomics, and human nutrition aimed at understanding and manipulating nutrient reactions and interactions at the molecular or genomic level. Dietary chemicals have been shown to alter gene expression in a number of ways. For example, they may act as ligands for transcription factor receptors, may be metabolized by primary or secondary metabolic pathways thereby altering concentrations of substrates or intermediates or serve as signaling molecules. There is a need for molecular data on the interaction between nutrition and genome.

Nutrient therapy can be very potent and does not involve side effects, since no molecules foreign to the body are needed. This therapeutic approach may eventually eliminate the need for most psychiatric medications.

References

Auwerx, J. (1992). Regulation of gene expression by fatty acids and fibric acid derivatives: an integrative role for peroxisome proliferator activated receptors. The Belgian Endocrine Society Lecture 1992. *Horm Res* 38: 269–277, 1992.

Barker, D.J., Gluckman, P.D., Godfrey, K.M., Harding, J.E., Owens, J.A., and Robinson, J.S. (1993). Fetal nutrition and cardiovascular disease in adult life. Lancet 341: 938-941.

Brown, Richard P. MD; Gerbarg, Patricia L. MD. (2001, March). Herbs and Nutrients in the Treatment of Depression, Anxiety, Insomnia, Migraine, and Obesity. Journal of Psychiatric Practice. 7(2): 75-91, March 2001.

Potera, C. (2004, May). Environmental Health Perspectives Volume 112, Number 7, May 2004).

Caspi A, Sugden K, Moffitt T, et al. Influence of Life Stress on Depression: Moderation by a Polymorphism in the 5-HTT Gene. *Science.*2003; 301:386-389.

Dauncey M.J.*; White P.; Burton K.A.; Katsumata M: Nutrition–hormone receptor–gene interactions: implications for development and disease , Proceedings of the Nutrition Society, February 2001, vol. 60, no. 1, pp. 63-72(10).

Egan MF, Goldberg TE, Kolachana BS, et al. Effect of COMT Val108/158 Met genotype on frontal lobe function and risk for schizophrenia. Proceedings of the National Academy of Sciences of the United States of America. 2001; 98:6917-6922.

Fairfield KM and Fletcher RH. Vitamins for chronic disease prevention in adults: scientific review. *JAMA* 287: 3116–3126, 2002.

Fergus Clydesdale-IFT expert report, Food Technology, VOL.58, NO.12. December 2004.

Francis, G. A., Fayard, E., Picard, F. & Auwerx, J. Nuclear receptors and the Control of metabolism. *Annu. Rev.Physiol.* 65, 261–311 (2002).

Handout written by Joseph M. Carver, Ph.D., a Clinical Psychologist. Private practice in Southern Ohio. Revised: January 2002, Dr. Joe Carver's Website.

Health Canada. A Report on Mental Illnesses in Canada. Ottawa, Canada 2002. http://www.cmha.ca/english/research/r_mic/index.html).

IFT expert report: Functional foods:Oppertunities and challenges.

IFT Export report: The intersection of food and genes.

Ordovas, J.M.Gene –diet interaction and plasma lipid responses to dietary interventions, JM USDA Human Nutrition Research Center on aging, Tufts University, Boston, MA 02111,USA. Biochemical society Transactions (2002) Volume 30, Part 2.

Jim Kaput and Raymond L. Rodriguez, Nutritional genomics: the next frontier in the post genomic era, *Physiological Genomics* 16:166-177 (2004).

John Ruskin, Forum: Environmental health perspective, Volume 112, Number 7, May 2004.

Kessler RC, Ahangang Z. The prevalence of mental illness. Horwitz AV, Sheid TL, ed., A Handbook for the Study of Mental Health - Social Context, Theories and Systems, (Ch. 3). Cambridge University Press, 1999.

Kliewer SA, Xu HE, Lambert MH, and Willson TM. Peroxisome proliferator-activated receptors: from genes to physiology. *Recent Prog Horm Res* 56: 239–263, 2001.

Kohen, Dora, Mental Health Needs of Women with Learning Disabilities, Tizard Learning Disability Review, Oct 2004.

Krauss RM. Dietary and genetic effects on LDL heterogeneity. *World Rev Nutr Diet* 89: 12–22, 2001.

Medical Science News, Reproductive hormones have effects on all of these stages of brain growth and development Published: Tuesday, 2-Nov-2004.http://www.news-medical.net/?id=6031

Meghan M. McKeough, PPT on mental illness: An Understanding of Depression, Mania and Schizophrenia, Linfield college School of Nursing.http://www.nationalserviceresources.org/filemanager/download/06_MultiState_Conf/B6m-illness1.ppt

Mental health: A report from Surgeon General, Chapter 4. http://www.surgeongeneral.gov/library/mentalhealth/toc.html

Michael Müller and Sander Kersten, Nutrigenomics: goals and strategies: NATURE REVIEWS | GENETICS VOLUME 4 | APRIL 2003 | 315).

Neumeister A, Praschak-Rieder N, Hesselmann B, Vitouch O, Rauh M, Barocka A, Kasper S: Effects of tryptophan depletion in fully remitted patients with seasonal affective disorder during summer.*Psychol Med* 1998, 28:257-264.

Patricia Griffin Kellicker, BSN: Genetics and Mental Illness: What's the Connection?, Swedish Medical Centre, http://www.swedish.org/16927.cfm

Reeta Hakkarainen[1], Timo Partonen[1], Jari Haukka[1], Jarmo Virtamo[2], Demetrius Albanes[3] and Jouko Lönnqvist[1] Food and nutrient intake in relation to mental wellbeing, *Nutrition Journal* 2004, 3:1, doi: 10.1186/1475-2891-3-14.

Reynolds EH: Folic acid, ageing, depression, and dementia. *British Medical Journal* 2002, 324:1512-1515.

Rogers PJ: A healthy body, a healthy mind: long-term impact of diet on mood and cognitive function, *Proc. Nutr. Soc.* 2001, 60:135-143.

Rotondo A, Mazzanti C, DellOsso L, et al. Catechol O-Methyltransferase, Serotonin Transporter, and Tryptophan Hydroxylase Gene Polymorphisms in Bipolar Disorder Patients With and Without Comorbid Panic Disorder. *American Journal of Pyschiatry.* 2002; 159:23-29.

Schwartz S. Biological approaches to psychological disorders. Horwitz AV, Sheid TL, ed., A Handbook for the Study of Mental Health - Social Context, Theories and Systems, (Ch. 4). Cambridge University Press, 1999.

Simopoulos AP, Ordovas JM (eds): Nutrigenetics and Nutrigenomics. World Rev Nutr Diet. Basel, Karger, 2004, vol 93, pp 1–28.

The Queensland transcultural mental health center multiliqual information series.http://www.health.qld.gov.au/pahospital/docs/mental_illness/mi-eng.pdf.

Tolmunen T, Voutilainen S, Hintikka J, Rissanen T, Tanskanen A, Viinamaki H, Kaplan GA, Salonen JT: Dietary folate and depressive symptoms are associated in middle-aged Finnish middle aged men. *J Nutr* 2003, 133:3233-3236.

Tsuang MT, Gilbertson MW, Faraone SV (1991) The genetics of schizophrenia: current knowledge and future directions. Schizophr Res 4:157–171.

University of Bristol, http://www.chm.bris.ac.uk /motm/serotonin/depression.htm

William Walsh, Ph.D. Nutrients Help Alleviate Mental Symptoms, Well Being Journal Vol. 11, No. 4 ~ July/August 2002

William Walsh, Ph.D. The Critical Role of Nutrients in Severe Mental Symptoms, Senior Scientist, Health Research Institute and Pfeiffer Treatment Center, 1804 Centre Point Circle, Suite 102,Naperville, IL 60563, www.hriptc.org

Society for Neurosciences 10/24/2004 http://www.sfn.org/index.cfm?pagename=news_102404d

Gender and Sex Hormones affect the Brain's Pain Response and more.

12

Effect of Iron Folic Acid Supplementation on the Physical and Mental Performance of Elderly Anemic Women

Pallavi Mehta, Komal Chauhan, Swati Khurana

Introduction

A demographic revolution is underway throughout the world. Today, worldwide there are around 600 million persons aged 60 years and above. Their numbers will double by 2025 and is likely to reach the two billion mark by 2025 and the vast majority of these people are in the developing world. With advancing age there is a reduced vitality and increased vulnerability to common diseases, both acute and chronic. At all ages over 65 years, there are more women than men. Despite their lower mortality rates, older women have greater morbidity, including more limitations in self-care. In India, it is common for women at any age to neglect their health, until the health problem begins to interfere in their daily chores. Since women on an average live longer than men, the health problems of older adults, in reality, are often those of older women. Nutritional problems are especially prevalent in the elderly women, requiring appropriate counseling for long-term management.

Anemia is common in the elderly and its prevalence increases with age (Lafuente et al., 2001). Anemia is defined as hemoglobin concentration below the normative cut off values that are based on age sex, physiological state and altitude.

Although the WHO has not defined the cut-off values of hemoglobin levels for elderly, most of the studies recommend use of reference values for hemoglobin concentration as suggested by WHO for adults. Prevalence of anemia in older individuals is about 50 per cent in developing countries and 12 per cent in developed countries (WHO 2000).

Iron deficiency anemia is the second most common cause of anemia in the elderly population. It usually results from chronic gastrointestinal blood loss caused by the non-steroidal anti-inflammatory drug induced gastritis, ulcer, colon cancer, diverticula or angiodysplasia. Older persons may become deficient in iron because of inadequate or poor absorption of iron (Smith 2000).

Age related disability and loss in physical function are growing public health priorities. Anemia is a risk factor for subsequent decline in physical and cognitive functions in older persons (Penninx et al., 1998), which compromises the independence and quality of life of the older people. Hence supplementation with medicinal iron is a short-term strategy to combat iron deficiency anemia. However, further research is required to study the effect of iron folic acid (IFA) supplementation on physical and cognitive performance of the elderly. This paper is based on a study of the effect of IFA supplementation on the hemoglobin levels, cognitive and physical performance of elderly women.

Methods and Materials

One hundred and eighty elderly women aged 60 years and above were selected from the free-living population of Vadodara city. As per their living arrangements they were distributed equally into three different groups: women living alone, women living with spouse and women living with their family.

The baseline data were collected using a semi-structured questionnaire. This included information on their socioeconomic and demographic characteristics (age, education, religion, income, living arrangements and marital status). Their nutritional status was assessed using anthropometric measurements like height, weight, body mass index (BMI) and mid upper arm circumference

(MUAC). Information on their dietary intake was obtained by 24-hour dietary recall method. Information on disease and morbidity was collected using a checklist and women were screened for iron deficiency anemia using the cynmethemoglobin method to estimate their hemoglobin levels.

Out of 180 subjects, 45 anemic women were randomly selected for the intervention, which comprised IFA supplementation for a period of 6 weeks. Pre and post data were collected on hemoglobin levels, cognitive function tests and physical performance tests administered to these women. Two aspects of mental functioning were assessed namely, attention and concentration test and memory tests. Physical performance was tested by measures of standing balance, walking speed and ability to rise from a chair. For tests of standing balance, the subjects were asked to maintain their feet in the side-by-side, semi-tandem (heel of one foot beside the toe of the other feet) and tandem (heel of one foot directly in front of the other foot) positions for 10 seconds each. An 8-feet walk (2.4m walk) at the subject's normal pace was timed and time of the faster of two time walks was used for scoring. Regarding rise from a chair, subjects were asked to fold their arms across their chest and to stand up from a sitting position once. If they successfully rose from the chair, they were asked to stand up and sit down five times as quickly as possible. Quartiles for the length of time required for this measure were used for assigning scores. The data obtained were subjected to appropriate statistical analysis.

Results and Discussion

The mean age of the anemic elderly women was 70 years, majority of them were Hindus and 46 per cent of the subjects had completed primary education only. About 55 per cent of the elderly women were married, 37 per cent were widowed and 8 per cent were single.

The data on the anthropometric measurements (table 1) of the subjects showed that all the subjects fell under the normal category and not much difference was found between the groups by their living arrangement.

Table 1: Mean anthropometric measurements of elderly women by living arrangement (Mean ± SD)

Indices	*Living arrangement*		
	living alone N=60	*living with spouse N=60*	*living with family N=60*
Height (m)	1.52±0.36	1.51±0.13	1.52±0.75
Weight(kg)	56.03±1.1	57.38±3.56	57.35±3.69
BMI (KgM)	24.00±4.32	25.88±11.22	24.40±5.38
MUAC (cm)	26.36±5.92	28.46±10.8	26.40±6.08

When nutrient intake was assessed, a significant difference ($P \leq 0.001$) was found in the energy and protein intake between the groups (table 2). The consumption of energy was less than the recommended daily allowance (RDA suggested by Natarajan (1991) in women living alone and the consumption of protein was less than the RDA in all three groups of women. There were little differences, albeit not significant, found in other nutrient intakes between the groups. The diet of all women, regardless of their living arrangement was found deficient in iron, β-carotene and vitamin C, whereas the intake of fat and calcium was more than the RDA.

Table 2: Nutrient Intake of the elderly women with different living arrangements (mean± SD)

Nutrients	*Living alone N=60*	*Living with spouse N=60*	*Living with family N=60*	*RDA*	*F-test*
Energy (kcal)	1250±356	1467±402	1494±383	1350	7.29*
Protein (gm)	34.9±10.7	39.5±9.09	41.98±9.57	50	7.41*
Fat (gm)	71.1±23	45.1±15.7	50.6±18.26	20	0.79
Calcium (mg)	540.8±233	607.5±190	593.8±194	400	1.70
Iron (mg)	14.3±9.4	17.5±9.3	15.0±7.57	28	2.20
T-Carotene (?g)	1159±111	1010±85.4	1166±94.1	2400	0.82
Vit- C (mg)	23.45±2.4	29.28±2.3	28.5±3.5	40	1.08

* Significant at $P \leq 0.001$.

The mean hemoglobin levels were 10.75gm/dl in women who were living alone, 11.08gm/dl in women who were living with their spouse and 11.44gm/dl in women living with their family. Overall, 80 percent of the women had some degree of anemia, from mild to severe. Nearly two-thirds were found to be mildly anemic, and among the rest, 10 and 4 per cent had moderate (Hb 7.1 – 9.9 gm/dl) and severe anemia respectively (Hb ≤ 7 gm/dl) (as shown in table 3). This may be attributed to the poor iron stores in women and their poor dietary intake after attaining menopause.

Table 3: Percent prevalence of anemia in elderly women

Degree of anemia	*Hemoglobin (gm / dl) Prevalence*	*Percent N=180*
Severe	≤ 7	3.8 (7)
Moderate	7.1 – 9.9	10.55 (19)
Mild	10 – 11.9	65 (117)
Normal	≥ 12	20.5 (37)

Figure in the parenthesis denote numbers.

The disease profile of the subjects revealed that minor health problems were reported more by women living alone (group-1) as compared to those living with their spouse (group-2) or their family (group-3) (table 4). The frequency of complaints like constipation (35 per cent), headache (23 per cent) and general weakness (32 per cent) were reported more by elderly women living alone. The frequency of reported complaints such as dental problems and dryness of skin was higher among women living with their spouse than among women living alone or with their family.

Among the major health problems reported by all three groups of women were: rheumatoid arthritis (most frequently reported by all groups – by 35 per cent women living alone, by 40 per cent women living with their spouse, and by 28 per cent women living with their family), followed by disability (reported by 12 per cent women living alone, 10 per cent women living with spouse and 5 percent women living with their family), hypertension (reported by

Table 4: Minor health problems of elderly women in different living arrangements

Problem	*Group 1*		*Group 2*		*Group 3*	
	Non-frequent	*Frequent*	*Non-frequent*	*Frequent*	*Non-frequent*	*Frequent*
Dental problems	39(65)	21(35)	35(58.3)	25(41.6)	41(68.3)	19(31.6)
Distention	47 (78.3)	13(21.6)	54(90)	06(10)	47(78.3)	13(21.6)
Constipation	39(65)	21(35)	47(78.3)	13(21.6)	47(78.3)	13(21.6)
Headache	46(76.6)	14(23.3)	50(83.3)	10(16.6)	51(85)	09(15)
Body ache	43(71.6)	17(28.3)	44(73.3)	16(26.6)	42(70)	18(30)
Sleep disturbance	50(83.3)	10(16.6)	49(81.6)	11(18.3)	43(71.6)	17(28.3)
Slow reflexes	49(81.6)	11(18.3)	44(73.3)	16(26.6)	55(91.6)	05(8.3)
General weakness	41(68.3)	19(31.6)	43(73.3)	17(28.3)	48(80)	12(20)
Dryness in mouth	44(73.3)	16(26.6)	47(78.3)	13(21.6)	51(85)	09(15)
Dryness in skin	39(65)	21(35)	37(61.6)	23(38.3)	39(65)	21(35)

Note: Figures in the parenthesis denote percentages.

33 per cent women living alone, 20 per cent women living with their spouse, and 28 per cent women living with their family) and diabetes mellitus (reported by 15 per cent women living alone, 20 per cent women living with their spouse, and 8 per cent women living with their family). Other major problems like asthma and heart disease were reported by less than 15 percent of the women from in all three groups.

From the total subjects, 45 anemic elderly women were selected and supplementation of IFA was given to them for a period of six weeks. Since all the subjects were not ready to perform physical and mental tests, only 30 subjects who were willing took the test before and after intervention. To compare their performance, their age and Hb matched counterparts were selected from the total subjects as control group. Women in the control group were not given any supplementation.

Data on the hemoglobin levels of the 45 women who were provided IFA supplementation for a period of six weeks are presented in table 5. As can be seen from the table, there has been a statistically significant ($P \leq 0.05$) improvement in the hemoglobin levels due to IFA supplementation. The hemoglobin levels of the subjects had increased by 0.9gm%, from 9.64gm% before the intervention to 10.56gm% after intervention.

Table 5: Mean hemoglobin levels of anemic women before and after intervention (Mean ± SE)

	Before intervention N=45	*After intervention N=45*	*Paired t-test*
Hemoglobin levels (gm/dl)	9.64 ± 1.24	10.56± 1.09	11.69*

* Significant at $P \leq 0.5$

Similarly, significant improvement was found in mental and physical performance tests of the elderly women after supplementation of IFA. As can be seen from table 6, the mean scores before intervention for the attention and concentration test of the control group was 5.10 and 4.6 for memory test as compared

Table 6: Mental function test scores of elderly anemic women, before and after intervention

Group	*N*	*Performance in Mental Function Tests* *Mean ± SE*					
		Attention and Concentration Test			*Memory Test*		
		Pre	Post	Paired 't'	Pre	Post	Paired 't'
Experimental	30	5.80±3.03	6.70 ± 2.83	3.80*	4.53±1.99	5.23±2.54	2.00
Control	30	5.10±1.62	5.466 ≤ ± 2.03	2.26	4.60±1.33	4.60±1.58	.00

Note: Significant at $P \leq 0.05$

Figure 1: Change in Physical Function Test Score before and after IFA Supplementation in elderly women

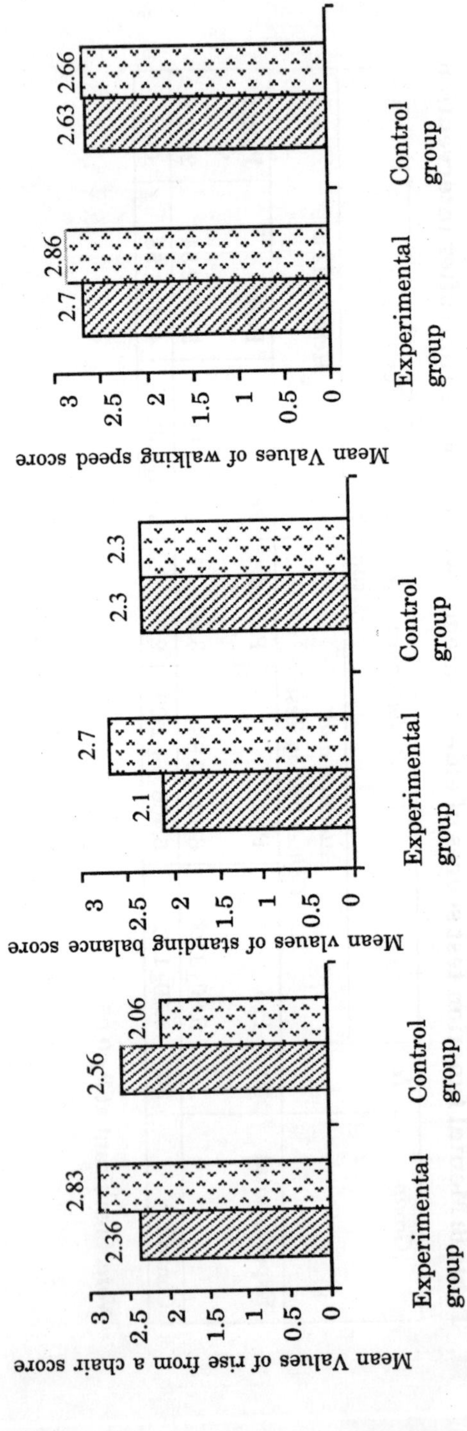

to 5.8 and 4.53 of the experimental group respectively. There was a rise in the mean scores after intervention but it was not significant for the control group whereas highly significant differences were found for the experimental group.

The physical performance test score for subjects belonging to experimental group were highly significant ($P \leq 0.001$) compared to control group (see Figure 1).

The mean increase in score level between the pre and post intervention data of experimental group was 0.53 for rise from a chair, 0.6 for standing balance, 0.16 for walking speed. The results thus reveal that anemia is associated with physical performance of the subjects. A similar finding has been reported by a cohort study of 1146 elderly subjects, age 71 years, which included assessment of standing balance, a timed 2.4m walk and timed test for five-chair rises combined into 0 to 12 summary scales. The study reported a decline of 2.3 in the mean score of subjects with anemia compared to subjects without anemia (Penninx et al., 2003).

Conclusion

In the present study, the mean age of the elderly women subjects was 70 years. The major important nutrients which were found to be deficient in the diets of these elderly women were energy, especially in the diet of women living alone, while protein, iron, β-carotene and vitamin C were found to be deficient in the diets of all women. Around 80 per cent of women were found anemic, of whom 65 per cent were suffering from mild degree of anemia, followed by 10 per cent who had moderate anemia and 8 per cent who had severe anemia. Significant differences in the intake were noted between the groups. Minor illnesses like headache, constipation and general weakness were reported more frequently. With respect to major health problems rheumatoid arthritis was the major problem among all the elderly women.

The intervention of IFA supplementation for a period of six weeks showed improvement in the hemoglobin levels of the elderly women; a rise of 0.9gm/dl was noted. Significant improvement was also observed in the physical and mental performance of the subjects.

From the findings of the present study one may conclude that supplementation of IFA for a period of six weeks to elderly anemic

women is an effective method for improving the hemoglobin levels which in turn reflects on their physical performance and mental function.

Acknowledgment

Authors would like to thank the staff and the Honorary Director of the Women's Studies Research Centre, M. S. University of Baroda, for their help and for providing partial funding for the study.

References

Lafuente, A., Fernandez-Burriel Tercero, B.J., Suarez Almenara, M., Betancort, J.L., Mastrangelo, C. C., and Guerra Hernandez, L. (2001). Anemia and functional incapacity at admission to a geriatric home. *An Med Interna, 18*(1), 9-12.

Bagchi, K., and Puri, S. (Eds.). (1999). *Diet and ageing: Exploring some facets.* New Delhi: Society for Gerontological Research and Helpage India.

Penninx, B.W., Guralnik, J.M., Onder, G., Ferrucci, L., Wallace, R.B., Pahor, M. (2003). Anemia and decline in physical performance among older persons. *Am J Med, 115*(2), 104-110.

Smith, D. L. (2000). Anemia in elderly. *Am Fam Physician, 62*, 1565-1572.

13

Physical and Mental Status of Geriatric Women of a District of Gujarat

Niraj Pandit, S. K. Choudhary, Jashmin Modi, Kalpesh Goswami

Introduction

Geriatric population is defined as the population aged 60 years and above (Elango, 1998).The phenomenon of population ageing (defined as increase in the median age of the population) (Bhende and Kanitkar, 1997), is already a major social and health problem in the developed countries. According to the 2001 census, the geriatric population constituted 7.45 per cent of the total Indian population and 6.9 per cent of the population of Gujarat (Office of the Registrar General of India, 2001a). The decadal rates of growth of the elderly population in India indicate that the elderly population has exploded in the 80 plus age range; this group has experienced a growth rate of above 50 percent in 1981-91 compared to 32 percent in 1971-81 (Gupta and Sankar, 2003). According to UN projections for 2050 the elderly would constitute 1,970 million of the world's population. Of these, 1,239 (63 per cent) would be in Asia (Dhar Chakraborti, 2005).

A long life does not necessarily mean a healthy life. People in the geriatric group have health problems that are unique from those of adults and children. Moreover, medical problems in the geriatric group show gender difference. Ageing is a time of multiple illness and general disability. Along with changes in biological constitution, life style factors are also important in the development of disorders and diseases in old age. Old age diseases are not always curable, implying a strain on financial as well as physical health infrastructure and resources, both at the macro and the micro levels.

Among the many factors, which affect the health of the elderly, is literacy. As per Census 1991, over all literacy among the elderly was 27.2 per cent; only 12.7 per cent of females were literate. (Office of the Registrar General of India, 2001b). Majority of the elderly in both rural (50.78 per cent) and urban (57.35 per cent) areas are totally dependent on others for economic support. About 15.20 per cent of the elderly in rural areas and 13.71 per cent of the elderly in the urban areas are partially dependent on others (Gore, 1992). Women constitute a significant majority of the older population and the sex ratio, with increase in age, rises in favor of women (Dhar Chakraborti, 2005).

Analysis of the National Sample Survey data for 1986-87 reveals that about 45 per cent of the rural elderly are chronically ill, among whom 45.01 per cent are men and 45.85 per cent are women. In the urban areas, 44.82 per cent of the elderly (45.49 per cent women and 44.34 per cent men) are chronically ill. Cough and problem of joints are the most common health problems. High blood pressure, heart disease and urinary problems are more common among the elderly in the urban areas (Kohli, 1996).

Ageing is not without mental problems. The psychological problems of elderly have roots in their personal, family, economic and social life. As life expectancy of women is greater than that of men at every age, an elderly woman is more likely than an elderly man to be living without a spouse and living alone. For providing care to an elderly woman it is important to establish how well she is functioning physically and cognitively and in what activities she may need assistance. Older women, are more likely to be depressed than older men, regardless of race, ethnic background, or economic status. The risk of suicide is however lower among older women than among older men. Late-life depression is treatable (Messinger-Rapport and Thacker, 2001), provided that it is diagnosed early.

The present study was undertaken with the aim to understand the physical and mental health problems of women living in urban and rural areas of Anand district, Gujarat.

Materials and Method

The present study was conducted in rural and urban field areas of the Department of Community Medicine, Pramukh Swami Medical College, Karamsad. It was a cross sectional, community based study. The geriatric age group was defined as 60 years and above. From each urban area and rural area 25 women in the geriatric age group were randomly selected. The house to house approach was used for data collection. A pre-tested proforma was used for recording personal details and socio-demographic information like, age, marital status, education, occupation past and current, income and type of family. The proforma also sought information regarding physical and mental health. In the section on physical health, information was elicited on chronic illness, visual impairment, hearing problems, sleep disturbance, and addiction. In the section on mental health the Yesavage Geriatric Depression scale was used (Stanford University Web Site). As per this scale, a score of 55 > 5 points is suggestive of mild depression and should warrant a follow-up interview, and scores > 10 are almost always depression. For the present study, the modified Prasad classification was used for the social classification of the study population (Prasad, 1961; Kumar, 1993). The data thus collected were analyzed and appropriate statistical tests were applied. The limitation of study was its sample size.

Results and Discussion

A significant percentage of the study population (38 per cent) was in the age group of 60-64 years. Almost 88 per cent of them were 'youngest old', that is 60-75 years of age. The mean age of rural women was 65.3 years and that of urban women was 67.5 years. Urban women seemed to live longer than rural women. The reason behind this may be the availability of good health care facilities in urban areas.

It was also observed that the level of education was higher among urban elderly women than among rural elderly women.

Table 1: Percentage distribution of the study population by age and level of education

Age	*Rural*				*Urban*				*Total (per cent)*
	Illiterate	*Primary*	*Secondary*	*Graduate*	*Illiterate*	*Primary*	*Secondary*	*Graduate*	
60-64	**7**	**2**	**1**	**0**	**0**	**5**	**4**	**0**	**19 (38)**
65-69	**2**	**4**	**0**	**0**	**0**	**3**	**4**	**3**	**16 (32)**
70-74	**3**	**4**	**0**	**0**	**0**	**1**	**0**	**1**	**9 (18)**
75-79	**1**	**0**	**0**	**0**	**0**	**0**	**2**	**0**	**3 (6)**
80+	**0**	**1**	**0**	**0**	**0**	**0**	**2**	**0**	**3 (6)**
Total	**13 (52)**	**11(44)**	**1 (4)**	**0 (0)**	**0 (0)**	**9 (36)**	**12 48)**	**4 (16)**	**50 (100)**

Fifty–two per cent of rural elderly women were illiterate whereas all urban elderly women were literate. The difference is statistically significant.

The modified Prasad classification was used for classification of the social status of the study population.[1] According to this classification, 44 per cent of the study population was from socio-economic class – II (table 2). Only 8 per cent of the urban study population belonged to socio-economic class IV and V, whereas 28 per cent of the rural elderly were from the same class.

Table 2: Percentage distribution of elderly women by socio–economic status

Socio-economic class	*Rural*	*Urban*	*Total (per cent)*
I	1	1	2 (4)
II	7	15	22 (44)
III	10	7	17 (34)
IV	6	2	8 (16)
V	1	0	1 (2)
Total	25	25	50 (100)

All rural women had been housewives in their past life and were presently also dependent on their children, whereas almost 52 per cent of the urban women had been working in the past. These findings support the fact that urban women have higher level of education and standard of living compared with rural women.

Over all 30 women (60 per cent) had one or the other type of chronic morbidity of over 1 month (table 3). A high percentage of self-reported morbidity, especially among females has been reported also by Yadava and colleagues (1997) in their study in rural Uttar Pradesh, in which 37 per cent of men and 70 per cent of women rated their health condition as "bad." Gurav (2002) has also reported same i.e., higher morbidity among females than males among the urban elderly.

In the present study, 33 per cent of elderly women had hypertension and diabetes mellitus and all were from urban area. Only one elderly rural woman had diabetes mellitus. Eight elderly

Table 3: Distribution of chronic morbidity and disability among elderly women by place of residence

Chronic morbidity and disability	*Rural*	*Urban*	*Total (per cent)*
Hypertension and diabetes mellitus	0	10	10 (33.4)
Hypertension	2	6	8 (26.6)
Diabetes mellitus	1	0	1 (3.3)
Osteoarthritis	3	0	3 (10)
Osteoarthritis and hypertension	2	0	2 (6.6)
Chronic obstructive pulmonary disease and breathlessness	1	2	3 (10)
Hypertension and breathlessness	0	1	1 (3.3.)
Breathlessness	2	0	2 (6.6)
Total	11	19	30

women had hypertension alone, 6 of them were from urban area. Gurav (2002) reported the almost 16 per cent of urban morbid elderly have hypertension. Five rural elderly had osteoarthritis and three had breathlessness. Yadava (1997) reported the most common morbidity among rural elderly as chest problems including asthma, tuberculosis, and bronchitis.

Only 8 per cent of rural women in the present study had sleep disturbance, whereas as high as 75 per cent of urban women had sleep disturbance. The findings from the present study indicate that rural women had morbidity as consequences of respiratory diseases and physical strain, whereas urban elderly women had diseases associated with modern life style. Disabilities like visual defects and hearing defects were reported among 78 per cent of the study population (table 4). Fifty–two per cent had hearing defects. Visual defects were higher among the rural elderly women (table 4).

Table 4: Distribution of visual and hearing disabilities among elderly women by residence

Disability	*Rural*	*Urban*	*Total (per cent)*
Vision defects	11	2	13 (26)
Hearing defects	5	21	26 (52)
Total	16	23	39 (78)

To assess the mental state of elderly women, Yesavage Geriatric Depression Scale was used. Sixteen per cent of the study population (all of them rural women) was found to be under severe depression on the Yesavage Geriatric Depression Scale, while 48 per cent had mild depression 36 per cent of study population was normal on the scale, and majority of them were from urban area (table 5). This difference in the level of depression among urban-rural population is statistically highly significant ($X^2 = 16.67$ $p<0.0001$ df= 2).

Table 5: Distribution of level of depression among elderly women by place of residence

Residence	*Level of depression*			*Total (per cent)*
	Normal	*Mild*	*Severe*	
Rural	3	14	8	25
Urban	15	10	0	25
Total	18 (36)	24 (48)	8 (16)	50 (100)

Note: Level of depression estimated on Yesavage Geriatric Depression Scale.

A similar finding has been reported in a study by Da Silva Pereira and colleagues (2002) conducted in Goa. The study reported nearly 44 per cent of geriatric population attending OPD as having psychiatric disorders. Depression alone contributed to 58 per cent of all the mood disorders and it was found to occur more in females. Also, higher level of depression was observed among rural elderly women compared to urban women.

Education seemed to have a positive effect on depression (table 6). All 14 per cent of severely depressed elderly women were illiterate, whereas all normal elderly women were educated. This difference is statistically highly significant ($X^2 = 24.37$ $p<0.0001$ df=6). Thus higher the level of education, lesser the chances of falling into depression.

Table 6: Association between level of education and level of depression in the study population

Level of education	*Level of Depression*			*Total*
	Normal	*Mild depression*	*Severe depression*	
Illiterate	0	6	7	13
Primary	9	10	1	20
Secondary	8	5	0	13
Graduate and above	1	3	0	4
Total (per cent)	18 (36)	24 (48)	8 (16)	50 (100)

The association between economic status and level of depression was observed, but it was not found significant, perhaps due to the small sample size.

The present study revealed that over half of the study population had one or more chronic physical illness and nearly two-thirds were affected by mild to severe depression. The study also revealed rural-urban differences in the prevalence of physical and mental health problems; urban geriatric women had more physical problems than rural women, but urban geriatric women were mentally healthier than rural women. As the sample size is too small to be representative of the elderly women, hence a study on a larger scale is required to corroborate the findings.

Conclusion

Old age is the last stage of human life cycle. This stage is also marked by low productivity and increased dependency. The problems of elderly have multiple dimensions.

The present study revealed that elderly women had more chronic morbidity and disability than other age groups. The level of depression was also higher. The pattern of morbidity and depression is also different in urban and rural areas. In light of this, the problems of elderly women need to be addressed through a multi-pronged approach – through medical, economic, social and mental health interventions.

The phenomenon of Ageing is established in developed world but developing countries have just started experiencing in last few years. Therefore program interventions and services for the elderly should aim to make them independent, and minimize medical and economic problems and thus reduce depression. Given the increase in the population of elderly, particularly women, it is high time that geriatric health is incorporated into the country's primary health care system. Geriatric morbidity and disability can easily be recognized at the primary health centre (PHC) level. By training medical officers, even mild depression can be diagnosed and treated by medical officers at the PHC level. Such an integrated approach can reduce work burden of specialists at the tertiary level.

India has very few social security schemes for the elderly like provident fund scheme, old age pension for government employees and a few others. These schemes are inadequate and do not cater to the entire old age population, especially women. Therefore, special social security schemes for elderly women need to be implemented.

Further research is required to consolidate the findings of the present study. State or country wide multi-centric studies on geriatric problems will help to get an in-depth understanding of the problems of elderly women.

References

Bhende, A., and Kanitkar, T. (1997). *Principles of Population Studies* (6th revised edition). Mumbai: Himalaya Publishing House, pp. 137-40.

Da Silva Pereira, Y., Estibeiro, A., Dhume, R. and Fernandes, J. (2002). Geriatric patients attending tertiary care psychiatric hospital. *Indian Journal of Psychiatry, 44*(4), 326-331.

Elango S. (1998). A study of health and health related social problems in the geriatric population in a rural area of Tamil Nadu. *Indian Journal of Public Health, 42*(1), 7-8.

Gore, M.S. (1992, April). Aging of the Human Being. *The Indian Journal of Social Work*, *3*(2), 212-219.

Gupta, I. and Sankar, D. (2003, June 24). Health of the Elderly in India: A multivariate analysis. *Journal of Health and Population in Developing Countries*. Retrieved from: http://www.jhpdc.unc.edu

Gurav, R.B. and Kartikeyan, S. (2002). Problems of geriatric population in an urban area. *Bombay Hospital Journal, 44*(1). Retrieved on February 25, 2005, from: http://bhj.org/journal/2002_4401_jan/org_47.htm

http://www.hindustantimes.com/news/181_ 839815, 00110 0040007 0006. htm

Kohli, A.S. (1996). *Social Situation of the Aged in India.* New Delhi: Anmol Publications Pvt. Ltd.

Kumar, P. (1993). Social classification: Need of constant updating. *Indian Journal of Community Medicine, 17*, 2.

Messinger-Rapport, B.J., Thacker, H.L. (2001, July). Prevention for the older woman. A practical guide to assessing physical and cognitive function. *Geriatrics, 56*(7), 24-6, 29-31, 35.

Office of the Registrar General of India. (2001a). *Census of India 2001, Population in five-year age group, Table C-14*. Retrieved on February 25, 2005, from: http://www.censusindia.net/agedata/DDWC-000014.xls

Office of the Registrar General of India. (2001b). *Census of India 2001, Literacy rate by important age groups and sex, Table 15*. Retrieved on February 25, 2005, from: http://www.censusindia.net/cendat/datatable15.html

Prasad, B. G. (1961). Social classification of Indian families. *Journal of Indian Medical Association*, *37*, 250-51.

Reserve Bank of India (RBI). (2003). RBI Bulletin, Jan 11, 2003. Retrieved on February 25, 2005, from: http://www.rbi.org.in/index.dll

Yadava, K.N., Yadava, S.S., Vajpeyi, D.K. (1997). A study of aged population and associated health risks in rural India. *International Journal of Aging and Human Development, 44*(4), 293-315

Yesavage Geriatric Depression Scale. Retrieved on February 25, 2005, from the Stanford University Website: http://www.stanford.edu/~yesavage/GDS.english.short.score.html

Notes

1. For the classification of the study population, per capita monthly income was used as the basis. Social classification by Prasad (1961)

was used with necessary modification as suggested by Kumar (1993). The formula used is as below:

Multiplication factor = $\frac{4.93 \times \text{value of CPI}}{100}$

Consumer Price Index for October 2002 was 408 (RBI, 2003)

14

Osteoporosis in Aging Women: A study of adult women in a local community of Gujarat[1]

Gayatree Jadeja and S. Rema

Introduction

Osteoporosis is a widespread health problem (Grissio et al., 1990; Wilkes and Meade, 1991). It is a generalized metabolic bone disease characterized by insufficient formation or increased resorption of bone matrix that results in decreased bone mass (Greenspan, 1984). The bone is quantitatively deficient but qualitatively normal (Rao, 1998). Thus osteoporosis is a disease of the skeleton in which the bones become brittle and prone to fracture. In other words, the bone loses density. Osteoporosis is diagnosed when bone density has decreased to the point where fractures occur with mild stress (Arden and Cooper, 1998).

Signs of the condition may include diminished height, rounded shoulders, evidence of bone loss from diagnostic tests; acute backache caused by pathologic vertebral compression fracture, etc. Thus bone will fracture under the slightest stress and heal poorly. In advanced stages of osteoporosis, any activity can cause fractures of the vertebrae (back bone) wrists and hips. In general, 75 per cent of the individuals who fracture a bone due to osteoporosis will suffer deformities and permanent disabilities which greatly decrease their quality of life (Seeley, 1991).

There are two types of osteoporosis. Type I occurs in 5 to 20 per cent of women, most often between the age of 50 to 75, because of the sudden postmenopausal decrease in estrogen levels which results in a rapid depletion of calcium from the skeleton. Type II is known as age related osteoporosis (Vergis, 1997).

The National Osteoporosis Foundation offers 5 steps which are important for preventing osteoporosis. (i) Calcium and vitamin D rich diet, (ii) Regular weight bearing exercise, (iii) Avoidance of smoking and excessive alcohol intake (iv) Talking to a doctor about bone health, and (v) Regular bone density tests and taking of medication if needed (Vergis, 1997).

Various bone mineral density (BMD) assessment devices have only recently been available in India and published data are based on assessments made by the use of dual energy X-ray absorptiometry (DXA), Quantitative Computed Tomography (QCT), Scanning and Quantitative ultrasound (QUS). It is to be noted that no normative reference database in the Indian population is available with any of these devices. In a study of 120 healthy Indian women aged between 20 and 70 years, QUS analysis revealed that 46 subjects were normal while 42 and 32 subjects had osteopenia and osteoporosis respectively (Chopra, 2000). The number of Indian women with low bone mass in this study was found to be 61.6 per cent. The author of this study has not mentioned the device or the normative reference database used (Chopra, 2000). It is therefore, likely that with the use of American database, the incidence of osteopenia and osteoporosis have been overestimated.

With the use of QCT in 100 Indian women between 20 and 60 years of age, the mean rate of trabecular bone loss was found to be 1.1 per cent in premenopausal women and 3.19 per cent in postmenopausal women (Suri and Khandelwal, 2000). Another study by Ravishankar (2000) involving 289 Indian women between 20 and 84 years of age showed that the peak BMD was reached in the third decade after which a slow decline of 0.6 per cent per year was noted. The study also revealed that the mean spinal and hip BMD in Indian women was lower as compared to the reference North American population. The authors of the last two studies did not report the prevalence of low bone mass in their study. There is evidence that BMD differs with ethnic origin and for the diagnosis of osteoporosis, the use of an appropriate reference database is essential (Genant et al., 1998). The Pronosco X-posure system uses the principle of Digital X-ray Radiogrammetry (DXR) and is the only system available in India, which has a normative reference database for Indian women and men (Pande, et al., 2001).

In this background the objective of the present study was to assess the bone mineral status of women of different age groups (26 to 60 years and above) compared to young controls aged (21-25 years) using the Pronosco X-posure System in order to assess the prevalence of osteoporosis in women of middle socioeconomic status residing in and around Anand and Vallabh Vidyanagar in Gujarat.

Methods and Materials

Pre and post menopausal women in different age groups of 21 to 60 years and above, belonging to middle socioeconomic status (SES) were selected using the snowball technique from in and around Anand and Vallabh Vidyanagar including Karamsad and Bakrol. A total of 240 females were selected, of these 25 subjects belonged to the age group 21 to 25 years and were considered as the control group. The remaining 215 subjects were divided into eight experimental groups of the age groups: 25-30 years (n=15), 31-35 years (n=20), 36-40 years (n=32), 41-45 years (n=55), 46-50 years (n=54), 51-55 years (n=15), 55-60 years (n=11), and 61 years (n=13). The subjects were explained about the purpose of the study before their selection. Only those willing to join the study were enrolled.

Both anthropometric measurement and radiographic techniques were used. Anthropometric assessment included measurement of standing height and weight. Height was measured in centimeters. The female subjects were asked to stand without shoes but with the heels together, and with the shoulders, buttocks and heels touching the scale. The individual was asked to look straight and make herself as tall as possible without raising her heels. Height was measured by keeping a straight ruler touching the scale on the head of the female subjects.

Weight was taken without shoes and in ordinary clothing on a weighing machine after adjusting the scale to zero.

The Pronosco X-posure System (Version V.2, Denmark) was used to calculate DXR- BMD, DXR-MCI (Metacarpal Cortical Index) and DXR- PI (Porosity Index) and it was based on radiogrammetry which needed digitally acquired x-rays of the left hand. These images were first acquired with the following parameters: filter 1.0, FFD 1 m, aluminium 80, tube voltage 42 kv, exposure 4 mAs, AGFA Scopix Laser 2 B (400).

The digital X-rays were subsequently printed and scanned into the system. The system itself checked the quality of the scanned images and aborted the examination in case of inadequate quality. The involved computer algorithms automatically defined regions of interest (ROI) around the narrowest bone parts of the metacarpals II, III and IV and subsequently found the outer and inner cortical edges of the included cortical bone parts. Not only was there no operator activity required for the location of the ROI, it is even not possible for the operator to modify or influence the size or location of the ROI. The analyzed image and the ROI were displayed on the monitor. The mean values of the cortical thickness and overall bone cortical thickness of the second, third and fourth metacarpal were estimated. Then for each bone the cortical volume per area (VPA) was calculated. Based on the mean VPA with a correction for the estimated porosity, DXR –BMD was computed. Porosity was derived from the area percentage of local intensity minima found in the cortical part of the bone relative to the entire cortical area. DXR-MCI expresses the mean cortical thickness normalized with the mean outer bone diameter (width). Due to an increase in bone width and the decrease in cortical thickness, the MCI decrease with age, especially in the years following menopause when accelerated cortical bone loss occurs. Detailed physical aspects of this technique and the mathematical models used are described by Rosholm and associates (2001).

For the available data, 't' scores were calculated for the subject population for further analysis. The WHO criteria were used to categorize the BMD into normal, osteopenic and osteoporotic.

Results and Discussion

The general and dietary information did not show any major differences. Medical history did not indicate any chronic illnesses in any of the subjects. Table 1 presents the anthropometric measurements of the different groups. As the age group of the

Table 1: Anthropometric measurements of experimental groups compared to control

Group	*n*	*Age (Years)*	*Height (cm)*	*Weight (kg)*
Control Group (21-25 years)	25	21.875 ± 1.035	156.875 ± 4.314	50.782 ± 6.984
Experimental Group I (26-30 years)	15	27.867 ± 1.356	155.167 ± 3.468	54.0 ± 9.899
Experimental Group II (31-35 years)	19	32.842 ± 1.642	156.605 ± 4.795	55.211 ± 8.728
Experimental Group III (36-40 years)	32	39.156 ± 1.081	153.913 ± 6.410	60.813 ± 11.40
Experimental Group IV (41-45 years)	55	43.055 ± 1.268	152.391 ± 6.792	58.036 ± 9.228
Experimental Group V (46-50 years)	54	47.778 ± 1.574	153.704 ± 5.782	60.50 ± 9.40
Experimental Group VI (51-55 years)	15	52.667 ± 1.291	153.0 ± 9.552	67.067 ± 13.193
Experimental Group VII (56-60 years)	11	58.273 ± 1.679	152.273 ± 7.023	57.455 ± 8.067
Experimental Group VIII (61 years & above)	13	64.231 ± 3.539	153.846 ± 3.625	61.538 ± 5.953

Note: Mean ± SEM.

subjects varied from 21 to 60 years and above, they were divided on the basis of age into eight age groups and their average age noted were 21.875, 27.867, 32.842, 39.156, 43.055, 47.778, 52.667, 58.273 and 64.231 years respectively. It is known that bone mass declines with age and is related to sex, race and ethnicity, menopause, family history and body weight. The age at which bone loss starts is uncertain but on the basis of cross sectional studies, it is generally believed to start during the thirties in both sexes (Buchanan, 1991).

Height of the subjects ranged between 152.273 and 156.875 cm. Body weight ranged between 50.782 and 67.067 kg and was lower in the younger age groups. Since every fracture of the

Table 2: Bone width, cortical thickness and metacarpal index of experimental groups compared to control.

Parameter	*n*	*D_1 (cm)*	*D_2 (cm)*	*D (cm)*	*D/D_1*
Control group (21-25 years)	25	0.716 ±0.006	0.367 ±0.012	0.348 ±0.011	0.486 ±0.015
Experimental group I (26-30 years)	15	0.736 ±0.014	0.357 ±0.019	0.379 ±0.016	0.516 ±0.021
Experimental group II (31-35 years)	19	0.727 ±0.011	0.341 ±0.013	0.386 ±0.008	0.532 ±0.013
Experimental group III (36-40 years)	32	0.751 ±0.008	0.347 ±0.013	0.404 ±0.011	0.539 ±0.015
Experiment Group IV (41-45 years)	55	0.731 ±0.006	0.347 ±0.009	0.384 ±0.007	0.528 ±0.011
Experimental group V (46-50 years)	54	0.745 ±0.005	0.386 ±0.009	0.359 ±0.007	0.488 ±0.009
Experimental group VI (51-55 years)	15	0.743 ±0.011	0.386 ±0.016	0.357 ±0.013	0.483 ±0.018
Experimental group VII (56-60 years)	11	0.760 ±0.013	0.426 ±0.017	0.334 ±0.019	0.422 ±0.027
Experimental group VIII (61 years & above)	13	0.758 ±0.016	0.477 ±0.022	0.281 ±0.016	0.384 ±0.020

Note: Mean ± SEM

n = number of subjects

D_1= Total width of the metacarpal

D_2= Marrow width of the same metacarpal

D = D1- D_2 Cortical thickness

D/D_1 = Metacarpal Index

vertebrae in the spine cause it to become a little shorter, as more fractures occur, the person experiences loss of height (Christiansen and Riis, 1990).

The normal spine age is 40 and osteoporotic changes start at ages 60 and 70. These changes can cause a loss of as much as 6 to 9 inches in height and result in the so called 'Dowager's Hump' (far right) in the upper thoracic vertebrae (Mcllwain et al., 1993).

Table 2 presents the bone width, cortical thickness and metacarpal index of the subjects. Bone width varied from 0.727 to

Table 3: Bone width, cortical thickness and metacarpal index of normal, osteopenic and osteoporotic subjects

Group		*Bone Width (D_1) (cm)*	*Cortical thickness (D) (cm)*	*Metacarpal Index (D/D_1)*
Control (21-25 years)	N = 17 OP = 5 O = 2	0.717 0.714 0.701	0.372 0.312 0.236	0.518 0.439 0.334
Exp. I (26-30 years)	N = 13 OP = 2 O = 0	0.741 0.707 -	0.389 0.313 -	0.527 0.449 -
Exp. II (31-35 years)	N = 18 OP = 1 O = 0	0.725 0.762 -	0.391 0.294 -	0.540 0.384 -
Exp. III (36-40 years)	N = 31 OP = 1 O = 0	0.728 0.726 -	0.407 0.312 -	0.543 0.428 -
Exp.IV (41-45 years)	N = 46 OP = 9 O = 0	0.735 0.704 -	0.398 0.320 -	0.544 0.458 -
Exp. V (46-50 years)	N = 45 OP = 9 O = 0	0.762 0.753 -	0.368 0.319 -	0.501 0.412 -
Exp.VI (51-55 years)	N = 10 OP = 5 O = 0	0.751 0.727 -	0.382 0.308 -	0.511 0.426 -
Exp.VII (56-60 years)	N = 6 OP = 2 O = 3	0.761 0.749 0.789	0.367 0.317 0.281	0.490 0.402 0.301
Exp.VIII (61 years & above)	N = 3 OP = 8 O = 2	0.772 0.744 0.792	0.359 0.264 0.233	0.471 0.374 0.297

Note: Exp. = Experimental, N = Normal, OP = Osteopenic, O = Osteoporotic

0.760 cm, while cortical thickness ranged between 0.281 and 0.404 cm. As age increased the cortical thickness of the bone decreased. Experimental group VIII showed the least cortical thickness compared to the control group.

The Metacarpal Index ranged between 0.384 and 0.539. As age increased the metacarpal index of the bone decreased. Women can lose up to 20 per cent of their bone mass within 5-7 years following menopause, making them more susceptible to osteoporosis (Seeman, 1988; Christiansen and Riis, 1990).

Table 4: BMD, T value and Z value of the normal, osteopenic and osteoporotic subjects

Group		*BMD (gm/cm²)*	*T value*	*Z value*
Control (21-25 years)	N = 17	0.549	0.166	0.523
	OP = 5	0.488	-1.397	-0.898
	O = 2	0.393	-3.089	-2.778
Exp. I (26-30 years)	N = 13	0.571	0.467	0.491
	OP = 2	0.486	-1.432	-1.525
	O = 0	-	-	-
Exp. II (31-35 years)	N = 18	0.571	0.167	-0.056
	OP = 1	0.475	-1.898	-1.898
	O = 0	-	-	-
Exp. III (36-40 years)	N = 31	0.589	0.744	0.433
	OP = 1	0.490	-1.351	-1.422
	O = 0	-	-	-
Exp.IV (41-45 years)	N = 46	0.588	0.315	0.242
	OP = 9	0.494	-1.376	-1.422
	O = 0	-	-	-
Exp. V (46-50 years)	N = 45	0.557	0.094	0.182
	OP = 9	0.488	-1.212	-1.054
	O = 0	-	-	-
Exp.VI (51-55 years)	N = 10	0.567	0.270	0.686
	OP = 5	0.484	-1.460	-0.964
	O = 0	-	-	-
Exp.VII (56-60 years)	N = 6	0.552	-0.311	0.923
	OP = 2	0.508	-1.045	-0.076
	O = 3	0.386	-3.210	-2.543
Exp.VIII (61 years & above)	N = 3	0.549	-0.299	1.087
	OP = 8	0.450	-2.075	-0.716
	O = 2	0.397	-3.021	-1.683

Note: Exp. = Experimental, N = Normal, OP = Osteopenic, O = Osteoporotic

Table 3 gives the bone width, cortical thickness and metacarpal index of the normal, osteopenic and osteoporotic subjects.

The data show that in each age-group the osteopenic and osteoporotic subjects showed lower bone width, cortical thickness and metacarpal index compared to normal subjects.

Normal subjects of the age group 31 to 45 years showed maximum metacarpal index which declined steadily with age.

Thirty per cent of postmenopausal Western women are known to suffer from osteoporosis (Pande et al., 2001). The present study revealed that 20.83 per cent of women over 55 years of age had osteoporosis and an additional 41.66 per cent had osteopenia. It is important to appreciate that the subjects in the present study were healthy adult women.

Table 4 gives the BMD, T value and Z value of the normal, osteopenic and osteoporotic subjects.

The T-score shows the number of Standard Deviations between the subjects' BMD and the average of the reference population at age of peak bone mass. The Z-score compares the subjects to the age-related reference population.

The database from which the present results were derived has confirmed a significant difference in the mean BMD between the control and all the eight experimental groups. BMD was lower in normal subjects belonging to the control age group compared to the normal subjects of the other groups, values ranging from 0.549 to 0.589. BMD ranged between 0.450 and 0.508 among the osteopenic women and 0.386 to 0.397 among the osteoporotic women and was lower compared to the BMD of normal subjects. Reports indicate an age dependent decrease in BMD in women over the age of 50 years (Kanis et al., 1994). Analysis of the normative reference data in women in the present study revealed that 20.61 per cent of the women above the age of 21 showed low bone mass.

Summary and Conclusion

The present investigation was conducted to evaluate the bone mineral status of adult women above 26 years and to compare them with younger women aged 20-25 years using radiographic studies of the wrist. For this study, the adult women subjects were selected and divided into nine groups, the first group was the control group

(20-25 years), and groups II-IX were experimental groups of women in the ages of 26-30 years, 31-35 years, 36-40 years, 41-45 years, 46-50 years, 51-55 years, 56-60 years and 60 years and above, respectively.

None of the subjects were suffering from any chronic illness. Body weight was higher in the age group of 51-55 years. Bone width did not show much variation whereas cortical thickness showed increasing mineralization with increasing age up to 45 years. After the age of 45 years a decreasing trend was observed in bone mineralization with increasing age. The differences were sharper between 41-45 years and the older age groups whereas the experimental groups I (26-30 years), II (31-35 years) and III (36-40 years) did not show any great differences between each other. Bone mineral status of female subjects was surprisingly inferior in the control group.

The data on bone mineral density also indicated that as age increased beyond 45 years bone mineral density showed a decrease. The number of osteopenic and osteoporotic subjects also increased as age increased beyond 40 years. Thus the findings of this study suggest that there is high prevalence of low bone mass in the aging women of middle socioeconomic status in a local community of Anand and Vallabh Vidyanagar, Gujarat.

Acknowledgement

The authors wish to thank: The University Grants Commission for funding the study; Dr. Janak Shah, Hari-om X-ray Centre, Anand, for providing the facility of x-ray machine along with the computerized software for all radiographic measurements; and Dr. Purohit, Orthopedist, Purohit Medical Centre, Anand.

References

Arden, M. and Cooper, C. (1998). Present and Future of osteoporosis epidemiology. In P. J. Meunier (Ed.), *Osteoporosis: Diagnosis and management* (1st edition) (pp.1-16). London: Moseby/Martin Dunitz.

Buchanan, J. P. (1991). Critical years and stages of puberty for spinal and femoral bone mass accumulation during adolescence. *Journal of Clinical Endocrinology and Metabolism, 73*, 555-563.

Chopra C. (2000). DEXA scan of forearm and quantitative ultrasound (QUS). In: B. Sankaran (Ed.), *Osteoporosis:* (pp. 144-52), World Health Organization.

Christiansen, C., and Riis, B. J. (1990). *Postmenopausal osteoporosis. A hand book of Medical Profession (The Silent Epidemic).* National Osteoporosis Society and the European Foundation for Osteoporosis and Bone Disease.

Genant H. K., Guglielmi, G., and Jergas, M. (1998). *Bone densitometry and osteoporosis.* Berlin: Springer Verlag.

Greenspan, A. (1984). *Orthopedic Radiology: A practical Approach* (3rd edition). Philadephia: Lippincott Williams and Wilkins.

Grisso, J. A., Baum, C. R., and Turner, B. J. (1990). What do physicians in practice do to prevent osteoporosis? *Journal of Bone and Mineral Research, 5*, 213-219.

Kanis, J. A., Melton, L.J., Christiansen, C., Johnston, C.C., and Kahltaev, N. (1994). The diagnosis of osteoporosis. *Journal of Bone Mineral Research, 9,* 1137-41.

Mcllwain, H. H., Bruce, D. F., Silverfield, J. C., Burnette, M. C. and Germain, B. F. (1993). *Winning with Osteoporosis* (2nd edition). John Wiley and Sons Inc.

Pande, K.C., Johansen, K.B., and Helboe, A.B. (2001). *Digital x-ray radiogrammetry; Establishment and comparison of Indian female and male normative reference data. Journal of Bone Mineral Research, 16*, S456.

Rao, P. P. (1998). *Osteoporosis* (pamphlet). Bombay: Rao Foundation (Medical Charitable Trust), Institute of Endocrinology, Hormone Hospital and Research.

Ravishankar U. (2000). Bone mineral content in normal Indian females: assessment by dual energy x-ray absorptiometry. In B. Sankaran (Ed.), *Osteoporosis* (pp. 120-31), World Health Organization.

Rosholm, A., Hylsdrup, L., Baeksgaard, L., Grunkin, M., and Thodberg H. H. (2001). Estimation of bone mineral density by digital X-ray radiometry: Theoretical background and clinical testing. *Osteoporosis, 12*, 961-969.

Seeley, D. G. (1991). Which fractures are associated with lower appendicular bone mass in the elderly women? *Annals of Internal Medicine, 115*, 837-842.

Seeman, E. (1988). The effect of early menopause on bone mass in normal and patients with osteoporosis. *American Journal of Medicine, 85*, 213-216.

Suri S. and Khandelwal B. (2000). Bone mineral content in normal Indian females: Assessment by quantitative computed tomography. In B. Sankaran (Ed.), *Osteoporosis* (pp. 132-7), World Health Organization.

Vergis, M. C. (1997). Osteoporosis in women. *U.A.E. Phamacist, 1*, 15-18.

Wilkes, H. C., and Meade, T. W. (1991). Hormone replacement therapy in general practice: A survey of doctors in the MRC's general practice research framework *British Medical Journal, 302*, 1317-1320.

15

Common Medical Problems in Elderly

Birenroy Chauhan, M.D.

Introduction

Older patients frequently have many comorbities in addition to cognitive and functional decline. For instance, in the United States, the average 75-year-old suffers from at least three chronic medical conditions and takes five or more medications (American Geriatric Society, 2000). The existence of comorbidities, atypical disease presentation in the elderly can result in misdiagnosis and inappropriate prescribing. Timely diagnosis and management of the diseases helps prevent adverse consequences and reduces sequelae of the diseases, and contributes to faster restoration to normal life. Therefore, understanding the complex medical illnesses in elderly persons, is important not only for health care providers so as to be able to provide effective treatment, but it is also important for the elderly persons and their caregivers to help them make timely presentation and proper description of the symptoms, and seek immediate care.

Older people however, often tend to resign themselves to a life of suffering and pain. They either are unable to or not particularly interested in changing and improving their medical conditions. They should be encouraged to lead a mentally, socially and physically healthy life.

This article is an attempt to impart information on the common medical problems of older people, which may have a bearing on their mental well-being. The five most common diseases in old age are: cardiovascular diseases (commonly referred to as heart diseases), cerebrospinal diseases, diabetes mellitus, gastrointestinal diseases, and respiratory diseases. This article gives an overview of these diseases and describes their symptoms, risk factors, complications and treatment and management options.

Cardiovascular Diseases

Cardiovascular disease (CVD) refers to the class of diseases that involve the heart and/or blood vessels (arteries and veins). While the term technically refers to any disease that affects the cardiovascular system, it is usually used to refer to those related to arterial disease (atherosclerosis). Cardiovascular diseases include arteriosclerosis, coronary artery disease, heart valve disease, arrhythmia, heart failure, hypertension, orthostatic hypo tension, shock, endocarditis, diseases of the aorta and its branches, disorders of the peripheral vascular system, and congenital heart disease. These conditions have similar causes, mechanisms, and treatment. Cardiovascular diseases are important components of chronic diseases worldwide. And chronic diseases are now the major cause of death and disability worldwide (WHO, 2005). Three most important cardiovascular diseases in older persons, are discussed in the following.

Hypertension

Blood pressure (BP) is the product of cardiac output and peripheral vascular resistance (BP = cardiac output × peripheral vascular resistance). Blood pressures ranging from 120 to 139 mm Hg systolic or 80 to 89 mm Hg diastolic are considered pre-hypertensive. For the general population, hypertension, i.e. an increase in blood pressure, is defined as a systolic BP of 140 mm Hg or higher or a diastolic BP of 90 mm Hg or higher. In developed countries, there appears to be a trend of increase in blood pressure with age. Diastolic blood pressure appears to plateau in the fifth decade and may decline thereafter, but systolic pressure continues to rise through the seventh decade. In persons younger than 50 years, diastolic pressure level is the major predictor of risk for strokes and other complications, whereas systolic blood pressure is the major predictor in those older than 60 years.

Individual risk is related to the level and duration of increased blood pressure, as well as to the presence of other cardiovascular risk factors and of injury to organs such brain, heart, kidneys, peripheral arteries, and retina.

Hypertension or increase in blood pressure, increases the risk of coronary events by causing direct vascular injury, increased left ventricular mass and myocardial oxygen demand. It increases the risk of peripheral vascular disease, especially in cigarette smokers and diabetic patients. It is the second leading cause of end-stage renal disease. Hypertension-related vascular disease causes loss of vision through a variety of mechanisms.

Lowering of blood pressure reduces the risk of death, stroke, heart failure, myocardial infarction, and other vascular events, especially in older patients with systolic hypertension.

Diagnosis

The diagnosis of hypertension relies on multiple office measurements of BP performed in a rigorous manner with a validated and well-maintained mercury sphygmomanometer and a cuff of appropriate size.

The patient is screened for a family history of hypertension, premature cardiovascular disease, and disorders that would increase the possibility of secondary hypertension. Factors which affect BP are lifestyle habits, level of physical activity, sodium intake, use of caffeine and alcohol, history of weight gain and tobacco use.

The physical examination includes at least two standardized measurements of blood pressure in the seated position in the opposite arm and in the standing position, especially in diabetic patients and older patients (to identify orthostatic declines). Height, weight, body mass index, and waist circumference (a potential cardiovascular risk factor) are recorded.

It is important to measure blood pressure in the elderly when they are in standing position, in addition to while they are sitting or lying. Elderly have tendency to develop postural hypotension in standing position, which may lead to fall and fracture.

Clinical and pathological investigations include: ECG, Lipid profile, Renal function test, Retinal examination, and Echocardiography.

Complications

Untreated hypertension can lead to premature death or disability from complications of cardiovascular diseases, atherosclerosis, and endothelial dysfunction, compounded by other factors (e.g., smoking, hyperlipidemia, and diabetes). Although the effect of hypertension on blood vessels is systemic, it expresses itself by characteristic effects on target organs—the heart, brain, kidneys, and eyes.

According to Eure (2005), blood pressure (elevated levels) among 80+ elderly is a major problem in US. Aggressive treatment is not possible in this age group people because they are reluctant and consider it as higher risk. According to the article, high blood pressure is treated by combination of medications (suitable to elderly), diet (weight loss if indicated and restricted salt intake) and exercise.

Hypertension causes a two-fold increase in the risk of myocardial infarction and sudden cardiac death. Hypertension in midlife is associated with an increased risk of cognitive dysfunction and dementia in later life. This may be a complication of multiple cerebral infarctions (multi-infarct dementia), but it also occurs in the absence of previous strokes. However, there appears to be an argument against aggressive management of blood pressure in the elderly. Stevens (2006) reported that dementia is not prevented in elderly by lowering blood pressure because very low BP causes impaired circulation in blood vessels of the brain.

Prevention and management of hypertension

The prevention and management of hypertension involves lifestyle modifications to lower risk, such as:

- Weight Management: If the Body Mass Index is greater than 25, weight management is advised.
- Restricting salt intake : For persons with sensitivity to salt (indicated by an increase in blood pressure with salt

consumption), a restriction of 2-4 grams is advised. For others, 3-4 gm of sodium (6g of salt) intake is advised.

- Maintaining adequate intake of potassium (90 mmol/day) ~ 2gm of potassium.
- Ingesting a diet rich in fruits and vegetables and low-fat dairy products which have reduced saturated and total fat.
- Increase aerobic exercise (30–45 min/day), brisk walking, etc. For the elderly, the recommendation is to continue to carry out the activities of daily living and increase mobility.
- Limiting alcohol intake to no more than 1 oz (30 ml; e.g., 24 oz of beer, 10 oz of wine, 2 oz of 100-proof whiskey) or to 0.5 oz for women and lighter-weight people.
- Discontinuation of tobacco use.
- Medical management with pharmaceutical agents under the supervision of a physician with treatment of associated diseases like ischemic heart disease (IHD), renal failure, and Left Visual Field (LVF) retinal injury.

Angina Pectoris

The coronary artery circulation normally supplies sufficient blood flow to meet the demands of the myocardium as it labors

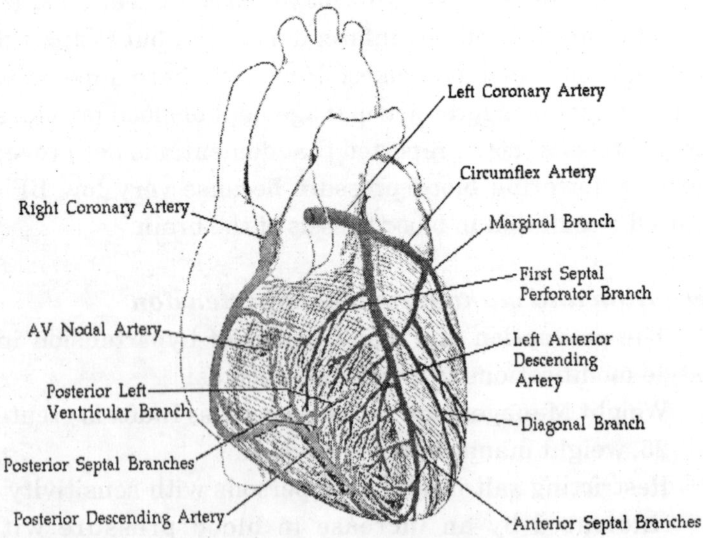

under a widely varying work load. An imbalance between coronary blood flow (supply) and myocardial oxygen consumption (demand) can precipitate ischemia, which frequently manifests as angina pectoris. When the imbalance becomes extreme, myocardial infarction, congestive heart failure, and electrical instability (arrhythmia) may result. Arrhythmia is probably the major cause of sudden death in ischemic heart disease. Narrowing of the cross-sectional area of a segment of a major coronary artery by more than 50 per cent (or narrowing of the diameter of a segment of an artery by more than 70 per cent) impairs nutrient blood flow under conditions of increased myocardial demand.

Clinical manifestations

Angina pectoris is typically a retrosternal chest discomfort, usually perceived as pain but often described as pressure or heaviness. The patient may clench a fist when describing the sensation. Discomfort often radiates to the neck, the left shoulder, the left arm, or the lower jaw and occasionally to the back, down the right arm, or down both arms. Although angina may be perceived as an epigastric discomfort resembling indigestion, the pain usually does not radiate far below the level of the diaphragm. Some patients describe their angina as shortness of breath, mistaking a sense of constriction for being out of wind. The patient's need to take a deep breath, rather than to breathe quickly, often identifies shortness of breath as an anginal equivalent. An anginal episode usually lasts several minutes. Chest discomfort is provoked by exertion or emotion, and is relieved by rest or nitroglycerin.

Diagnosis

Electrocardiogram is a critical tool in the diagnosis of angina pectoris. It can show firm evidence of an old myocardial infarction or an ST-segment depression which is a characteristic sign of subendocardial ischemia. Many patients with angina have a normal ECG in the absence of pain. Thus, an ECG taken when a patient is free of pain may misdirect the effort to diagnose the cause of the patient's chest pain.

Another tool for diagnosis is the Stress Test. The Stress Test will be more a useful test when at rest there is no chest pain and no

ECG finding. It has good sensitivity and specificity, if the patient has chest pain during the test.

Echo-cardiography can help, however it cannot rule out cardiac chest pain, if it is normal, but has good specificity if it shows regional wall motion abnormality. It can also pick up any other valvular heart disease, and systolic and diastolic dysfunction.

The Stress dobutamine echo is more specific for peeking up regional wall motion abnormality. It is useful when the patient is unable to walk due to other reasons.

Radionuclide assessment of coronary perfusion is usually performed after either exercise or after administration of dipyridamole or adenosine. Myocardial perfusion may be assessed, although at considerably greater cost. The radionuclide techniques can also identify the area of hypoperfusion and thereby identify the abnormal coronary artery

Coronary angiography is gold standard for diagnosing coronary heart disease. It will show the lumen of vessels and obstruction in the coronary.

Prevention and treatment

Controlling the risk factors for atherosclerosis is essential for the prevention and treatment of angina pectoris. This can be done by controlling high blood pressure, and making lifestyle changes such as increasing exercise to control excess weight, eating a heart-healthy diet to control cholesterol levels, and stopping smoking. High blood pressure, and high cholesterol can be treated with medications. Anti-platelet agents (low dose Aspirin and clopidogrel) can prevent blood-clots with cause heart attacks.

The most commonly used medication to treat people with angina are beta blockers (because they decrease the heart rate, blood pressure, and myocardial oxygen consumption). Long-acting calcium channel blockers are also prescribed because they cause the blood vessels to relax and allow blood to flow freely to the heart, lowering blood pressure and relieving anginal pain. Nitrates (such as amyl nitrite and nitroglycerin) are used to treat angina. These help alleviate pain by widening the blood vessels, thereby allowing more blood flow to the heart muscle and decreasing the work load of the heart.

Revascularization surgery, either coronary artery bypass or angioplasty, may be necessary, if there is significant narrowing of the coronary arteries.

Acute Myocardial Infarction

Acute myocardial infarction, commonly known as heart attack occurs when the myocardial blood supply is completely hampered. The heart is a muscle pump that delivers blood to the body each time it beats. It is fueled by blood from the coronary arteries. A blood clot may form and block one of these arteries. If the blockage is not promptly relieved, the heart muscle supplied by that artery will die. This is known as heart attack or myocardial infarction. Atherosclerotic plaques are formed in the blood vessels when the macrophages in the blood ingest the lipids in blood (and are now called foam cells) and sit in the lining of the blood vessels. These atherosclerotic plaques are susceptible to sudden rupture and hemorrhage into the vessel wall, which may result in the sudden partial or total occlusion of the coronary artery.

Risk factors

The risk factors for developing atherosclerosis (narrowing of the arteries) include: male gender, age, cholesterol, smoking, high blood pressure, diabetes, obesity, stress and family history.

Diagnosis

Heaviness, pressure, squeezing, or tightness in the chest, and that has persisted for more than 30 minutes, is the sign of a heart attack. A heart attack may start at rest or when a person is exerting. It is a typical sensation of tightness or pressure behind the sternum (breast bone). It may also be felt in the arm, between the shoulder blades, neck or jaw. The pain is similar to that of angina, but it is not relieved by tablets or spray placed under the tongue. Other symptoms include cold skin, shortness of breath, faintness and nausea.

Many patients with acute myocardial infarction, particularly those with inferior infarction, have perspiration; nausea and vomiting are common as well. Breathlessness is also a common associated symptom. Giddiness with transient unconsciousness may occur and is more frequent with inferior than anterior infarction, in part because of the more frequent occurrence of irregular and slow pulse rate, heart block, and irregular and high pulse rate with inferior infarction.

Elderly patients with infarction often present with symptoms that differ from the symptoms of infarction in younger patients; more than half of elderly patients present with shortness of breath as their main complaint, and many others present with dizziness or symptoms of arrhythmia rather than the classic symptoms of acute myocardial infarction.

Approximately two thirds of patients describe the new onset of angina or a change in their anginal pattern in the month preceding infarction. However, in approximately one in every four patients, myocardial infarction is associated with only mild symptoms or no symptoms at all.

The ECG (Electrocardiogram) is a valuable tool both in confirming the diagnosis of acute myocardial infarction and in selecting the most appropriate therapy for the patient. The serum cardiac marker - creatine kinase (CK) and an isoenzyme, creatine kinase-myocardial band (CK-MB), will be raised after 3 hours to rise and confirming myocardial infarction.

Echocardiography may be useful in identifying patients with myocardial infarction in the emergency department. Regional wall motion abnormalities occur within seconds of coronary occlusion and well before myocyte necrosis, and most patients with acute myocardial infarction have regional wall motion abnormalities readily seen on echocardiography. However, echo cardiographic evidence of myocardial infarction is not required in patients with symptoms and electrocardiographic evidence typical of acute myocardial infarction, and treatment should not be delayed, so that an echocardiogram can be performed. Similarly, wall motion abnormalities are not specific for acute myocardial infarction and may be caused by ischemia or prior infarction.

Treatment

The Emergent Therapy for myocardial infarction consists of the administration of oxygen by nasal prongs, I.V. analgesia (most commonly morphine sulfate), oral aspirin, and sublingual nitroglycerin if the blood pressure is greater than 90 mm Hg. Continuous ECG monitoring is must for all patients. High-risk patients should be admitted to a coronary care unit. Aspirin should be given to all patients as soon as a diagnosis of myocardial infarction is made.

The Reperfusion Therapy in the treatment of myocardial infarction which takes longer to initiate (e.g., primary coronary angioplasty) may actually be superior if it achieves reperfusion more rapidly than another therapy that can be initiated more rapidly (e.g., thrombolytic therapy). At institutions where a skilled catheterization team is on call 24 hours a day and can be rapidly assembled, coronary angioplasty would most likely be able to restore coronary blood flow in more patients more rapidly, than thrombolytic therapy. Elsewhere, thrombolytic therapy may be preferable.

Other drugs are clopidogrel, heparin, low molecular weight heparin, atorvastatin, beta blockers, ramipril intravenous nitroglycerin and magnesium have good role to play in acute myocardial infarction. Glycoprotein IIb/IIIa Inhibitor Therapy like abciximab, tirofiban are the newer drug for platelet inhibition.

Surgery or other interventions in the treatment of myocardial infarction include:

- **Angiography:** Coronary artery X-rays will outline blockage that may be relieved by angioplasty or surgery.
- **Angioplasty:** This procedure is similar to an angiogram, being done by passing thin tubes up from the groin while the patient is mildly sedated. A tiny balloon is passed down the narrowed vessel and inflated to clear the blockage.
- **Coronary Artery Bypass Surgery:** This is a procedure that splices healthy blood vessels taken from elsewhere in the body to the affected coronary arteries so that the clogged areas are bypassed

Emergency coronary artery bypass surgery should generally be reserved for patients in whom immediate angiography reveals coronary anatomy that precludes primary coronary angioplasty; for patients in whom angioplasty has failed; and for patients with a ventricular septal defect, severe mitral regurgitation, or myocardial rupture. It has been reported by Mclaughlin et al. (1999) from Agency for Health Care Research and Quality that elderly heart attack patients with multiple health problems who are most in need of thrombolytic (clot-busting) medications, do not receive it as promptly as other patients, because elderly have a higher risk of bleeding, particularly intracranial hemorrhage with thrombolytic treatment.

Diabetes Mellitus

Diabetes mellitus is a metabolic disease characterized by hyperglycemia that results from defects in insulin secretion, insulin action, or both. It is caused by deficiency of insulin or failure to convert sugar into energy for storage, resulting in high blood glucose and sugar in the urine. Important abnormalities in fat and protein metabolism are also present.

A variety of pathogenic processes are involved in the development of diabetes. These processes range from autoimmune destruction of the beta cells of the pancreatic islets with consequent insulin deficiency to mutations in the insulin receptor gene with consequent resistance to insulin action.

As per its etiology, Diabetes is classified into: a) Type 1 diabetes mellitus, which is insulin dependant; b) Type 2 diabetes mellitus, which may range from predominantly insulin resistance with relative insulin deficiency to a predominantly insulin secretory defect with insulin resistance; c) Genetic defects in insulin action, Genetic defects of ß cell function Disease of the exocrine pancreas Pancreatitis, Neoplasia, Endocrinopathies, Acromegaly, Cushing syndrome, Glucagonoma, Drug- or chemical-induced-nicotin acid glucocorticoids and thizides' infections, congenital rubella, cytomegalovirus, etc.

The symptoms of poorly controlled hyperglycemia include polyuria, polydipsia, blurred vision, weight loss, polyphagia, stunting of growth, and vulnerability to infections or susceptibility to a more virulent or chronic course when infected (poor wound healing). Acute life-threatening consequences of diabetes mellitus are ketoacidosis and nonketotic hyperglycemic hyperosmolar coma. Overtreatment of hyperglycemia can lead to hypoglycemia, which may be severe enough to cause seizures and loss of consciousness.

The chronic hyperglycemia of diabetes mellitus is specifically associated with long-term damage, dysfunction, and failure of various organs, especially the retina and lens of the eye, the kidneys, and both somatic and autonomic nervous systems. The heart, arterial system, and microcirculation are also adversely affected.

The specific long-term complications of diabetes include (1) retinopathy with potential loss of vision, (2) nephropathy leading to end stage renal disease (ESRD), and (3) neuropathy with risk of foot ulcers, amputation, Charcot joints, sexual dysfunction, and potentially disabling dysfunction of the stomach, bowel, and bladder. Numerous mechanisms have been discovered that may mediate the specific tissue damage caused by hyperglycemia. Diabetic patients are also at increased risk for atherosclerotic cardiovascular, peripheral vascular, and cerebrovascular disease. These conditions may be related to hyperglycemia as well as to hypertension and abnormal lipoprotein profiles that are often found in diabetic patients.

Diabetes Mellitus is more common with age, although prevalence estimates for elderly people (above 65 years) vary widely from 8-9 per cent to 16.6 per cent (Manton, 1993; Wilson et. al., 1986). A prospective cohort study to determine the relationship between risk factors and the development of non-insulin dependent diabetes mellitus in the elderly, showed high body mass index and low physical activity among elderly as significant risk factors for the development of diabetes mellitus (Gurwitz et al., 1994)

Applying proven processes of care to prevent, diagnose and treat diabetes could significantly reduce morbidity and mortality among the elderly.

Management of Diabetes

The blood glucose level can be maintained either with the administration of insulin or with oral hypoglycemic drugs (OHA). Insulins are of different types: ultra short acting (lispro), short acting (actrapid) intermediate acting (mixture of actrapid and NPH) and long acting (NPH).

OHA include: insulin sensitizer (glitazones and metformin) and insulin secretor-sulphonamides. Each drug has different pharmacokinetics and hence different dose intervals and doses.

The doses should be adjusted in such way that they: 1) maintain preprandial capillary whole blood glucose levels at 80 to 120 mg/dl, bedtime blood glucose levels at 100 to 140 mg/dl, and postprandial peak blood glucose levels at less than 180 mg/dl, and (2) maintain an HbA_{1c} of less than 7.0 per cent.

Nutritional therapy and exercise

Intensive and conventional insulin treatment will produce unsatisfactory results unless it is appropriate for the nutrient intake. To facilitate the matching of insulin doses to meals and to prevent hypoglycemia, patients with type 1 diabetes mellitus should eat consistent regular meals comprising about 50 per cent carbohydrate calories, less than 30 per cent total fat calories, and less than 300 mg cholesterol a day. Exchange categories are bread, meat, milk, fruit, fat, and vegetable. For optimal instruction and reinforcement of diet therapy, a dietitian should be part of the diabetes care team.

Exercise is another important component of diabetes care because it helps maintain cardiovascular conditioning, insulin sensitivity, and general well-being. However, patients must be instructed how to adjust their meals, their insulin doses and timing, or both, so as to prevent hypoglycemia during, immediately after, or even 6 to 12 hours after exercise as muscle glycogen stores are replenished from plasma glucose. High-impact sports are contraindicated for patients with advanced retinopathy who are at risk for vitreous hemorrhage or for patients with peripheral neuropathy or vascular disease who are at risk for foot trauma, because such sports can be hazardous.

Complications of Diabetes

The following is a description of the complications of diabetes, their symptoms and treatment options.

Diabetic Ketoacidosis (DKA)

DKA is the ultimate result of insulin deficiency which is aggravated by stress-induced elevations of glucagon, cortisol, growth hormone, epinephrine, and norepinephrine. DKA are precipitated by infection. Sepsis, myocardial infarction, and other major intercurrent illnesses are more often the cause of death than the metabolic disequilibrium itself.

DKA presents with signs and symptoms of dehydration secondary to osmotic diuresis and vomiting and diarrhea, hyperventilation to eliminate CO_2; and of various degrees of depressed mentation or decreased consciousness and seizures.

Treatment of DKA requires volume repletion, insulin therapy, correction of electrolytes, treatment of infection and acidosis. It is preferable to treat patients with DKA in an intensive care unit to ensure close monitoring.

Hypoglycemia

Hypoglycemia is a more common emergency and is dangerous. Clinical hypoglycemia can range from tachycardia, tremulousness, anxiety, and sweating, confusion, seizures to coma.

The most common causes of hypoglycemia are missed meals and snacks, insulin dosage errors, exercise, alcohol, and drugs such as beta-adrenergic blockers- all very common in elderly.

In older people, the first symptom of hypoglycemia may occur only at glucose levels as low as 35 mg/dl (as opposed to 55 to 60 mg/dl) and may consist of confusion or loss of judgment, which interferes with self-treatment.

Patients recognize most episodes of hypoglycemia quickly and can effectively treat themselves with a promptly absorbed oral carbohydrate. Approximately 15 g of carbohydrate is sufficient to restore blood glucose levels to normal. This amount is provided by approximately 6 oz of orange juice, 4 oz of a cola drink, 3 to 4 tsp of table sugar, five Life Savers candy, or three glucose tablets (each containing 5 g of glucose). The use of complex carbohydrates and foods with a high fat content, such as chocolate, may delay digestion and absorption of the glucose and are not first choices for treatment of hypoglycemia. If the patient cannot swallow or cooperate, a gel form of glucose and simple carbohydrates can be administered by mouth, applying it between the gums and cheeks, from where it slowly and generally safely trickles down into the stomach. Glucagon (1 mg administered subcutaneously or intramuscularly) will also usually raise blood glucose levels sufficiently within 15 to 30 minutes, when the patient can then take oral carbohydrates. Glucagon comes in emergency kits, and it should always be on hand for patients with a history of severe hypoglycemic episodes. When all else fails, intravenous glucose must be given by emergency medical service personnel or in an emergency room, whichever is quicker. Patients with severe hypoglycemia usually respond rapidly to treatment, although patients who are postictal or in a prolonged coma may require days to regain normal mental status and cognitive function. Quite often, there is amnesia for such extended episodes, including a period preceding the onset of hypoglycemia. In rare instances, neurological deficits can be permanent.

Hyperosmolar coma

In Type 2 Diabetes Mellitus, hyperosmolar hyperglycemic nonketotic coma (HHNC) is a common and feared acute complication in older persons. It is characterized by extreme hyperglycemia (>600 mg/dl) and serum hyperosmolarity (>320 mOsm/L) but with little or no ketosis. The CNS effects of extreme hyperosmolarity range from somnolence or confusion to coma, but notably can also include focal or generalized seizures as well as focal neurological deficits that disappear with treatment. HHNC is marked by extreme dehydration, in which the deficit of free water is prominent and the circulatory volume is often seriously compromised. Thus, hypotension; extremely dry skin and mucous membranes; and gross elevation of hematocrit, urea nitrogen, creatinine, and albumin are frequent. However, stroke and myocardial infarction, along with pancreatitis and sepsis, may also precipitate the syndrome.

Elderly patients living in nursing homes are particularly vulnerable to HHNC because their thirst mechanisms are less sensitive to a rising serum osmolality and because dementia, increasing obtundity, or institutional conditions may combine to reduce water intake to less than urinary and insensible water losses. At presentation, serum sodium level is usually elevated or surprisingly normal in the face of extreme hyperglycemia.

Fluid replacement is the most important component of therapy. Total fluid deficits of as much as 12 L may have to be replaced. In insulin treatment, Potassium must be added to intravenous fluids to prevent hypokalemia caused by insulin action. It may take days of fluid replacement, the tonicity of which must be carefully adjusted to achieve a gradual steady decrease in serum osmolality and sodium levels, before the central nervous system function returns to normal or at least to baseline. The mortality in HHNC is still quite high.

Diabetic neuropathy

It causes numbness or tingling in the toes and feet. When neuropathy becomes more severe, hypoesthesia or anesthesia takes the place of paresthesias and dysesthesias (abnormal painful sensation). Ultimately, the insensate feet become very vulnerable to trauma, and neuropathic foot ulcers are frequent causes of hospitalization and even amputation. In some instances, neuropathy is manifested by severe pain that can interfere with sleep and normal daily activities. Involvement of the autonomic nervous system is also common and can become debilitating.

Manifestations of diabetic neuropathy include male impotence and female anorgasmia, difficulty voiding and urinary retention, impaired gastric emptying with early satiety and emesis, diarrhea, orthostatic hypotension, and decreased sweating and vasomotor tone in the lower extremities. The combination of decreased sympathetic tone and loss of vagal control of the heart rate can produce persistent resting sinus tachycardia; sudden death can result.

A form of diabetic neuropathy called amyotrophy occurs most commonly in elderly men with diabetes. It is manifested by severe, unremitting pain and weakness in the thigh muscles. Severe depression, cachexia, and weight loss may mark the 1 to 2-year course of this form of neuropathy.

Diabetic nephropathy

Diabetic nephropathy is the complication associated with the highest mortality- between 35 and 45 per cent in type 1 diabetes mellitus and a somewhat smaller percentage in type 2 diabetes mellitus patients. Histologically, the earliest change is thickening of the capillary basement membrane. Excretion of low but abnormal levels of albumin in the urine is a marker of the incipient phase of nephropathy. Albuminuria increases and eventually gross proteinuria appears. Microalbuminuria is defined as excretion of 30 to 300 mg of albumin a day or an albumin-creatinine ratio between 30 and 300 in a random urine specimen. Clinical proteinuria is defined as excretion of more than 0.5 g of total protein a day. This level of excretion can be detected by a positive dipstick urine test for protein. The nephrotic syndrome may also eventually occur.

Early in type 1 diabetes mellitus, kidney size and glomerular filtration rate (GFR) may actually be greater than normal. However, in both types of diabetes, GFR begins to decline, and after clinical proteinuria develops, GFR almost inexorably falls to the level of end stage renal disease (ESRD). Unlike the risk of retinopathy, the risk of nephropathy does not continue to rise with increasing duration. The incidence of nephropathy peaks at approximately 15 to 17 years and declines somewhat thereafter. If the dipstick test has not revealed proteinuria by 25 to 30 years of diabetes duration, the risk of ESRD decreases.

Diabetic retinopathy

It occurs in almost all patients with type 1 diabetes mellitus and in most patients with type 2 diabetes mellitus, who are on conventional treatment that does not come close to normalizing glycemic levels. It begins with loss of capillary pericytes, the supporting cells of the retinal vasculature to microaneurysms - Small dot hemorrhages form when microaneurysms leak blood – and loss of vision. Capillary closure leads to ischemia of the retina. Infarctions of the retinal nerve result in loss of vision (soft exudates – cotton wool appearance in fundoscopy).

Coe (2001) reported the link between Type 2 diabetes and poor cognitive performance and suggested that older people with diabetes should be routinely screened for changes in brain functions. Croxson and Jagger (1995) in their study revealed that subjects with known diabetes were more likely to have low Mini Mental Status Examination (MMSE) scores compared to newly found diabetic subjects.

Gastrointestinal Diseases

Malabsorption and constipation are among the two most commonly occurring disorders in the elderly.

Malabsorption

Malabsorption refers to the impaired intestinal absorption of nutrients. It can result from congenital defects in the transport of nutrients, or from acquired defects in the absorptive surface of the intestinal epithelium.

Maldigestion, another factor in nutrient absorption, refers to the impaired digestion of nutrients within the intestinal lumen. Although these two processes are pathophysiologically distinct, they are interdependent; and in clinical practice, malabsorption has come to signify derangements in both processes. Malabsorption is clinically defined as impaired absorption of fat (steatorrhea); other substances such as iron, calcium, bile salts may be poorly absorbed in elderly.

Causes of malabsorption in older people

Radiation enteritis, Amyloidosis, Mastocytosis, Ischemic bowel disease (most common), short bowel syndrome, cirrhosis/ parenchymal liver disease, Cholestasis due to extrahepatic obstruction, Chronic Pancreatitis, cancer of the Pancreas, Hyperthyroidism, Diabetes Mellitus (autonomic dysfunction) and Carcinoid syndrome are among the causes of malabsorption in older people.

The treatment of malabsorption varies as per the diagnosis. However in many disorders, no specific treatment is available, except symptomatic.

Constipation

The most common syndromes associated with disorders of motility are non-ulcer dyspepsia, irritable bowel syndrome (IBS), functional constipation and outlet obstruction to defecation (evacuation disorders). The prevalence of gastroparesis and chronic intestinal pseudo-obstruction is far lower. These disorders result from impaired neurologic or muscular control of the gut or from incoordination of defecation dynamics. Motility disorders are sometimes caused by a process that influences the extrinsic autonomic nerves that supply the gut. Motor function of the gut depends on the contraction of the smooth muscle cells and their integration and modulation by enteric and extrinsic nerves. The enteric nervous system plays essential role in controlling peristalsis and the migrating motor complex. Derangement may lead to altered gut motor function.

Volvulus of the stomach, small bowel loops, cecum, and sigmoid colon may present as acute or sub-acute symptoms caused by mechanical obstruction.

Drugs also cause constipation. Drugs like Tricyclic antidepressants, narcotics, anticholinergics, antihypertensives, vincristine, cause constipation.

The diagnosis of slow-transit constipation should be made only after exclusion of mucosal diseases, such as tumors and strictures.

Treatment of slow-transit constipation consists of increasing dietary bulk or fiber and administering osmotic laxatives (e.g., magnesium salts when not contraindicated) and stimulant laxatives or colonic prokinetic agents.

Intestinal tumors

Intestinal tumors are common in elderly and are manifested with either constipation and or loose motion. Usually it is associated with low grade fever anorexia and weight loss. Ultrasonography (USG) will diagnose most of the tumors either benign or malignant. Sometimes endoscopy, colonoscopy and CT scan is necessary.

Treatment of intestinal tumors is usually symptomatic, surgical and at times radiation is necessary.

Respiratory Diseases

Infections (Pneumonias) are common due to poor immunity and poor cough reflex in old age. Etiological organisms such as Gram-positive cocci, bacilli, Gram-negative cocci, bacilli, Mixed flora (aspiration pneumonia), mycobacteria (*Mycobacterium tuberculosis,* Fungi, Parasites Viruses) also cause infections.

Fever, cough with expectoration, chest pain, dysponea on exertion are the common symptoms of respiratory infections.

Diagnosis

A Chest X- ray will diagnose almost all pneumonias. Sometimes culture and gram stain of sputum is necessary to find out the etiological organism for better selection of antibiotics, particularly in the case of non-resolving pneumonias.

In rare instances CT scan is needed to r/o alveolar cell carcinoma and other malignancy. Sometimes thorascopic biopsy also needed for confirmation and culture of the organism. Bronchoalveolar lavage may rule out tumor and infection.

Lipoid pneumonia is a noninfectious, inflammatory lung disorder caused by the aspiration of mineral oil or other oily substances. It is most common in elderly patients and others with impaired swallowing. The most common symptom is a chronic cough, which may be caused by coexisting lung disease rather than lipoid pneumonia; fever is uncommon. Often, the disease is discovered on a routine chest radiograph that shows a focal, dense infiltrate, usually in a lower lobe or in the right middle lobe.

The only specific therapy is avoidance of exposure to mineral oil and other lipid-containing agents.

Chronic obstructive diseases of the lung (COPD)

Chronic Bronchitis and Emphysema are COPDs. Chronic bronchitis is defined by the presence of cough and sputum on most days for at least 3 months of the year for a minimum of 2 years in succession.

Emphysema is defined in pathologic terms on the basis of findings of abnormal permanent enlargement of air spaces distal to the terminal bronchiole accompanied by the destruction of the alveolar walls without obvious fibrosis.

In cigarette smokers, the prevalence of chronic bronchitis increases with age and the number of cigarettes smoked. More than 50 per cent of middle-aged men who smoke at least one pack of cigarettes a day report having chronic productive cough. Although occupational dust exposure is also associated with the development of chronic bronchitis, the effect of cigarette smoking overwhelms the occupational effect.

Clinical manifestations

The hallmarks of COPD are chronic productive cough and persistent, progressive exercise limitation because of breathlessness in the context of prolonged cigarette smoking. Patients with predominant chronic bronchitis present with chronic productive cough, whereas patients with predominant emphysema complain of dyspnea. Cough with expectoration develops 10 to 12 years after smoking begins. The symptom is often dismissed as a simple smoker's cough. However, persons with established chronic bronchitis commonly produce 2 oz or more of mucoid sputum a day.

Transient periods of sputum discoloration caused by purulence commonly occur, often in association with respiratory tract infections. The patient may become breathless during activities of daily living such as making the bed or bathing.

Orthopnea (breathlessness in supine position) is often present in patients with advanced airway disease. The orthopnea of COPD must be differentiated from the paroxysmal nocturnal dyspnea of chronic heart failure.

Diagnosis

In the early stages, physical examination may yield entirely normal results. With more advanced disease, tachypnea and a prolonged expiration. Breath sounds may be reduced by decreased airflow, and wheezes are heard in 40 per cent of patients.

The pathological investigations for diagnosis are: 1) pulmonary function tests (including arterial blood gases); 2) chest radiography; 3) CT of the chest.

In Pulmonary function tests, Spirometry reveals a reduction in the FEV_1/FVC, decline in the forced expiratory flow between 25 and 75 per cent of vital capacity.

Measurement of lung volumes uniformly reveals an increased residual volume (RV) and a normal to increased functional residual capacity (FRC). Residual volumen may be two to four times higher than normal because of slowing of expiratory flow and trapping of gas behind prematurely closed airways. As a result, tidal breathing may take place at lung volumes as high as 1 to 2 L above normal levels.

In Chest imaging, radiographic abnormalities may be minimal, even in cases of advanced COPD. Three types of radiographic abnormalities exist: Arterial deficiency in the lung periphery, hyperinflation, and Bullous diseases. If a bulla is present it is virtually diagnostic of emphysema.

CT scan of the chest can be useful in the differential diagnosis of COPD.

Treatment of COPD

Helping a patient to quit smoking is probably the single most important intervention; effective methods include counseling by physicians and nurses, use of nicotine chewing gum or patches, behavior intervention (e.g., individual or group therapy), and several pharmacologic interventions (e.g., bupropion and nortriptyline).

Reduction in morbidity and mortality in patients with COPD can be achieved with yearly vaccinations against influenza, pneumococcal vaccine with *Haemophilus influenzae* vaccine.

A variety of other therapies offer potential relief of symptoms in patients with chronic airflow obstruction (CAO). These include the use of bronchodilators; anti-inflammatory therapy; administration of antibiotics during acute purulent exacerbations; pulmonary rehabilitation programs, including physical exercise and respiratory muscle training; and, for patients with cor pulmonale, the use of diuretics.

- Bronchodilators: The first line of therapy is inhaled atropine derivatives (e.g., ipratropium bromide tiotropium). If an inadequate response is seen with anticholinergic therapy, an inhaled beta2 agonist can be substituted or added.
- Corticosteroids: Given the underlying pathophysiology of emphysema, corticosteroids would be expected to provide little benefit, because tissue destruction is the basic disease mechanism. Corticosteroids should be reserved for acute exacerbations of disease or, if required on a regular basis, given in the lowest possible dose, preferably on alternate days. Analyses of large databases have suggested that inhaled corticosteroids, especially when used with long-acting beta2 agonists, may also improve survival.
- Antibiotics: Intermittent antibiotic administration is indicated for acute episodes of clinical worsening marked by increased dyspnea, excessive sputum production, and sputum purulence. The duration of symptoms and the risk of serious deterioration in lung function can be reduced by a 7- to 10-day course of broad-spectrum antibiotics.
- Diuretics and Vasodilators: Diuretics are administered for symptomatic relief of peripheral edema; they may also reduce pulmonary arterial pressure by decreasing intrapulmonary blood volume. Digoxin and aminophylline are only weak inotropic stimulants of the right ventricle.

- Pulmonary Rehabilitation: Physical training programs, such as treadmill walking, significantly increase the exercise capacity of patients with even far-advanced chronic bronchitis and emphysema. Much interest has focused on the possibility that resistive or endurance exercises (Yoga and Pranayam) aimed at strengthening the inspiratory muscles might increase respiratory muscle strength and endurance and thereby improve exercise capacity.
- Long-term Oxygen Administration: Probably the single most important advance in recent years in the treatment of advanced COPD has been the widespread home use of supplemental oxygen. Chronic hypoxemia causes secondary erythrocytosis and contributes to exercise limitation, pulmonary hypertension and right heart failure, and impaired neuropsychiatric function. Each of these consequences of chronic hypoxemia can be ameliorated or even corrected by the administration of oxygen at levels that are sufficient to maintain the arterial oxygen saturation at values exceeding approximately 90 per cent. In general, patients should receive long-term home oxygen supplementation if the P_aO_2 is 55 mm Hg or less or if the P_aO_2 is 59 mm Hg or less, presence of peripheral edema (cor pulmonale), a hematocrit of 55% or greater, and P pulmonale on the ECG. Oxygen for home use can be stored in cylinders as compressed gas or as liquid oxygen, or it can be generated from oxygen concentrators and Portable tanks of oxygen can provide supplemental oxygen for several hours of use outside the home.
- Surgery: Emphysematous lung tissue can be removed by several approaches. The purpose is to remove over distended, poorly functioning emphysematous regions, thereby allowing more-normal or less-affected regions to expand with a decrease in the functional residual capacity (FRC) and an improvement in inspiratory muscle function. The surgery can be performed on many patients who are not candidates for lung transplantation, instead of lung transplantation, or as a bridge to transplantation. In younger patients with far-advanced COPD, lung transplantation is a therapeutic option.

Having discussed the various common health problems of elderly people, it may be concluded that healthy physical state leads to a healthy mind, positive attitude and pleasant moods. Therefore understanding the pathology of disorders, proper diagnosis and timely treatment play an important role in mental well being. Public awareness programmes about common health problems of the elderly, their diagnosis and treatment are needed to educate the elderly, so that they can take their health in their own hands.

References

Coe, M. C. (2003). Older adults with diabetes: Staying smart about mental status changes,. *Health and Age.* (on-line). Available: http://www.healthandage.com/Home/gid2=1173

Croxson, S. C. M. and Jagger, C. (1995). Diabetes and cognitive impairment: A community based study of elderly subjects. *Age and Ageing, Vol. 24* (5), 421-424.

Dale, D. C. and Federman, D. D. Dale and Federman (2004). *ACP Medicine, 2004-2005 (, A publication of the American college of Physicians).* New York: WebMD.

Eure, M. (2005). Blood pressure among elderly. *Journal of American Medical Association, 3*:23.

Gurwitz, J. H., Field, T. S., Glynn, R. J. , et al. (1994). Risk factors for noninsulin-dependent diabetes mellitus requiring treatment in the elderly. *J Am Geriatr Soc, 42*, 1235–40.

Kasper, D. L., Braunwald, E., Fauci, A., Hausen, S., Longo, D., and Jamsen, J. L. (2004). *Harrison's Principles of Internal Medicine* (16th edition). New York: Mc-Graw-Hill Professional.

Lloyd Jones. (2000). *Differential control of systolic and diastolic blood pressure: Factors associated with lack of blood pressure control in the community. Hypertension, National Heart, Lung and Blood Institute, Framingham study.* Lippincott, Hagerstown, MD< ETATS_UNIS

Manton, K. G., Stallard, E., and Liu, K. (1993). Forecasts of active life expectancy, policy and fiscal implications. *Jr Gerentol, 48* (Special Issue), 11-26.

Mclaughlin, D., Jerry H, Gurwitz, J. H., Donald, M. D., and Wilson, J. (1999). Thrombolytic therapy for eligible elderly patients with acute myocardial infarction, *Jr of Am Geriatric Soc., 47* (10), 1222-1228.

Stevens, L. M. (2006, May 23). Lowering Blood Pressure Doesn't Prevent Cognitive Impairment, Dementia. *Health Behavior News Service*. Availablehttp://www.cfah.org/hbns/get Document. cfm? document ID=1279

Wilson, P.W., Anderson, K.M. and Kannel, W. B. (1986). Epidemiology of diabetes mellitus in the elderly. The Framingham Study. *Am J Med, 80 (Suppl 5A)*, 3-9.

WHO. (2005). Preventing chronic diseases: a vital investment. Geneva: WHO. Available: http://www.who.int/chp/chronic_disease_report/full_report.pdf

16

Oral Care for Elderly People

Amit Parekh

Introduction

Average life expectancy has increased in most parts of the world, including India, on account of improvement in health care. As a result the population of old people is increasing. For a long time now, oral hygiene in India has been a neglected area of health. It is only with advancing age, when people start experiencing dental problems more acutely that they begin to take care of their oral hygiene. As such old age or aging does not cause any problem in maintaining the oral hygiene. There are several other factors that underlie poor oral hygiene in old age. As medical problems increase with advancing age, it makes a person less caring about his or her oral hygiene. Physical and cognitive impairment in older adults can interfere with their ability to perform oral hygiene procedures. Also, various illness and medications change the composition of saliva and reduce the salivary flow, causing deterioration of oral health in old age. Harmful habits like chewing or smoking tobacco and lack of knowledge about oral care, exacerbates the deterioration of oral health.

Oral health is directly associated with mental health. Individuals having oral problems such as broken teeth, pyorrhea, and so forth, often suffer from inferiority complex and poor social life. Edentulous state (without teeth) or ill-fitting dentures also can cause depression because of the deprivation of certain foods and malnourishment. On the other hand, mental illnesses are responsible for poor dental hygiene and oral cavity problems leading to overall poor health. With this background, this article on "oral health" giving general information about oral cavity problems and care has been presented here.

Common Dental Problems of the Elderly

The following is a brief overview of the commonly found dental problems of old people, their causes, risk factors and treatment. Gum diseases (pyorrhea) and tooth decay are major dental problems of Indians. These are also the two main reasons for loss of teeth.

Pyorrhea (periodontitis)

Small particles of food and bacteria (called plaque) stick to the tooth, which gets calcified gradually and forms the tarter. When the tarter goes between the tooth and gums, it causes irritation to gums. In the initial stage of pyorrhea there is swelling and bleeding from the gums. If care is not taken at this stage, tarter and bacteria start causing damage to the bone and bone gets resorbed, and gradually the affected tooth starts shaking.

Various diseases and medicines used for their treatment can enhance the risk of pyorrhea. For instance, in persons who are diabetic, sugar enriched blood provides a good cultivating medium for bacteria to grow in the gingival margin. This causes damage to the gums and the underlying bone. The drugs used for treating hypertension (Amlodipine) and epilepsy (Phenytoin) cause enlargement of gums.

Treatment

The best treatment option for pyorrhea is removal of plaque and tarter (scaling). If pyorrhea is treated at the early stage it gives excellent results. Sometimes when the tarter gets deposited at a deeper level, from where it cannot be removed easily, Flap surgery is required.

The best way to prevent pyorrhea is regular cleaning of the teeth (scaling). If this preventive care is taken at an early age, one will have better gums and good oral hygiene in one's advancing years.

Dental caries

Dental caries or tooth decay is the second most common disease after common cold. It is also the most important cause of tooth loss. Bacteria, acid, food debris, and saliva combine in the mouth to form a sticky substance called plaque that adheres to the teeth. Plaque is most commonly found on grooved chewing surfaces of the back molars, just above the gum line on all teeth, and at the edges of fillings.

The acids in plaque dissolve the enamel surface of the tooth and create holes in the tooth (cavities). Cavities are usually painless until they grow very large inside the internal structure of the tooth (the dentin and the pulp at the core) and can cause death of the nerve and blood vessels in the tooth. If left untreated a tooth abscess can develop.

With the decrease in salivary flow caused by disease (Sjogrean's syndrome), use of certain medicines (antidepressants) or post radiotherapy and chemotherapy, the rate of caries (decay of tooth) increases.

Treatment

Once the outer layer of the tooth (enamel) is destroyed it can never regenerate. Dental caries in this early stage is painless. Decayed portion of tooth is removed and is filled with various materials like silver, gold or composite resins.

When decay crosses the second layer (dentin) of the tooth and reaches the nerves of the tooth (pulp) it causes severe pain. Root canal treatment is recommended in such a case. In the root canal treatment, the decay, nerves and blood vessels of the tooth are removed and the canal is filled with sealing materials.

Regular check up and early treatment is the best way to prevent dental decay. All patients of oral cancer should undergo florid application prior to radiotherapy as a preventive measure against dental decay.

When teeth loss is not preventable. The lost teeth should be replaced by removable prosthesis (partial denture), fixed prosthesis (bridge) or implants. Replacement of tooth not only prevents further deterioration of adjutant teeth and maintains good chewing surface, but it also helps in the digestion of food, which is very important, especially in old age.

When there is more then 60 to 70 per cent loss of natural teeth and partial prosthesis is not possible full denture or complete denture is given. In order to have a good, complete denture person should have good compliance.

Ill-fitting dentures however, can cause problems. If there is constant irritation or ulcer formation on account of the dentures, one should ask for medical advice. Dentures should be cleaned everyday with soap or appropriate denture cleansers available in the market. Partial dentures and complete denture should be removed in the night so that the underlying oral mucosa and the jaw bone get enough rest. Food debris collected beneath the denture on the mucosa will get flushed with saliva which prevents fungal infection.

The Caretaker's role in Maintenance of Oral Hygiene of the Elderly

As mentioned earlier, physical and cognitive impairment in older adults can interfere with the patient's ability to perform oral hygiene procedures. It is the caretaker's responsibility to take care of the elderly patient's oral hygiene, like brushing the patient's teeth, cleaning the patient's mouth after every meal. If the elderly patient is unable to gargle his /her mouth should be cleaned with cotton gauze. The elderly patient's mouth should be examined regularly.

It is advised that elderly people be accompanied by a caretaker when they visit a dentist. The Dentist should be informed about the medical problems of the elderly patient and the medicines being used for their treatment. Certain medicines, like aspirin should be stopped two to three days before and after extraction of the tooth or any other surgery. In case of certain heart disease, prophylactic antibiotics should be given. And sometimes, a physician's reference may be needed. It is caretaker's duty to know patient's medical history and to inform the dental surgeon of the same before treatment.

Conclusion

Simple, preventive measures at an early age can help us maintain oral hygiene, and to keep in check gum diseases and tooth decay, even in old age. If old age or physical impairment does not permit a person to perform the daily care for the oral hygiene it is the caretaker's moral responsibility to take care of that person. Following are the preventive measures one must take to maintain good oral health at any age.

1. Regular Brushing of teeth -twice in a day with proper method.
2. Regular flossing of teeth
3 Filling of decayed teeth
4. Cleaning (scaling) of teeth once a year.
5. Replacement of teeth should be done after removal of teeth.
6. Self examination of mouth (oral cavity)
7. Regular check up by a dentist (every six months)
8. Dentures should be removed every day at night and it should be cleaned with appropriate denture cleansers.

Regular care and follow up will keep us smiling forever.

References

Cohen, S., and Burns, R.sC. (1994). *Pathways of the pulp* (6th edition). St. Louis, Missouri: Mosby-Year Book.

Carranza F. (1990). *Glickman's Clinical Periodontology* (7th edition). Philadelphia: WB Saunders Company.

Little, J. W., Palace, D., Rhodus, N. L. (2002). *Dental management of medically compromised patients*. St. Louis, Missouri: Mosby.

17

Psychological and Social Aspects of Breast Cancer: Some observations from Clinical Practice

Jayshree Mehta

Breast Cancer is one of the common cancers among women. The incidence of breast cancer is increasing worldwide. Currently the lifetime risk of developing breast cancer varies from 1 to 7 in the United States (SEER 2004), 1 in 8 in the United Kingdom to approximately 1 in 30 in India. The incidence is rising in developing countries, and in India, it is the commonest cancer in women in urban areas of the country. Although the increasing incidence is alarming, there is a silver lining to the dark cloud. Today, more women survive breast cancer because of early detection and improved treatment.

Cancer is a word that immediately evokes a negative image with far reaching implications. It is an illness that unleashes disequilibrium in the affected individuals and in the lives of the persons who are from their immediate environment. For Indian women, this illness brings with it severe emotional stress. The emotional destabilization occurs at two levels: in the patient and in the people with whom the patient interacts. It is important to recognize these complex set of reactions. There is ample evidence to show that negative emotions such as worry, anxiety, deferred hope, disappointment and depression when allowed to grow, can increase susceptibility to disease (Lock and Callgan 1986), whereas positive emotions such as optimism, humor and fighting spirit can protect health and help in the process of healing (Wiseman).

When cancer strikes, there are some day to day issues to be faced. The individual has to immediately face the stress of undergoing various medical examinations, arranging for finance and the physical implications of the tests as well as treatment. It is at this stage that the patient is unable to discharge daily responsibilities. Patients who are employed may be required to go on leave and their work suffers. These experiences dissipate and sap one's energies and one may find oneself at the brink of an emotional breakdown. This psychological framework may thus be characterized by lingering diffidence. One experiences a tentativeness, a nagging sense of doubt, difficulty in facing the inescapable and inevitable negative consequences of one's illness. Thus the diagnosis and initiation of treatment may result in low self-esteem. However, in the case of some persons it could lead to reinforced determination.

Doctors treating cancers often observe two reactions from patients immediately after the diagnosis of breast cancer. Grief reaction and depression. Knowledge about the diagnosis of one's breast cancer is followed by grief reaction which manifests in three phases as follows:

1. **First Phase:** Shock and denial characterized by a sense of disbelief about the diagnosis, or feeling of numbness.
2. **Second Phase:** Acute anguish. Once the seriousness of the diagnosis sinks in, the patient experiences intense negative feelings, like physical distress, social withdrawal, and preoccupation with the illness and its imagined consequences. She might experience anger towards the treating doctor or who-so-ever she holds responsible for her illness. She might also experience a feeling of guilt for having "indulged" in a lifestyle which increased the risk of development of the cancer.
3. **Third Phase:** Resolution. Over a period of several weeks or months, the patient comes to terms with her illness, resumes her daily routine, and may start re-experiencing pleasure in appropriate situations.

The duration of these phases varies from person to person, and all three phases may not necessarily be seen in a single individual.

Women who are diagnosed with cancer experience depression, which becomes evident in the form of psychological symptoms like low mood, thoughts of guilt, feeling of hopelessness or worthlessness, loss of interest in the surroundings, psychomotor agitation or retardation, irritability, social withdrawal, and suicidal thoughts. These women often also show characteristic physical symptoms like anorexia, weight loss, insomnia and fatigue. Almost all patients with cancer at some point, fall into the "Depressive Spectrum" one end of which is formed by the milder "grief reaction" and other by intense Depressive Disorder".

While treating a patient, health professionals need to consider factors several which might impact on the treatment. One can begin by a looking at the environment of the patient. On the one hand there are physical, psychological and financial pressures that the patient is trying to deal with. On the other hand are significant others in the environment of the patient, like the doctor; oncologist, paramedics, family and colleagues (if the patient is employed).

One of the most important factors in cancer treatment is the attitude of the doctor. Has the doctor given up or is the doctor fighting for the patient's life? The approach of the doctor will have a significant impact on the patient. If the doctor's interaction with the patient reinforces the positive attitude - "you are too good to be ill we will fight together and not give up" - it will make a difference to the patient's motivation to fight cancer. Doctors must bear in mind that the person may be the 1000th patient for the doctor, but the patient has only one life. Thus the manner in which oncologists and paramedics deal with the patient is very important. Equally important is the setup of the hospital. Does the setup facilitate easy interaction with providers, provision of services or does it make it more difficult? It is imperative for the hospital administration to attempt to strike a balance between the availability of services and the needs of the patients and be more supportive. A strong will to live (fighting spirit) prolongs survival of breast cancer patients (Wiseman).

The degree of support provided by the family, the financial status and degree of responsibility on the patient are the other important factors. The family must avoid reflecting that the patient is going to die soon and make the patient dependent. Rather, the patient should be encouraged to do small jobs and undertake activities that are of interest to her. This would develop the ability to cope with problems. Goodwin et al. (1987) emphasizes the protective impact of marriage and says that it affects every stage of cancer care. The best odds for survival seem to lie with those who are married. This view is supported by Neale, Tilley and Vernon (1986).

If the patient is working she may be required to deal with the reaction of her colleagues. The patient needs to gear up to the situation and deal with it. In fact the attitude of others may be taken up as a challenge to fight the situation and get well soon. Helplessness and hopelessness affect negatively the survival of patient. Therefore patients must come out of such negative feelings and should develop a fighting spirit.

Perhaps the most important aspect is the patient's state of mind. It is important to look at the emotional dynamics. As mentioned earlier, with grief reactions there will be sudden feeling of inadequacy. The patient might feel as though her whole world is crumbling and everything seems suddenly to have come to an end. It is at this time that the patient's expectations from others increase to the point of being unrealistic. The patient starts experiencing self pity accompanied by a feeling of utter helplessness. There starts a search for sympathy from everyone around. The person becomes very sensitive. Thoughts like "nobody wants me", "everyone is rude", "I am useless, now of no use of the people", "they do not respect me any more" and so on constantly trouble the patient. These emotional dynamics become pricking reminders and also lead to a state of general tentativeness in the patient.

From the therapeutic perspective, it is important for the patient to develop a proactive approach to life rather than a reactive one. It is necessary that one trains oneself to look for support from within rather than develop a dependence on external support.

Wisdom gained from an experience of being close to death leads to some pertinent observations.

First of all, there should be a focus on "nowness". Death is inevitable for every human being. Illness needs to be looked at as a notice given to us. One can use this notice period to do what one desires and enjoy as much as one can. The psychological framework must emphasis equality of life rather than quantity. Each day must to be looked at one at a time. One must realize that living 10 days of life doing constructive, productive work has greater value than living 10 years. This attitude to life would help the patient to move ahead.

The clock provides only a technical measurement of how long we live. Far more real than ticking of the minutes is the way we spend the minutes and invest them with meaning.

It has been observed that family neutrality can have a positive impact on the patient's motivation to fight illness and recover. When the family avoids treating the individual as a patient, the patient is forced to do the things for oneself. At this time, in the initial phase, the patient is likely to feel neglected. But as there is pressure to undertake one's own activities, successful execution slowly helps develop confidence in the patient. Branden (1997) has rightly said that "we stand in the midst of an almost infinite network of relationships; to other people, to things, to the universe. But the most intimate and powerful of all relationships and one we can never escape is the relationship to ourselves. No significant aspect of our thinking, motivation, feelings or behavior is unaffected by one's self evaluation". Treating the patient as capable would enhance self esteem.

Another important factor providing support to the patient is spirituality. Having faith would help in instilling hope, which goes a long way in motivating the individual to believe in quality of life, accept death and yet fight against the illness.

Psychological factors affect the strength of the immune system and thereby play a role in the occurrence as well as persistence of illness. Some studies at the University of Pennsylvania have reported that animals in the "stressed" group that had control over the stressors immunologically rejected cancer 63 per cent of the time compared to 28 per cent of the "victim" group. It appears therefore, the ability to deal with stress, and to gain a sense of control (Hafen et al., 1996), is more important in fighting against illness. Thus the mind plays an important role in determining health.

References

Branden, N. (1997). *The art of living consciously*. Needham Heights, MA: Simon & Schuster.

DeVita, V. T., Hellman, S., and Rosenberg, S. A. (Ed.). (2004). *Cancer: Principles and Practice of Oncology* (7th edition). Philadelphia, Pennsylvania: Lippincott Williams & Wilkins.

Goodwin, J. S., Hunt, W. C., Key, C. R., and Samet, J. M. (1987). The effect of marital status on stage, treatment and survival of cancer patients. *Journal of the American Medical Association, 258,* 3125-30.

Hafen, B., Karren, K., Frandsen, K., and Smith, N. (1996). *Mind, Body, Health; the effect of attitudes, emotion and relationships*. Needham Heights, Massachusetts: Allyn and Bacon.

Holland, J. C. (1997). Preliminary Guidelines for the Treatment of Distress. Oncology (Huntingt), 11, 109-114

Neale, A.V., Tilley, B.C., Vernon, S.W. (1986). Marital status, delay in seeking treatment and survival from breast cancer. *Social Science and Medicine,* **23,** 305–312.

Spiegel, D., and Giese-Davis, J. (2003). Depression and cancer: mechanisms and disease progression. *Biological Psychiatry, 54*(3), 269-282.

Wiseman, A. D. *Cancer, the behavioral dimensions*, p. 331.

18

Depression and Comorbid Anxiety in Older People: Diagnosis and Treatment Options[1]

Anand B. Khorana

Diagnosis of Depression in Older People

Depression is often present in less obvious and straight forward ways in older people (age 60 years and above) than in earlier life (age 18-59), as shown in table 1. Several studies show that older people are less likely to present with complaints of low mood. Hypochondriacal bodily complaints for which no adequate cause can be found such as intractable sleep disturbances, various aches and

Table 1: Differences in symptom pattern between older and younger depressed patients

Found MORE frequently in older patients	*Found LESS frequently in older patients*
Sleep disturbance	Sadness
Hypochondriasis	Expressed suicidal intent
Agitation	
Alexithymia	

pains, may, however, occur relatively frequently. This may be understood in terms of older depressed patients being more likely to be "alexithymic" or unable to express feeling in words, and instead, express their feelings in terms of pain and bodily symptoms (Downes et al., 1988; Oxman et al., 1990; Prince et al., 1999).

Gender differences in depression in older people

In 1988 in Finland, a large community based study by Kivela and Pehkala found that older depressed men had more marked sleep disturbances and loss of interest, whereas guilt, anxiety, diurnal mood disturbances and hypochondriacal complaints were more common in depressed women (Table 2).

Table 2: Gender differences in symptom pattern

More common in women	*More common in men*
Guilt	Sleep disturbance
Anxiety	Loss of interest
Somatic symptoms	
Worrying	
Tearfulness	
Feelings of hopelessness and helplessness	
Thoughts of suicide	

Depression and cognitive impairment

Another important source of diagnostic difficulty is the frequency of depressive symptoms and cognitive impairment in older people. The clinical features of depressive pseudo-dementia include: Apparent dementia, marked self-neglect, rapid onset, preserved insight, indifference to poor performance and biological features of depression. Patients with depressive pseudo-dementias usually have good insight into their poor performance but appear curiously indifferent to it. Patients with dementia cannot comprehend appearance, loss of memory, etc. There is a real deficit with those with dementia unlike those with pseudo-dementia (extreme clinical depression).

Depression and Comorbid anxiety

Anxiety symptoms are commonly found in association with depression. A community survey found that both generalized and phobic anxiety each occurred in over 20 per cent of the people aged 65 and above with depression. Seventy five per cent of the older patients with generalized anxiety and almost 50 per cent of those with phobic anxiety also fulfilled the criteria of depression (Manda et al.). This suggests that generalized anxiety at least should be regarded as indicative of depression unless proved otherwise.

Clinical pointers towards depression – Worsening physical complaints in the absence of objective changes in physical health, loss of interest and of the ability to enjoy, recent onset of sleep disturbances and self-neglect are particularly helpful pointers (Table 3).

Table 3: Pointers to depression in the older surgery attendees

Unexplained physical worsening
Loss of interest
Anhedonia (inability to enjoy)
Recent intractable sleep disturbance
Depressive cognitions
Self as useless
World as hostile
Future as hopeless
Overgeneralization
Misattribution

How common are depression and comorbid anxiety in older people?

The comprehensive review by Beekman and colleagues (1999) found point prevalence rates ranging between 0.4 per cent and 35 per cent depending on the diagnostic criteria used. The weighted average prevalence was 1.8 per cent for major depression, but was as high as 10.2 per cent for minor depression and 13.5 per cent for all clinically relevant depressive syndromes. A comparison of nine

European studies using Geriatric Mental State Schedule (GMS) – Automated Geriatric Examination for Computer Assisted Taxonomy (AGECAT) – a standardized diagnostic interview and computerized diagnostic algorithm for psychiatric epidemiology studies in older people. The overall prevalence of depression was 12.3 per cent with a constant patter for higher rates in woman than in man (Averaging 14.2 per cent versus 8.6 per cent or 2:1) (Copeland et al., 1999).

Comorbid anxiety has been extensively studied. Flint and Rifat (1995) found that the prevalence of anxiety disorders in general in older people is about 10 per cent. Again there were significant associations between depression and anxiety; 22 per cent of subjects with depression also meeting criteria for generalized anxiety and the same proportion meeting the criteria for phobic disorders.

Assessment of Depression and Anxiety in Older People

Depression is all two frequently undetected and/or untreated in older people. In 1997, Katona and colleagues found that only 10 out of 103 older people identified as depressed in a community survey were receiving antidepressants. One important factor is that depression is understandable and inevitable in the face of the multiple adversaries and losses that older people have to face. Epidemiological studies are remarkably consistent in showing community rates of depression of 12-15 per cent in older people, indicating that such depression cannot justifiably be seen as a "normal" consequences of the aging process (Gallo et al., 1999). Table 4 lists some of the barriers to recognition and treatment of depression and anxiety in older people.

Table 4: Barriers to recognition and treatment

Ageist assumptions
Depression inevitable consequence of ageing and associated loss
Older people unable to achieve psychological change
Older people too frail for physical treatment
Diagnosis more difficult
Stigmatizing effect of diagnosis
Constraints of brief consultation

One option for increasing recognition rate in primary care is the use of screening questionnaires.

Apart from the usual diagnostic criteria, the Geriatric Depressive Scale (GDS) of Yesavage and associates (1983) has probably been evaluated most extensively in the primary care centre (Table 5), answers score 1 point each, scores of >4 suggest possible depression.

Table 5: Geriatric Depression Scale

Are you basically satisfied with your life?	Yes/No
Have you dropped many of your activities & interests?	Yes/No
Do you feel that your life is empty?	Yes/No
Do you often get bored?	Yes/No
Are you in good spirits most of the time?	Yes/No
Are you afraid that something bad is going to Happen to you?	Yes/No
Do you feel happy most of the time?	Yes/No
Do you often feel helpless?	Yes/No
Do you prefer to stay at home rather than going out and doing new things?	Yes/No
Do you feel that you have more problems with memory than most people?	Yes/No
Do you think that it is wonderful to be alive now?	Yes/No
Do you feel pretty worthless the way you are?	Yes/No
Do you feel full of energy?	Yes/No
Do you feel that the situation is hopeless?	Yes/No
Do you think that most people are better off than you?	Yes/No

Management of Depression and Anxiety in Old Age

Depression and anxiety in old age are very frequently untreated. Much of the research concerning their management has been carried out in specialist settings these are outlined in Table 6.

Table 6: Consensus statement on recognition and management of depression in late life in general practices

Depression is more difficult to diagnose in old age
Its prevalence is higher in general practice surgery attendees than in community
Risk is increased by poor health and adverse life events
Ageist attitudes may impede appropriate management
Physical and psychological treatments are as effective as earlier in life
Depression in old age is a relapsing condition and must be monitored closely.

The first step towards the successful management of depression in late life is, therefore, to identify and break down the barriers preventing appropriate treatment being instituted and maintained.

The main treatment modalities, drug treatments, electroconvulsive therapy, and psychological treatments should not be considered in isolation but be integrated.

Table 7: Newer antidepressants

Drug class	*Drug*	*Recommended daily dose range in older people*	*Comments*
SSRI	Fluoxetine	20-40 mg.	Long half-life
	Paroxetine	20-40 mg.	
	Sertraline	50-150 mg	
	Citalopram	20-40 mg	
	Fluvoxamine		

(Contd.)

(Contd.Table 7)

Drug class	*Drug*	*Recommended daily dose range in older people*	*Comments*
	Nefazodone		Also blocks SHT2 receptors
SNRI	Venlafaxine	75-225 mg.	
NARI	Reboxetine	2-4 mg	Not indicated for use in old age
RIMA	Moclobemide	150-600 mg	
NASSA	Mirtazapine	15-45 mg.	

Antidepressant drugs: A wide range is available including "older" anti depressants such as tricyclic antidepressants (TCAS) and related heterocyclic (Mianserin) and the monoamine-oxidase inhibitors (MAOIS) and a wide variety of "newer" antidepressants (Table 7).

Age related pharmacokinetic and pharmodynamic changes seem less clinically important for newer antidepressants than for the TCAS.

Psychological Therapies: These therapies tend not to be considered in the treatment of depression and anxiety in older people lack the physiological flexibility to respond well to such approaches.

The evidence base attesting to the efficacy of cognitive approaches in older people is, in fact, surprisingly strong (Koder et al., 1996)

Interpersonal psychotherapy (IPT), widely used in the United States and increasingly so in Europe, has been shown to be effective by the studies by Reynolds and associates. Cognitive and behavioral approach (CBT) are also useful in managing coexisting anxiety symptoms

Electroconvulsive Therapy (ECT) is indicated where depressive delusions are present, where retardation is marked and where suicide risk is high.

Conclusion

Depression is common in older people, particularly those with chronic physical illness and those in institutional care. It is associated with markedly increased health and social service use. All too often, such depression is significantly disabling and persistent, partly because it usually goes untreated or is treated inadequately. Doctors, patients and caregivers tend, wrongly, to think of depression as inevitable in view of the multiple adversities and losses experienced by older people. Such depression should rather be seen as abnormal and potentially treatable.

Depression may be difficult to recognize in older people. Overt sadness is often absent and many of the symptoms characteristic of depression overlap with those associated with the ageing process and with the range of physical illnesses often found in this age group. Both phobic and generalized anxiety, often coexist with depression in older people, reducing the chances of spontaneous recovery and making treatment more challenging. The distinction between depression and dementia is also sometimes difficult to make, but is critically important for appropriate management.

The prognosis of depression in older people, particularly when associated with comorbid anxiety, may be less favorable than for depression earlier in life. If detected early and treated rationally, however, such depression and anxiety respond well. Response to antidepressant drugs is as good as that found earlier in life. Newer antidepressants have fewer adverse effects and are better tolerated and, therefore, may have particular advantages in this patient group. Response to psychological treatments (particularly cognitive behavioral therapy) is also similar to that found in younger depressed patients, contradicting the widely held view that older people are too set in their ways of thinking to respond to talking treatments. The primary care team is ideally placed both to achieve high rates of detection and (with specialist support where appropriate) to provide appropriate treatment.

References

Beekman, A.T.F., Copeland, J.R.M., Prince, M.J. (1999). Review of community prevalence of depression in late life. *British Journal of Psychiatry, 174*, 307-311.

Copeland, J.R.M., Beekman, A.T.F., Dowey, M. E. et al. (1999). Depression in Europe. Geographical distribution among older people. *British Journal of Psychiatry, 174*, 312-321.

Downes, J.J., Davies, A.D.M., Copeland, J.R.M. (1988). Organization of depressive symptoms in the elderly population: hierarchical patterns and Guttman scales. *Psychological Aging, 3*, 367-374.

Flint, A., and Rifat, S. (1995). Augmentation strategies in refractory depression. *International Journal of Geriatric Psychiatry, 10*, 137-146.

Gallo, J.J., Ryan, S.D., Ford, D.E. (1995). Attitudes, knowledge and behavior of family physicians regarding depression in late life. *Archives of Family Medicine, 8*, 249-256.

Katona, C.L.E., Freeling, P., Hinchliffe, K. et al. (1995). Recognition and Management of depression in late life in general practice: a consensus statement. *Primary Care Psychiatry, 1,* 107-113.

Katona, C.L.E., Hunter, B.N., Bray, J. (1998). A double-blind comparison of the efficacy and safety of paroxetine and imipramine in the treatment of depression with dementia. *International Journal of Geriatric Psychiatry,13,* 100-108.

Katona, C., and Judge, R. (1996). Antidepressants for elderly peoples: Can the use of selective serotonin reuptake inhibitors (SSRIs) be justified? *Primary Care Psychiatry 1996, 2*, 123-128.

Katona, C., and Livingston, G. (2002). How well do antidepressants work in older people? A systematic review of number needed to treat. *Journal of Affective Disorders, 69*(1-3), 47-52.

Katona, C.L.E., Manela, M., Livingston, G. (1997). Comorbidity with depression in clder people: the Islington Study. *Aging and Mental Health, 1*, 57-61.

Kivela, S.L., Pahkala, K., E. (1989). Depressive symptoms and signs that differentiate major and atypical depression from dysthymic disorder in elderly Finns. *International Journal of Geriatric Psychiatry, 4*, 79-85.

Koder, D.A., Brodaty, H., and Anstey KJ. (1996). Cognitive therapy for depression in the elderly. *International Journal of Geriatric Psychiatry, 11*, 97-107.

Oxman, T.E., Barrett, J.E., Barrett, J., et al. (1990). Symptomatology of late-life minor depression among primary care patients. *Psychosomatics, 31*, 174-180.

Prince, M.J., Peischies, F., Beekman, A.T.F. et al. (1999). Development of the EURO-D Scale-a European Union initiative to compare symptoms of depression in 14 European Centres. *British Journal of Psychiatry, 174*, 330-338.

Reynolds, C.F., Jupfer, D.J., Houck, P.R., et al. (1988). Reliable discrimination of elderly depressed and demented patients by electroencephalographic sleep data. *Archives of General Psychiatry, 45*, 258-264.

Reynolds, C.F., Frank, E., Perel, J.M. et al. (1992). Combined pharmacotherapy and psychotherapy in the acute and continuation treatment of elderly patients with recurrent major depression. *American Journal of Psychiatry, 149*, 1687-1692.

Reynolds, C.F., Frank, E., Perel, J.M. et al. (1999). Nortriptyline and interpersonal psychotherapy as maintenance therapies for recurrent major depression: a randomized controlled trial in patients older than 59 years. *Journal of American Medical Association, 281*, 39-45.

Yesavage, J.A., Brink, T.L., Rose, T.L. et al. (1983). Development and validation of a geriatric depression screening scale: a preliminary report. *Journal of Psychiatric Research, 17*, 37-49.

SECTION - V
Intervention Strategies

19

"Pancha-Kosha" Purification in Mental Health Management: With Reference to Aging Women

B.M. Palan

Introduction

The spiritual teachings of *Vedanta* describe a concept, *"Pancha-kosha"*. It is suggested that the "I", the consciousness, is constantly operating from or identifying with one of the five sheaths (*Pancha-kosha*). Purification of these sheaths by the use of several techniques suggested in the system of eight fold *Yoga (Ashtang Yoga)* and by remaining aware about certain spiritual concepts can contribute to breaking the vicious cycle of stress and aging and thereby reduce the risk of development of age-related biological changes – the rate of aging.

Relation between stress and aging in general (Selye, 1956) and cellular aging in particular (Epel et al., 2004), the theory of *Pancha-kosha* with its relevance to perception of stress and various *Pancha-kosha* purification techniques have been discussed in this paper.

Biomarkers of Biological Aging

Chronological age is simply the number of years since the person was born. The WHO classifies those aged 65–75 as the 'Young

Elderly', those aged 75–85 as 'Old' and those over 85 years as 'Oldest Old'. Generally, the young elderly are physiologically similar to those in the younger age group.

The biological age, which is more important, can be calculated from the scores on a battery of tests of biomarkers of aging. The tests measure aging in four broad categories: (1) Motor functions (muscle movements), (2) Sensory functions (perception of various senses like, vision or hearing), (3) Cognitive functions (higher functions of brain like, thinking, decision making or memorizing) and (4) Pulmonary functions (lung functions are one of the earliest biomarkers to deteriorate predictably with aging).

More recently, biomarkers of 'Cellular Aging' are identified. They are telomeres and telomerase enzyme. Telomeres are the caps at the ends of chromosomes. With every cell division, the length of telomeres is reduced. The enzyme telomerase helps rebuild telomeres but its level naturally declines with advancing age. So, in the natural aging process, telomeres eventually get so short that cells can no longer divide and they then die. As more and more cells die, the inexorable process produces the signs of aging, like, weakening of muscles, wrinkling of the skin, fading eyesight and hearing and diminishing thinking ability.

Stress and Aging

Hans Selye (1950), the father of stress physiology, explained that stress is cumulative and it affects aging. He demonstrated that with every exposure to a stressor (a demand for adjustment), the individual's adaptability – stress coping ability is reduced if it happens to be a distress (unhealthy stress wherein the person fails to cope up with the demand), as shown in the following diagram. But if it happens to be a eustress (healthy stress wherein the person is successfully able to cope up with the demand, i.e., s/he is able to make the necessary psychological and biological adjustment), the adaptability increases.

Whenever a person is exposed to a stressor, some of the reserve of adaptability is utilized. When the stress period is over, the system will come ***almost*** back to the baseline, but not exactly to the baseline. Certain amount of adaptability is exhausted. Upon exposure to a stressor next time, the person will utilize his/her adaptability

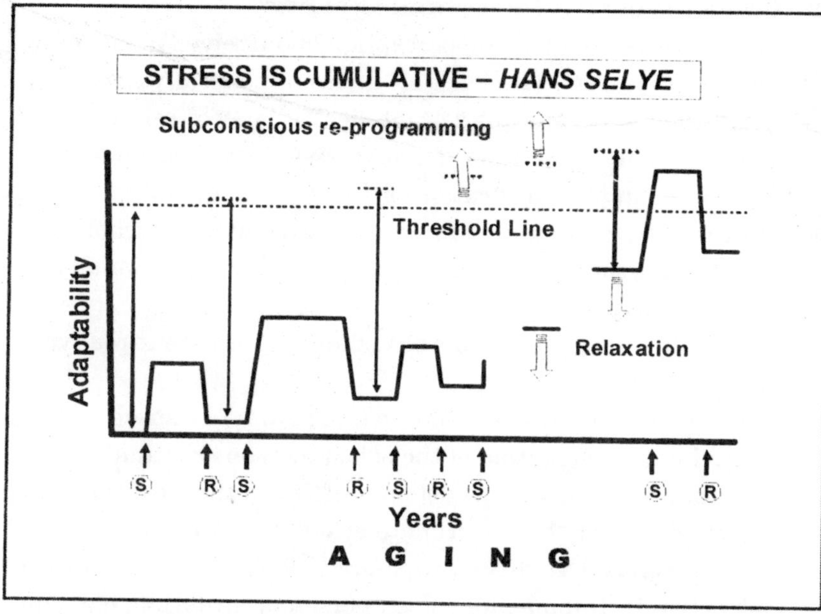

from the new baseline. At the end of the stress period s/he will again come ***almost*** back to the base line. Like this, over a period of time the person's adaptability is reduced. This is called aging by Selye. (Along with the base line, the threshold line is also raised. If it happens to be a eustress, the threshold line rises more than the base line and ultimately adaptability is increased).

Recently, Elissa Epel and her colleagues (2004) have demonstrated that chronic stress – and especially, how a person perceives stress – reduces telomerase activity with a significant impact on the length of telomeres in immune system cells indicating cellular aging.

Mental Health of Aging Women

The aging women face increasing obstacles to their mental health due to a number of factors like, their life course medical history and present physical health, lifestyle, work, social protection, care-giving responsibilities, socio-economic status, marital status, access to health services, dependence on other family members and their long-term exposure to gender-based violence, unremunerated labor and discrimination. In turn the mental health and perceived stress will influence their aging process.

The Concepts of "I", "I-ness" and "Reality"

The impression of or the perception of ourselves in our mind is called ego or "I-ness". The sense of "I-ness" is generally associated with (identified with) our mind or intellect or body or relationship/ social status. The sense that "I am stressed" or "I am aging" is actually the result of identification of "I-ness" with the mind or with the body respectively. Sigmund Freud explains that the psychological aspect of our personality which helps us in thinking rationally on the basis of ***reality*** is ego.

According to the teachings of Vedanta, there are three types of realities or *satta*:

(1) The perceptual reality (*Aanubhavik satta*) is based on the individual's perception of the object, person or situation, e.g. "the sun is rising in the east and setting in the west" or "I am good or bad" or "I am fortunate or unfortunate".

(2) The empirical reality (*Vyavaharik satta*) is based on the objective fact about the object, person or situation, e.g. "the earth is moving around its axis and whichever part of the earth is coming in front of the sun there a person will sense that as though the sun is rising" or "I am tall" or "I am aging".

(3) The absolute reality (*Parmarthik satta*) is "I am (and also the whole universe is) a pure, absolute, eternal and blissful consciousness". So acceptance of absolute reality means realizing that the consciousness is manifested in the form of the sun over there, it is the same consciousness manifested in the form of this earth and also I, by myself (the witness of the sun and this earth) am the same consciousness.

The Concept of Pancha-kosha

The pure, absolute, eternal blissful consciousness – I, always remains identified with (or operates from) one of the five *koshas* (sheaths).

Annamaya kosha **(Food sheath):** This includes the external physical body. When a person thinks (says or believes), "I am tall" or "I am beautiful or handsome", s/he is operating from her/his *Annamaya kosha*. S/he assumes that s/he is the body which actually is tall or beautiful or handsome.

***Pranamaya kosha* (Vital sheath):** This includes biological processes and their consequences (instincts or diseases). When a person senses that "I am thirsty" or "I am hungry" or "I am weak" or "I am suffering from diabetes", s/he is operating from her/his *Pranamaya kosha.* (Actually reduction in fluid volume or increase in electrolyte concentration in the body is causing activation of 'thirst center', situated in the hypothalamus of brain, and it is sensed by the individual as thirst.)

***Manòmaya kosha* (Mind sheath):** This refers to the mind or thoughts and feelings. When a person says or perceives that "I am angry" or "I am sad" or "I am frightened", s/he is said to be operating from her/his *Manomaya kosha.* The anger or sadness or fear is a feeling created in her/his mind. But the person identifies with this emotion and gets totally indulged into the particular feeling.

***Vigyanamaya kosha* (Intellect sheath):** This is the knowledge. When a person says that "I know" or "I don't know" or when a person is using intellect or knowledge in performing any task, s/he is operating from the *Vigyanamaya kosha.*

***Anandmaya kosha* (Bliss sheath):** This is the presence of pleasure, joy or ecstasy in the mind. Generally an individual will identify with this *kosha* when s/he gets the object, person or situation which s/he desired to have or when s/he is able to get rid of an object, person or situation which s/he wanted to get rid of.

Originally the concept of *Pancha-kosha* was utilized by the *shastras* or the *Guru* for explaining to the disciple the real nature of the 'self', the consciousness, the absolute reality by negation of each of the five *koshas.*

Purification of Koshas

The mental health of a woman is the outcome of interplay among her identification with different *koshas* under different circumstances.

While she is identified with her *Annamaya kosha* she is "the physical I". Another functional part of the 'physical I' is identification with *Pranmaya kosha.* She would like to have a good looking, active, alert and healthy body. Consumption of *shuddha, satvik* and vegetarian diet, observing the five *Niyamas,* practicing *Yogasana, Pranayama* and *Satkarma* are the recommendations by the *shastras* for purification of *Annamaya and Pranmaya koshas.* Ultimately understanding (in the *Vigyanmaya* kosha) the illusion (*maya*) and thereby thinking that "it is the body which is growing old and as I love my body, it is the tool by which I am living my life in this world, I wish to take loving care of my body" will make her proactive (for better care of her body) but prevent her from going into depression.

When the woman is identified with her *Manomaya kosha,* she is 'the mental or emotional I'. One would like to be calm, secure, content (in the present), ambitious (for a brighter future), confident and cheerful mentally. Practice of *Yoganidra* (which include *shavasana, pratyahara, dharana and dhyana*) gradually brings this kind of mental state in a person under most situations of life. By subtle observation of her own and other's lives one can realize (in the *Vigyanamaya kosha*) that the life is actually a journey for becoming more mature emotionally; every event and situation is a well designed incident for serving this purpose only.

The 'intellectual I' is identification of 'I ness' with *Vigyanamaya kosha.* One would like to be achieving and remaining open to learn with sharp and subtle intellect. Learning and internalizing the knowledge of *shastras* by a continuous process of *shravan* (listening the spiritual discourses from an able teacher), *manan* (introspection or contemplation) and *nididhyasana* (meditation or self-hypnosis) gradually purifies the *Vigyanamaya kosha.* Inculcation of rational and empowering knowledge will make the person objective while considering achievements in the empirical life. One may slowly then observe the natural order – the laws of nature (physical order, biological order, psychological order and social order) to be the manifestations of the ultimate absolute reality.

In a normal ordinary human being, generally identification with the *Anandmaya kosha* takes place upon acquiring the object, person or situation which the individual wanted to possess or upon getting rid of the object, person or situation which one did not like. This is the 'social I'. One would like to be loving, caring, non-projecting and non-judgmental socially. Surrendering to God and having value of moral values (following *Yamas*) will make the *Anandmaya kosha pure* and then it is possible for a person to accept the objects, persons or situations gracefully and with understanding.

Yogadarshan recommends having specific types of attitude towards four different types of people: sharing happiness with the happy, having compassion towards the unhappy, developing friendship with the gentleman and indifference towards a bad man.

With consistent practice of recommended techniques and wisdom, a woman can develop a healthy state of dissociation (internally) of herself from the issues related to her body, mind, intellect or relationships and yet remain proactive (externally) towards each one of them. This kind of attitude will then convert stressors and problems into events or rather opportunities of growth for the individual. The present life situation and experiences of past – which were interpreted as good or bad – are now understood as the stepping stones for her growth and maturity. They now no more cause distress. This will in turn lead to reduction in the rate of development of age related biological and psychological changes – reduction in the rate of aging.

References

Selye, H. (1956). *The Stress of Life*. New York: McGrawHill (revised edition, 1976).

Epel, E. S., Blackburn, E. H., Jue Lin, Dhabhar, F. S., Adler, N. E. Adler, Morrow, J. D., Cawthon, R. M. (2004, December 1). Accelerated telomere shortening in response to life stress (on-line). *Proceedings of the National Academy of Sciences of the United States of America (PNAS), 101*(49), 17312-17315. Available at: http://www.pnas.org/cgi/reprint/101/49/17312 ?ijkey=35ccad81f7308bb149a872be5 444a 8d8e27c0f4b

20

Dealing with Depression During Menopause: Recommendations from Praxis[1]

Monali Desai

"It is sad to grow old, but nice to ripen."
- Brigitte Bardot

Association between Depression and Menopause

Menopause, 'meno' meaning menses and 'pause' meaning stops, occurs due to loss of follicles in the ovaries of women. During the menopause, the process of ovulation stops and estrogen hormone levels decline. This brings about a range of short and long term effects. Among the short term complaints are primarily hot flashes, night sweats, irritability, mood swings and depression. Though most researchers disagree about the link between menopause and depression and believe that menopause itself does not induce depression, it is commonly acknowledged that a definite change does occur in a woman's mental health during menopause. In the brain, estrogen is believed to increase the concentration of serotonin, which helps transmit "feel good" messages to the brain. Low estrogen levels during menopause may be responsible for depression or "feel low" factor.

The Melbourne Women's Midlife Health Project, the New England Research Institute study, and similar other studies have found that depression is associated more with stressful life events, life changes or 'midlife crisis' than to hormonal changes during menopause. The Melbourne Women's Midlife Health Project found prior negative mood, history of premenstrual complaints, negative attitudes toward aging or menopause, poor health, and daily hassles to predict depressed mood (Dennerstein et al., 2004). The New England Research Institute study found that menopausal women are no more depressed than the general population (Bacarat, et al., 2002).

Research has shown that women with a history of depression are at a greater risk of relapse during perimenopause. Also, studies indicate that depressed women begin perimenopause earlier than non-depressed women. Hay in 1994 carried out a six-month study in Edinburgh on 95 women, of whom 78 were in the perimenopausal stage. Of these 78 women, 63 per cent suffered from depressive disorder at some time in their life and 37 per cent of all episodes occurred within the period of perimenopause.

Mild to moderate depression, which may not be diagnosed gets aggravated during menopause resulting in a high number of women presenting it during this period. Among the 20 depressed patients between 40-50 years of age studied recently at Vadodara in 2004, 10 per cent had severe depression and 60 percent had moderate depression and 30 per cent had mild depression as per the Beck's Depression Inventory (Desai and Mehta, 2004).

Dealing with Depression during Menopause

In Indian women, menopause occurs at an average age of 47 years. Indian society being a male dominated one, a woman's experiences during menopause may be influenced by other life changes, such as: children leaving home, changes in domestic, social and personal relationships, anemic status and poor diet, divorce or widowhood, retirement, increased anxiety about illness, aging and death, lack of financial security, increased responsibility for aging parents.

Life style modification is the most important option to treat depression during menopause. The main changes that need to be advocated are: a positive attitude, dietary changes and regular exercise.

Adopting a positive attitude

Ask a woman – How do you view menopause? Is it the end of the book or the beginning of a wonderful new chapter? If she describes it as the end of a book then she is probably going to suffer a number of perimenopausal and menopausal complaints, ranging from hot flashes to depression. But if she describes it as the beginning of a new and wonderful chapter in her life, then all 'hot flashes' will be 'power surges' and the energy derived from them will keep her miles away from depression. Instead of menopause being the end of fertility, it will be an invitation to a thousand other ways of being productive. Indeed, it is all about adopting a positive attitude!

Positive attitude is a subjective concept, depending on one's family history, nutrition, general health, life circumstances and several other factors. However, by making healthy lifestyle choices all women can acquire it. Large multicentric studies have shown that women who had a more positive attitude towards menopause were less likely to be concerned about body changes or looking older, and they were also less likely to report depression.

There are also great achievers among Indian women to look up to for inspiration. Their achievements, for the most part, have happened during their menopausal age. Indira Gandhi, the former Indian Prime Minister, has discussed at length in her biography, the difficulties that she faced during her menopausal period and how she turned to yoga to overcome them. Another example is from Kolkatta, Mother Theresa, who continued to work tirelessly for society long after her menopause. Here spirituality and strong inner drive to do something are highly visible. And then there are Lata Mangeshkar, the nightingale of India, and M. S. Subbalakshmi, who, though well past their prime, continue to enthrall audiences with their dedicated work. It becomes the foremost duty of health care providers and primary physicians to women to encourage a positive attitude in women.

Some of the common situations faced by menopausal women are lack of creativity, widening generation gap, declining interest in sex, and loneliness on account of their children leaving home. These can be dealt with a positive change in their attitude by:

Being creative: Art can be a key to the door of the inner mind, externalizing thoughts and feelings and thus giving insight into hidden concerns that may be preventing a person from achieving full potential in life.

Higher education, marriage, career and children can be a continuously draining experience for a woman in her middle age. But then comes menopause. This can bring an empty void to some or a whole lot of time for creative things and opportunities to take up creative work that was never taken up due to other familial or career preoccupations. Menopause must be viewed as a time to sit back and relax, as a time for oneself.

Unfortunately human nature tends to fall into inertia. That should be recognized. If women are coaxed into cooperativeness, if spontaneity exists and they are made to realize how great they felt in times of creativity, each woman can create a work of art.

A housewife engaged in daily routines of cleaning, cooking, looking after children and the elderly can do the same as a daily challenge in a creative sense. One's daily life presents creative opportunities continuously, and if a woman can be part of the creative process going on all around her in nature, she develops a sense of fulfillment which is very essential for her mental health. A living example is Tarla Dalal, the celebrity chef, who has revolutionized Indian cooking. Similarly, a woman's experience and her creative ability can make her the most sought after senior at her work place and prevent her from falling into depression.

Narrowing the generation gap: As India is becoming younger, with a growing population of young people, menopausal women may seem invisible or undesirable to the young. This should never depress menopausal women because old wisdom never dies. Modern menopausal women should be ready to recognize their role, adapt themselves to it and use their wisdom to gracefully teach and handover the responsibilities to the next generation.

Enjoying the increased libido: Night sweats, hot flashes, trouble sleeping, irritability, anxiety about looking older, and tendency for weight gain, these unpleasant symptoms are commonly considered as obstacles to desire. On the contrary, many women may experience increased interest in sex (Morokoff, 1988), especially a there is no fear of pregnancy. However, there are reservations of sexual activity after a certain age, which may depress women. Women must adopt a positive attitude to in this regard.

Letting the young ones fly: Just as mother birds let their little ones fly to build their own nests and find their own food, and their own mates, children leaving home must be seen as the biggest achievement for a parent. It signifies good parenting and support that has helped the child to now move ahead towards better life prospects and higher goals.

Making diet alterations

High fiber, low fat, high calcium and food rich in soya isoflavones help in countering menopausal depression. Soya is a source of phytoestrogen isoflavones. The mild estrogen effect of soya can ease menopausal symptoms for many women, without creating estrogen related problems. Soyabeans are the richest food source of phytoestrogen. Other sources of phytoestrogens, which are sufficiently strong to help limit menopausal symptoms, are linseeds, chickpeas, whole wheat and oats. There are around 300 different plant foods which give us protection and a diet rich in vegetables, grains and pulses, as well as soya and linseeds is likely to be the answer to many menopausal problems. Soyabean works like an anti-aging pill. It contains isoflavones like genistein, diadzein that have a positive effect on bone health, sex drive, heart disease, vaginal dryness, depression, insomnia (sleep disturbances), etc. Genistein in soya is a potent antioxidant with anticancer properties. A recent study has demonstrated that isoflavones have potent antioxidant properties comparable to that of vitamin E. The anti-oxidant powers of isoflavones can reduce the long term risk of cancer by preventing the free radical damage to DNA. Genistein is the most potent among antioxidants among soy isoflavones, followed by daidzein. Soya helps lower cholesterol, triglycerides and regulates blood sugar levels. Patel and Mehta (2003) conducted a study on 20 institutionalized elderly age 60 years and above in Baroda. A significant ($p<0.005$) reduction was obtained in Tc, TG, HDL-C, LDL-C, TC/HDL and LDL/HDL ratio after supplementing 25 gm of soya bean for a period of 6 weeks. Therefore it plays a definite role in heart disease prevention in post menopausal women. Phytoestrogens in soya have a direct benefit on bone health (Potter et al., 1998).

In another study on soya supplementation in depressed women in Vadodara (Desai and Mehta, 2004), 60 mg/day soya isoflavone in tablet form was given as supplement to 20 depressed menopausal women for 6 weeks and has shown encouraging results. Severe depression was reduced from 10 per cent to zero, moderate depression was reduced from 60 per cent to 10 per cent, and the number of women having mild depression was reduced from 30 to 50 per cent. In case of life satisfaction, a majority of the subjects were rated as fully satisfied. A significant change (0.05) was observed in serum cholesterol, which reduced from 203.8± 37 to 176 ± 29.8 mmole/L with a t-value of 4.92 indicating the lipid lowering effect of soya isoflavone. A larger study with longer study period may show a profound improvement in the mental health of women on soya supplements.

A four-month controlled trial reported in the Journal of Obstetrics and Gynecology March 2002 (Han et al., 2002) examined 80 postmenopausal women between 45 and 55 years, who were assigned to receive either 100 mg of soy isoflavones per day or placebo. Frequency and severity of 11 different menopausal symptoms were measured by questionnaire before and after treatment. Blood cholesterol and sugar levels, blood pressure, body mass index (BMI, a measure of obesity) and reproductive hormones were measured at the same intervals. The results showed a significant decrease in menopausal symptoms and improvement of mental health from the beginning to the end of the study in women taking soya isoflavones. In addition, menopausal symptom scores in women taking soya isoflavones were 40 per cent lower (indicating less severe symptoms) than in those taking a placebo, a statistically significant difference. Compared with the placebo group, the soya group had a significant reduction in total cholesterol and LDL ("bad") cholesterol, suggesting that soya has heart-health benefits as well.

Improving physical strength with exercise

Regular yoga for enhancing both bodily flexibility and mental health, combined with 40-minute walks daily to improve cardiovascular fitness are essentials for all menopausal women. Physical fitness helps develop inner confidence to deal with existing situations keeping the women away from depression.

Conclusion

If a woman is depressed, then from time to time, she may experience agitation, irritation, disharmony, and suffering. And when a woman suffers from agitation, she cannot keep this misery limited to herself. She passes it on to others around her as well. The agitation permeates the atmosphere around the woman who is feeling miserable. Everyone who comes into contact with her, especially family members closest to her, also becomes irritated, agitated. This is certainly no way to live life. As medical practitioners and physicians treating women, we must emphasize positive attitude, diet alterations and physical fitness to help them deal with menopause and prevent depression.

The key message therefore must be: "Life is sacred. Celebrate life. Care for others and share whatever you have with those less fortunate than you. Broaden your vision, for the whole world belongs to you."

References

Baracat, E. C., Soares Jr., M. D, and Bang, A. (2002). Benefits of soy isoflavone therapeutic regimen on menopausal symptoms. *Obstetrics and Gynecology, 99*, 389-394.

Cassidy, A. et al. (1988). Biological effects of a diet of soy protein rich in isoflavones on the menstrual cycle of premenopausal women. *Journal of American Medical Association, 280*, 60-113.

Dennerstein L, Guthrie JR, Clark M, Lehert P, Henderson VW. (2004 Sep-Oct). A population-based study of depressed mood in middle-aged, Australian-born women. *Menopause, 11*(5):563-8.

Desai, M. and Mehta, P. (2004). *A study on diet, health and nutritional status of adult depressed women (40-50yrs) with and without soya isoflavone supplementation*. Unpublished master's dissertation, Department of Foods and Nutrition, The Maharaja Sayajirao University of Baroda, Vadodara, India.

Han, K. K., Soares, J. M., Haider, M. A., Rodrigues, de Lima, G., and Baracat, C. (2002). Benefits of soy isoflavone therapeutic regimen on menopausal symptoms. *Obstetrics and Gynecology, 99*, 398-94.

Hay, A., Bancroft, J., and Johnstone, E. (1994). Affective symptoms in women attending a menopause clinic. *British Journal of Psychiatry, 64*, 513-516.

Matthews, K. A., Wing, R. R., Kuller, L. H., Meilahn, E. N., Kelsey, S. F., Costello, E. J., and Caggiula, A. W. (1990). Influences of natural menopause on psychological characteristics and symptoms of middle-aged healthy women. *Journal of Consulting and Clinical Psychology, 58*, 345-351.

Morokoff, P. J. (1988). Sexuality in perimenopausal and postmenopausal women. *Psychology of Women Quarterly, 12*, 489-511.

Patel, N., and Mehta, P. (2003). Effects of soya feeds on health and nutritional status of institutionalized elderly. Unpublished master's dissertation, Department of Foods and Nutrition, The Maharaja Sayajirao University of Baroda, Vadodara, India.

Potter, S.M., Baum, J., Teng, H., et al. (1998). Soy protein and isoflavones: Their effects on blood lipids and bone density in postmenopausal women. *American Journal of Clinical Nutrition, 68*(suppl),1375S-9S.

21

Brahmi: An Alternative Therapy for Depression in Elderly Women

Pallavi Mehta, Tejal Vasavda, Arpita Shah and Komal Chauhan

Introduction

Mental disorders are diseases that affect cognition, emotion, and behavioral control and substantially interfere both with the ability of children to learn and with the ability of adults to function in their families, at work, and in the broader society. Mental disorders tend to begin early in life and often run a chronic recurrent course. They are common in all countries where their prevalence has been examined. Because of the combination of high prevalence, early onset, persistence, and impairment, mental disorders make a major contribution to the total disease burden.

Depression is the most common of mental disorders. Ranked as the fourth leading cause of disease burden globally, it represents the single largest contributor to nonfatal burden (Ustun et al., 2004). In the year 1990, depression ranked fourth among the ten leading causes of the total worldwide disease burden, measured in disability-adjusted life years. By the year 2020, depression is projected to rank second, accounting for 5.7% of the total disability-adjusted life years, compared to 2.6% for HIV. Furthermore, depression is expected to become the number one cause of disease burden among females in developing countries (Lopez and Murray, 1998).

Depression can be caused by many factors both genetic and biological. Individuals may have a genetic makeup that makes them prone to depression, or stressful events like the loss of a close one, could also be a cause. The depletion in the levels of neurotransmitters in the brain (Serotonin and other chemicals like dopamine, acetylcholine, norepinephrine largely act as antidepressants and tranquilizers), which are responsible for maintaining a sense of well-being that a person feels, is said to cause depression.

Clinical depression affects mood, mind, body, and behavior. Treatment can alleviate the symptoms in over 80 percent of the cases. Yet, because it often goes unrecognized, depression continues to cause unnecessary suffering.

Depression in Elderly Women

Depression is a pervasive and impairing illness that affects both women and men, but women experience depression at roughly twice the rate of men (Blehar and Oren, 1995). While researchers continue to explore how special issues unique to women—biological, life cycle, and psychosocial—may be associated with women's higher rate of depression, difference in female and male prevalence rates reflect the greater vulnerability of females to depression. Approximately 10 percent of women experience depression within a given year, compared to 6 percent of men; this gender differential continues across the lifespan (WHO Fact Sheets, 2004b).

Older age has been established as a major predictor for depression with 45.2% of women and 26.9% of men being afflicted by it by age 70 (Gottfries and Karlsson, 2004). As people age they become biologically vulnerable to depression. This is because of dysregulation of brain neurotransmitter secretion. Depression in the elderly could be a result of chronic illnesses. Certain medications have also been linked to depression in the elderly.

Depression in the elderly is often overlooked because the physical symptoms of depression are thought to be age related. Diagnosing depression may be difficult in late life due to the complex relationship between depression, serious physical illnesses and drug interaction in the older persons. Therefore an accurate diagnosis in this group is important.

Brahmi: A Treatment Option for Depression

Antidepressants, which are currently the most widely used treatment option, essentially enhance neurotransmission simultaneously increasing the levels of the neurotransmitters, especially serotonin. These drugs however are not free of side effects. Medication coupled with natural remedies has been known to be very effective in treating depression.

Herbal intervention is thought to be one of the treatment options to reduce the signs of depression and improve the cognitive function. Ayurveda, the most ancient medical system in the world with a wide acceptance, makes use of herbs such as Brahmi, Ginkgo biloba, Jiaogulan, Pumpkin seeds, Ashwagandha, and Ginseng for mental illnesses.

Brahmi (*bacopa monniera*), one of the common Ayurvedic herbs used for mental health related problems. Known as a 'brain tonic', as an effective "brain food", Brahmi is believed to nourish the brain and improve intelligence and memory. It has traditionally been used as an Ayurvedic *rasayana* or rejuvenative which helps to slow down to process of aging, particularly of the brain, as it increases mental clarity and brain functioning.

Brahmi contains saponins which have been shown to strengthen the nervous system, and decrease insomnia. It also has marked hypotensive and diuretic properties. It has been clinically proven and documented to be effective in improving cognitive function and promoting mental alertness (Roodenrys et al., 2002; Fitoterapia, 1995). It has also been fcund effective in reducing psychosomatic stress levels in patients suffering from anxiety neurosis, leading to lowered secretion of stress hormones (Singh and Singh, 2005).

As life expectancy continues to rise in virtually all populations throughout the world, the number of people reaching old age is increasing. There are currently 580 million peopie in the world who are aged 60 years or older. This figure is expected to rise to 1,000 million by 2020 – a 75% increase compared with 50% for the population as a whole. Older women will outnumber older men. Women, particularly in patriarchal social structures like in India, often lack necessary resources to maintain a healthy physical and mental status. In old age, these problems get compounded with deterioration in physical condition and unsupportive social environment.

Maintenance of physical and mental health is vital for well-being and quality of life in old age, so that older people may continue to make active contributions to society. Therefore it is important to implement appropriate interventions to address the common mental illnesses such as depression in the elderly population, particularly women.

As Brahmi has been traditionally used as a brain tonic and has proven results in clinical studies, it was thought worthwhile to undertake an intervention to study the effect of the herb on women, wherein Brahmi capsules were administered to the older women having depression with cognitive impairment.

Methods and Materials

The present intervention was a part of a larger community-based study of the physical and mental health of depressed aging women. The study examined the nutritional and health status of moderately depressed adult and older women (≥50 years of age) residing in Baroda city.

The community-based study was carried out in two phases:

In the phase I, 150 middle-income group women were selected from the free living population of Baroda city. The subjects were selected by purposive sampling technique and were screened for depression using the Beck's Depression Inventory (BDI). They were grouped into 3 categories (with 50 subjects in each) on the basis of their age as follows:

a) 50 – 59 years

b) 60 – 69 years

c) ≥70 years of age

The BDI used for diagnosis of depression comprises a scale having 21 questions with 4 options each as answer. Each answer has a score from 0-3. The total of all answers gives the extent of depression. Respondents who obtained scores in the range of 20-28, indicating moderate depression, were selected as subjects (Amin et al., 1996).

In Phase II, out of the 150 subjects, 30 (≥60 years of age) were selected for the intervention of brahmi supplementation. Further, they were categorized into experimental group (n =15 subjects) and control group (n =15 subjects) and the selection criteria were matched with respect to age, income (middle-income) and moderate BDI score.

Baseline data were collected from the selected subjects of the study with a pre-tested questionnaire. This included information on their socio-demographic background, activity and addiction pattern, mental health status, nutritional status, diet profile and disease profile. Clinical parameters – blood pressure and hemoglobin - were also measured. Intervention with brahmi supplementation was carried out for a period of 6 weeks, following which the post intervention data were collected.

Brahmi was given in the form of soft gel capsules (supplied by Soft Health Creations Pvt. Ltd.Vadodara to a group of 15 elderly female subjects having moderate depression along with impaired cognitive function. One capsule contained 250 mg of Brahmi extract (20 per cent bacoside content) in it. Three such capsules per day were given to the subjects for a period of 6 weeks. Thus women were given 750 mg of Brahmi extract (60 per cent bacoside content) per day for 6 weeks.

Besides the procedure mentioned above, an attempt was made to assess the mental health of the selected subjects by Mini-Mental Status Examination (MMSE) (Folstein et al., 1975), Cognitive Impairment Test (CIT) (Katzman et al., 1983), and the Self Esteem Rating. The MMSE is a test used to assess orientation, registration, attention, calculation, memory, language and visuospatial abilities of the subjects. The total of all the answers gives the extent of mental health. The cut-off was 23-25 and those who scored above 26 were considered normal (Folstein et al., 1975). The CIT test is used to assess the cognitive function of subjects. The score of 1 is given for each incorrect response, the maximum weighed error score is 28. A score of 0-11 indicates normal and 11-28 indicates abnormality (Katzman et al., 1983).

The Self Esteem Rating Scale contains 40 questions, each with 5 options and each having a score of 1-5. Out of 40, 20 questions are positive and 20 are negative. The total of all the answers gives the extent of psychological well-being. If the score is positive the subject is rated as having high self esteem, and if the score is negative, the subject is rated as having low self esteem.

Appropriate statistical tests were applied on the compiled data; Mean ± SD or percent responses were calculated for all the parameters expressed numerically. Paired t-test was applied to note the differences for the purpose of comparison.

Results and Discussion

Socio – demographic profile

A pre-tested questionnaire was used to obtain the socio-demographic information such as age, marital status, education, occupation, religion, ethnic group, per capita income, economic status and living arrangement of the 150 study subjects.

As can be seen from table 1, the number of widows is greater among women over the age of 60 (54 per cent women age 70 and above, followed by 32 per cent women aged 60-69). Almost all the subjects (97 per cent) were literate, with 76 per cent of women age 70 and above, and around 50 per cent each of the women between the ages 50-59 years and 60-69 years having completed at least school education. In the case of elderly women in the age groups of 50-59 yrs and 60-69 years, only 28 per cent and 18 per cent respectively were working, whereas among women age 70 years and above, only 12 per cent were working.

Table 1: Socio-demographic characteristics of the subjects belonging to three different age groups.

Sr. No.	*Characteristics*	*Age groups*			*Total N = 150*
		50 – 59 yrs n = 50	*60 – 69 yrs n = 50*	*70 + yrs n = 5 0*	
1.	**Age (Mean±SD)**	53.80 ± 2.9	63.26 ± 2.83	74.72 ± 5.39	63.93 ± 9.41
2.	**Marital Status (%)**				
	Unmarried	2 (1)	6 (3)	6 (3)	5 (7)
	Married	88 (44)	62 (31)	40 (20)	63 (95)
	Widow	6 (3)	32 (16)	54 (27)	31 (46)
	Divorced	4 (2)	0 (0)	0 (0)	1 (2)
3.	**Education (%)**				
	Illiterate	0 (0)	2 (1)	6 (3)	3 (4)
	School	50 (25)	56 (28)	76 (38)	61 (91)
	College	50 (25)	42 (21)	18 (9)	36 (55)

(Contd.)

(Contd.Table 1)

Sr. No.	*Characteristics*	*Age groups*			*Total N = 150*
		50 – 59 yrs n = 50	*60 – 69 yrs n = 50*	*70 + yrs n = 5 0*	
4.	**Occupation (%)**				
	Working	28 (14)	18 (9)	12 (6)	19 (29)
	Non-working	72 (36)	82 (41)	88 (44)	81 (121)
5.	**Religion (%)**				
	Hindu	100 (50)	92 (46)	94 (47)	95 (143)
	Muslim	0 (0)	2 (1)	0 (0)	1 (1)
	Others	0 (0)	6 (3)	6 (3)	4 (6)
6.	**Ethnic group (%)**				
	Gujarati	82 (41)	74 (37)	80 (40)	79 (118)
	Non-Gujarati	18 (9)	26 (13)	20 (10)	21 (32)
7.	**Per Capita Income (Rs.) (%)**				
	500 – 2000	24 (12)	46 (23)	28 (14)	33 (49)
	2001 – 3500	40 (20)	28 (14)	40 (20)	36 (54)
	3501 – 5000	36 (18)	26 (13)	32 (16)	31 (47)
8.	**Economic Status (%)**				
	Lower-middle	24 (12)	46 (23)	28 (14)	33 (49)
	Middle-middle	40 (20)	28 (14)	40 (20)	36 (54)
	Upper-middle	36 (18)	26 (13)	32 (16)	31 (47)
9.	**Living arrangement (%)**				
	Alone	0 (0)	4 (2)	10 (5)	5 (7)
	With spouse	10 (5)	20 (10)	20 (10)	17 (25)
	With family	90 (45)	76 (38)	70 (35)	78 (118)

Note: Figures in the parenthesis denote number of subjects.

The majority of the subjects were Hindu and all belonged to the middle income group. Regarding living arrangement, over three-fourths (78 per cent) of the subjects lived with their families. However, the number of women living alone was found to be higher among women in the older age groups.

As mentioned in the methodology, information was gathered on the mental health status of the subjects with the help of Beck's Depression Inventory Scale (BDI), Mini-Mental State Examination Scale (MMSE), Cognitive Impairment Test (CIT) and Self-Esteem Rating Scale.

The BDI scores of all the selected subjects from all the three age groups showed that they were moderately depressed. The MMSE found that out of 150 women, 65 per cent had moderate depression. The number of such women was greater in the 60-69 years age group (76 per cent).

Women who had severe depression were found in the age group of 70 years and above (10 per cent). Findings of the CIT showed that 65 per cent of women fell in the 'normal' category. However, as many as 52 per cent of women aged 70 years and above were found to be abnormal as per the CIT. The test showed that abnormality increased with increase in age, showing association between aging and decline in cognitive functioning. Thus all the tests administered to women to assess various aspects of their mental health strongly indicated a deterioration of mental health status with increase in age.

As mentioned earlier, in Phase II of the study, out of the 150 subjects, 30 (≥60 years of age) women with moderate depression, from the middle income group, were selected for the intervention of Brahmi supplementation. These 30 women were further categorized into experimental group (n=15 subjects) and control group (n=15 subjects). Women in the experimental group were given 750 mg of Brahmi extract (60 per cent bacoside) daily for a period of 6 weeks. Prior to the intervention, these women were assessed for their mental health status, nutritional status (in terms of anthropometric measurements – height, weight, mid-upper arm circumference, body mass index- and blood pressure, hemoglobin levels), their dietary intake, and physical health status, i.e. diseases they had. After 6 weeks of administration of Brahmi to the women, post intervention data were collected on these parameters to study the effect of the herb. The results are presented as under.

Impact of the Brahmi intervention on the mental health status of elderly women

Figures 1, 2 and 3, and Table 2 present the mean scores of the various tests conducted on women to assess their mental health status (BDI, MMSE, CIT and Self Esteem) before and after the intervention.

Figure 1: Percentage of depressed subjects showing degree of depression according to BDI scale before and after intervention

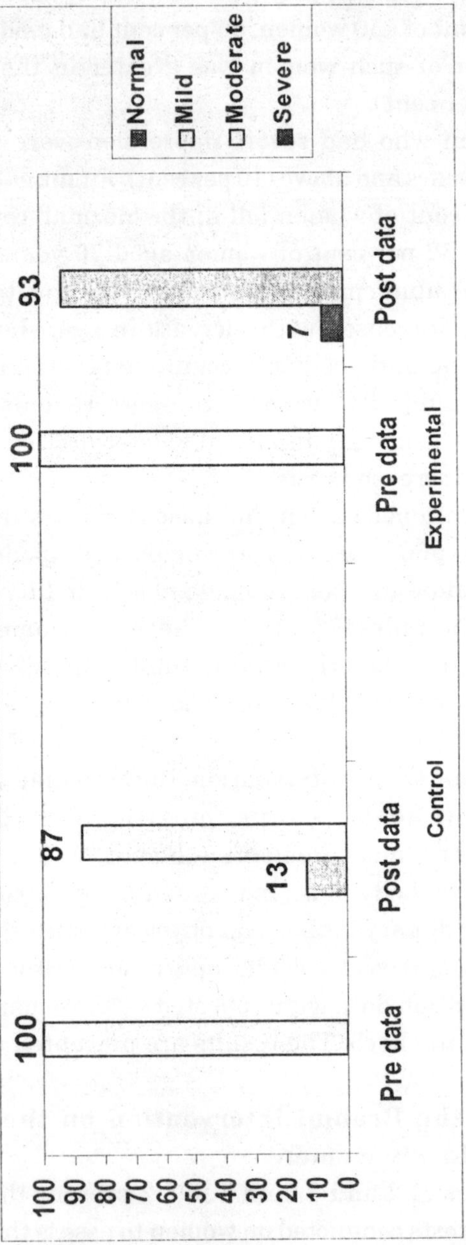

Figure 2: Percentage of depressed subjects showing degree of performance according to MMSE scale before and after intervention

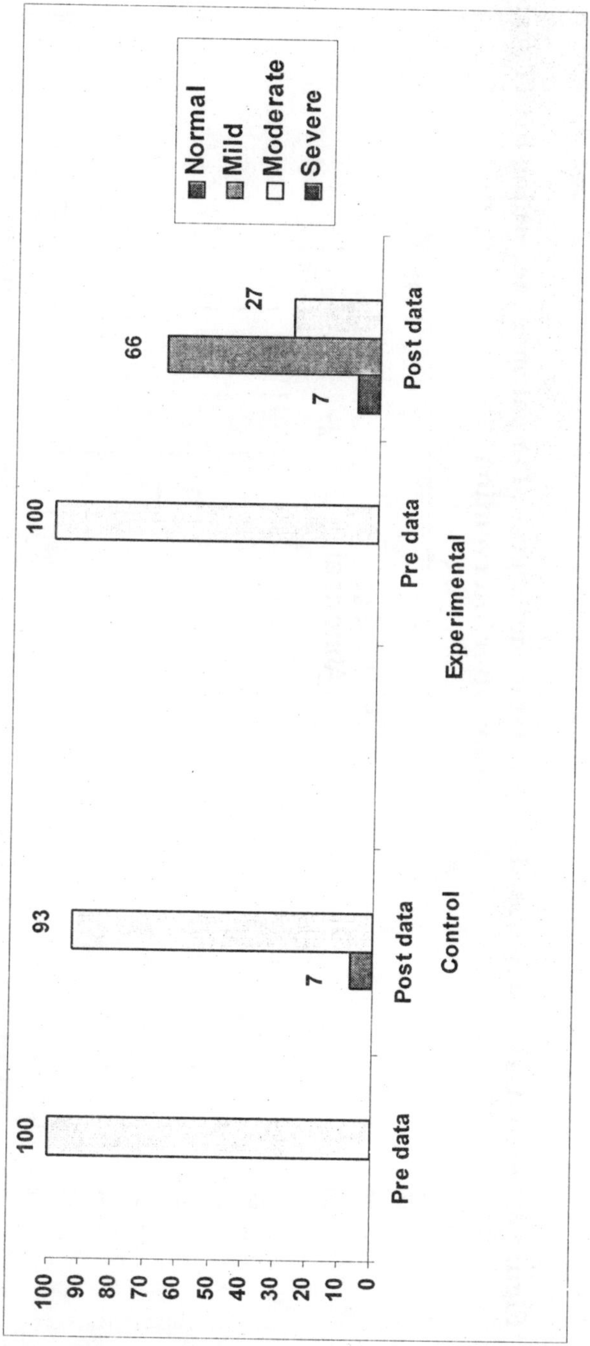

Figure 3: Percentage of depressed subjects showing degree of impairment according to CIT scale before and after intervention

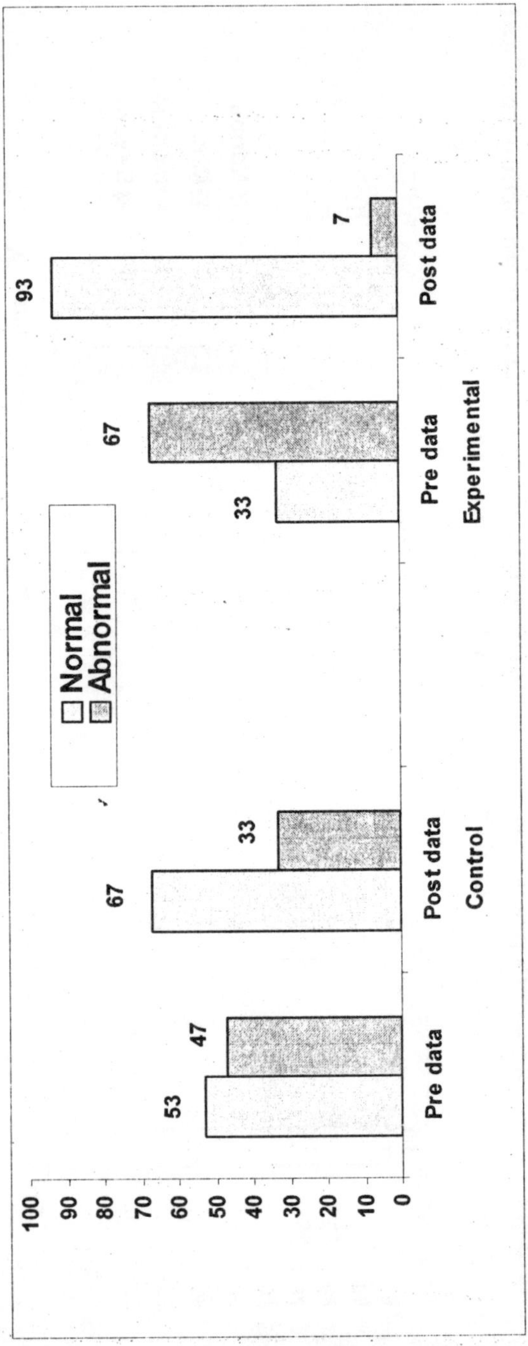

Figures 1, 2, and 3 indicate that there was an improvement in the level of depression in the subjects. Depression levels appear to have decreased significantly; as per BDI scores and MMSE scores showed that there was a shift of subjects from moderate levels to mild and normal levels of mental performance after the intervention. In case of CIT too, the percentage of subjects with cognitive impairment decreased and shifted to normal scores of CIT post intervention. Table 3 shows the mean scores of various tests for mental status of subjects.

Table 2: Mean scores of various tests for mental status of depressed subjects before and after intervention

Scale	*Control group (n = 15)*			*Experimental group (n = 15)*		
	Pre data	*Post data*	*'t' value*	*Pre data*	*Post data*	*'t' value*
Self Esteem	15.47 ±19.36	17 ± 17.49	0.482	17.06 ± 24.27	24.26 ±19.63	1.73

* $P \leq 0.05$

As can be seen from Table 2, there was a significant (p<0.05) improvement among the experimental group with regard to Self-esteem, where improvement in the scores of Self-esteem (significantly increased levels) were observed. Decrease in degree of depression (BDI score) shows improvement in other mental health parameters, indicating improvement in health of the elderly after intervention with Brahmi. These improvements were found with respect to significant changes in scores of MMSE and CIT (See Figures 2, 3 and 4).

Although such type of improvement was also seen among the control group in some parameters, however it was not very evidently significant. Thus one may conclude that the intervention with Brahmi showed a better impact on the elderly subjects.

A study conducted by Stough and others (2001) on 85 healthy volunteers using a dose of 300 mg Bacopa monniera standardized to 55% bacosides for a period of 12 weeks found a significant improvement in the speed of visual information processing, learning rate and memory consolidation.

Impact of Brahmi intervention on the nutritional status of elderly women

The nutritional status of the 30 elderly women selected for the intervention was assessed in terms of anthropometric measurements and biochemical estimation. The anthropometric measurements such as weight, height, mid-upper arm circumference (MUAC), body mass index (BMI) were taken using bathroom scale and measuring tape. The biochemical/ clinical parameters of nutrition were measurement of systolic and diastolic blood pressure levels and hemoglobin values of the subjects.

The results of Brahmi intervention for a period of 6 weeks did not show any significant impact on the physical health of the elderly subjects. In the experimental group however, a minor weight gain was observed. Not much change was seen in the control group. Thus intervention with Brahmi appeared to have had a more significant impact on the mental health of the elderly than on the physical health, suggesting the need for a long-term intervention.

Data on mean systolic and diastolic blood pressure levels and hemoglobin values of the 30 elderly women before and after the intervention showed a significant decrease in the level of systolic ($p<0.05$) and diastolic blood pressure of elderly subjects belonging to experimental group. No significant change was noted in the hemoglobin levels of experimental group on completion of the intervention. No changes were observed in regard of these two parameters among women in the control group.

Impact of Brahmi intervention on the dietary intake of elderly women

The dietary intake was assessed in terms of nutrient intake using 24-hour dietary recall for depressed subjects before and after intervention. The nutrient intake has been assessed in terms of energy, protein, fat, choline, folic acid, tryptophan, methionine, vitamin B6, vitamin B12 and vitamin C. Table 3 depicts the mean nutrient intakes of depressed subjects before and after intervention.

From the above table it can be seen that women in the experimental group showed a significant increase in the mean nutrient intakes in terms of choline, folic acid, tryptophan, vitamin B6 and vitamin C, whereas marginal increase was also found in the

Table 3: Mean nutrient intake of depressed subjects before and after intervention (n = 15, Mean ± SD)

Nutrient	*RDA*	*Control group*		*t-value*	*Experimental group*		*t-value*
		Pre	*Post*		*Pre*	*Post*	
Energy (kcal)	1875	1252 ± 207.1	1119± 201.4	1.18	1265 ± 205.1	1357± 141.8	2.023
Protein (gm)	50	25.40± 10.68	21.67± 4.98	1.39	28.33± 11.07	30.66± 8.02	1.22
Fat (gm)	20	23.13± 5.64	22.80± 5.52	0.16	25.40± 9.43	25.50± 7.84	0.07
Choline (ug)	30	20.13± 5.48	18.13± 5.22	1.32	22.67± 7.2	27.06± 6.25	2.98*
Folic acid (ug)	100	59.00± 25.15	47.67± 22.81	2.12	67.00± 33.66	85.00± 25.83	2.38*
Tryptophan (mg)	200	131.10± 27.29	131.33 ± 21.75	0.028	128.20± 25.5	144.70± 17.46	3.22*
Methionine (mg)	650	365.60± 121.3	319.30± 113.0	0.93	404.87± 81.68	435.47± 115.3	1.00
Vitamin B6 (mg)	2	1.15± 0.52	1.04± 0.25	0.73	0.77± 0.42	1.09± 0.38	2.44*
VitaminB12 (ug)	1	0.34± 0.3	0.43± 0.45	0.95	0.35± 0.299	0.45± 0.36	1.77
Vitamin C (mg)	40	25.26± 7.06	20.73± 7.72	2.48*	22.60± 5.28	29.46± 7.13	3.46*

* Significant at ≤ 0.05

intake of other nutrients such as energy, protein, methionine and vitamin B12($p< 0.05$). Low intake of majority of nutrients was found in the control group even after a period of six weeks. There was a significant ($p< 0.05$) decrease in the mean nutrient intake of vitamin C in the depressed elderly women subjects of the control group, whereas there was a marginal decrease in the mean nutrient intake of other nutrients such as energy, protein, choline folic acid, methionine, vitamin B6 and vitamin B12 which are the important nutrients for mental health.

A study conducted on 137 elderly volunteers who were studied for six years, found that those with higher intake of B complex and vitamins A, C, and E had better scores on tests of abstract reasoning and visual-spatial function (Rue et al., 1997).

As reported earlier in this section, the intervention with Brahmi for a period of 6 weeks showed a positive impact on the mental health of the elderly. Therefore it is likely that the decreased level of depression might have increased the appetite of the elderly women in the experimental group. Liking for foods like pulses, milk products, citrus fruits and green leafy vegetables showed significant increase intake of choline, typtophan, vitamin C, vitamin B6 and folic acid. These nutrients are found to be associated with mental health.

Brain neurotransmitters require choline as acetyl choline for normal functioning in the body. Therefore these nutrients act in the mechanism of the pathway enhancing the mental performance of the depressed subjects.

Thus in the present study, Brahmi intervention was found to have beneficial effect on the dietary intake of depressed elderly women subjects in the experimental group.

Impact of Brahmi intervention on the disease profile of elderly women

Data on the health and disease profile of the elderly women were collected using an exhaustive check-list. The prevalence of major and minor health problems of depressed elderly subjects before and after intervention is shown in Table 4.

From the above table, it can be observed that there was a slight reduction in the major health c   laints of the depressed

Table 4: Comparison of health profile in terms of number of health complaints of depressed subjects before and after intervention.

Disease profile	*Control group (n = 15)*			*Experimental group (n = 15)*		
	Pre data	*Post data*	*t value*	*Pre data*	*Post data*	*t value*
Major health problems	3.133 ± 1.64	3.133 ± 1.40	–	2.40 ± 1.50	2.00 ± 1.19	1.19
Minor health problems	11.87 ± 4.82	10.86 ± 4.53	0.92	12.20 ± 4.42	4.50 ± 2.10	7.33*

*** Values on ± S.D.**

elderly women from the experimental group. With regard to minor health problems, there was a significant ($p \leq 0.05$) reduction in the number of minor health complaints, thereby showing a positive impact of Brahmi. Compared to this, among the control group, a very slight reduction in the number of minor health complaints was observed.

Conclusion

From the present study, one may make the following concluding remarks:

- Age and severity of depression are the two major determinant factors for cognitive impairment in the old age.
- With the increase in age and level of depression the nutrient intake decreases.
- The disease profile showed deterioration in the health of depressed elderly women.
- Brahmi intervention seems to have beneficial effect in reducing level of depression, cognitive impairment and minor health complaints among elderly women.
- Deficiency of nutrients contributing to improvement in mental health can be considered as a risk factor for depression and cognitive impairment.

Beneficial effects of Brahmi were observed after intervention for a period of 6 weeks with respect to state of depression (as shown by BDI score), cognitive function (as shown by MMSE and CIT score), consumption of food intake and nutrient intake and health profile (as shown by reduction in number of health complaints and improvement in systolic blood pressure).

Thus this study indicates Brahmi Supplemented in as a part of an alternative therapy, Brahmi (supplementation of 60 per cent bacoside, 750 mg of Brahmi extract) has proven to be effective in improving the mental health status of moderately depressed elderly women.

References

Amin, G., Shah, S., and Vankar, G. K. (1998). The prevalence and recognition of depression in primary care. *Ind J of Psychiatry, 40*, 364–369.

Beekman, A. T., Deeg, D. J., Geerlings, S. W., Schoevers, R. A., Smit, J. H., and van Tilburg, W. (2001).Emergence and persistence of laie life depression: a 3-year follow-up of the Longitudinal Aging study, Amsterdam. *J.Affect.Disord., 65*, 131-138.

Bhatia, M.S. (2000). Psychiatric morbidity: An issue overlooked. *J Clin Psychiatry, 61*, 473-476.

Blehar, M.C. and Oren, D.A. (1995). Gender differences in depression. *Medscape Women's Health,* 1997; 2:3. Revised from: Women's increased vulnerability to mood disorders: *Integrating psychobiology and epidemiology. Depression,* 1995; 3:3-12.

Brown, M.N., Lapane, K.L., Luisi, A.F. (2002). The management of depression in older nursing home residents. *J Am Geriatric Soc 50*(1), 69-76.

Diane, M.E. and Susan, G. (2003).Gender differences in depression and response to antidynenant treatment. *Psychiatric Clinics, 26,* 581-594.

Federal Interagency Forum on Aging-Related Statitics. (2004). *Older Americans 2000: Key Indicators of Well-Being*. Washington DC: U.S Government Printing Office.

Fitoterapia. (1995). *Role of brahmi*. Italian journal, Vol. LXVI, No.3, pp. 216-222.

Folstein, M.F., Folstein, S.E. and McHugh, P.R. (1975). Mini-mental state. A Practical method for grading the cognitive state of patients for the clinician. *J Psychiatry Res, 12*(3), 189-98.

Gottfries, C. G. and Karlsson, I. (2004). *Depression in Later Life*. Oxford, UK: Sterling Press.human memory. *Neuropsychopharmacology, 27*(2), 279-81.

Jorm, A. F. (1987). Sex and age differences in depression: a quantitative synthesis of published research. *Aust N Z J Psychiatry 21*(1), 46-53.

Katzman, R., Brown, T., Field, P. et al. (1983). TITLE??. *American Journal of Psychiatry, 140*, 734-9.

Lebowitz, B. D., Pearson, J.L., Schneider, L.S. et al. (1997). Diagnosis and treatment of depression in late life. Consensus statement update. *JAMA 278*(14), 1186-1190.

Lopez, A. D. and Murray, C. C. (1998). The global burden of disease, 1990-2020. *Nat.Med, 4*, 1241-1243.

Mazure, C.M., Keita, G.P., Blehar. M.C. (2002). *Summit on women and depression: proceedings and recommendations*. Washington DC: American Psychological Association.

Nolen-Hoeksema, S. (1995). Epidemiology and theories of gender differences in unipolar depression. In M. V. Seeman (Ed.), *Gender and Psychopathology* (pp. 63-88). Washington, D.C.: American Psychiatric Press.

Prabhu, G.G. and Raghuram, A. (1987).*Mental Health in India in India. Encyclopaedia of Social Work in India, 2*, 188-189 (published by Ministry of Welfare, New Delhi).

Roodenrys, S. et al. (2002) Chronic effects of Brahmi (Bacopa monnieri) on

Rue, A., Koehler, K.M., Wayne, S.J., et al. (1997). Nutritional status and cognitive functioning in a normally aging sample: a 6 year reassessment. *Am J Clin Nutr,65*(1), 20–9.

Singh and Singh (2005). Bacopin: An alternative to antidepressants, cited Article from a magazine Sabinsa Corporation 2001 last Update 8-3-2005.

Stewart, D. E., Rondon, M., Damiani, G., Honikman, J. (2001). International psychosocial and systemic issues in women's mental health. *Arch Women's Mental Health, 4*: 13.7.

Stough, C., Lloyd, J., Clarke, J., Downey, L., Hutchison, C., Rodgers, T., and Nathan, P. (2001). The chronic effects of an extract of Bacopa monniera (Brahmi) on cognitive function in healthy human subjects. *Psychopharmacology (Berl), 156*(4), 481 – 484.

Ustun, T. B., J. L. Ayuso-Mateos, S. Chatterji, C. Mathers, and C. J. L. Murray. (2004). Global Burden of Depressive Disorders: Methods and Data Sources. *British Journal of Psychiatry, 184* (5), 386–92.

WHO. (2004). *Gender in mental health research*. Geneva: World Health Organization (WHO/HSC/SAB/04.11).

WHO. (2004b). *Mental and Neurological Disorders. Fact Sheet number 265.* Geneva: WHO

Epilogue

Some years ago, I told an Indian politician gaining national attention that his party's slogan, taking after former US President Harry Truman who campaigned with a slogan, "A chicken in every pot", should be, "A tap in every kitchen". I argued not only on the grounds of health, i.e. availability of potable water, but also that such ready access to a mainstay of life would free up untold hours of women, both rural and many urban, who toil in rain or heat. Given the controversy kicked up recently by the possibility of an Indo-US nuclear deal, I'd suggest that not just for the sake of the industrial economy but more importantly to relieve women from the tiresome hours spent in collecting fuel for their hearths, and cooking in smoke filled kitchens, the nation should embrace the option of generating electricity by nuclear energy.

This brings me full circle back to health and mental health of women. Here we have two elements, Water and Fire; add to that a third, the Wind and we have the three *doshas, Vata, pitta, and Kapha,* the principles of Ayurvedic pathophysiology. In both cases, that is the availability of water and supply of energy, my argument went farther in suggesting that the time saved by women, free from the physical and emotional drudgery, will improve their health, mental attitude, and relationships, with their husbands in marital intimacy, and their children improving the quality of childcare. Ergo, a solution to a complex set of psychosocial issues of the Indian family.

The volume at hand delves into many issues that plague the health and mental health of women. I had a very peripheral and insignificant role in the design of these studies, but nevertheless I'm pleased to add my two cents as an afterthought because I'm convinced that the principal and primary, nay, I shall say, single overriding objective of preventive mental health should be women's freedom from toil and emancipation from oppression in Indian society.

And this volume gives us a few good and close glimpses of the tasks ahead. From domestic abuse to the problems of aging, from depression to psychoses, from the adverse gender ratios to life style issues, the project conceived at the Maharaja Sayajirao. University's Women's Study Center and undertaken over the last several years. Both quantitative as well qualitative investigations and culling from the National Family Health Survey and the National Sample Survey have enriched our insights into the psychosocial problems of women, young and old, rural and urban. Investigators have also collected data on psychiatric illnesses from regional hospitals and independently analyzed them. To the best of my knowledge this is the only kind of attempt made to study the problem in such detail, at least in Gujarat.

The volume also contains several articles that are more of self help, health education, and doctorly advice. These attempts to be comprehensive makes me think of the Mahabharata or the Indian Cinema in the need to not leave too many questions unanswered. It is hoped that future volumes and I am confident that the Women's Study Center has a robust future, will separate these two aims, viz. in-depth investigation and self help advice.

Where might we go from here? Clearly there is a need to expand research efforts in many directions, and to bring together academics and researchers from wherever one might find them. While quantitative analyses offer a wide panoramic view of the problem, well knit individual narratives might offer an in-depth view of working of women's minds. It might even be useful to analyze characters in literature or the silver screen, from newspaper accounts to criminal court testimonies, of victims of domestic abuse and that of communal riots; there is gold in them hills there. Veena Das's "Language and Body: Transactions in the Construction of Pain" (Daedalus, Winter 1996, pgs 67-91) is a case in point.

A lot has been said about the mother-son dyad in India, but there is never enough. If the family nexus of both health and pathology from one generation to the next revolves around this central core we need case studies to focus on all the varied implications of where things go right and where they go wrong. Not only in Indian studies but in depth psychological literature worldwide, there is scant evidence of how the father-son relationship plays into the unfolding family drama, esp. in India where the father is a reported figure of distant authority for the son, and how this particular wrinkle affects women's lives. Another area that cries out for attention is the way young women confront choices of education, work- professional or otherwise, partners and lovers, their sisterhoods, their widowhoods and so on and so forth. The study of severe mental illness and the psychosocial implications of these illnesses might best be left to the psychiatric profession and centers like the one sponsoring this volume better save its scant resources for the way every day life of an *aam aurat,* to borrow and adapt from the current political lexicon, is lived.

Finally, let us welcome this singularly important attempt at giving us glimpses of lives of women in Gujarat with its focus on mental health and aging. I hope that the material presented here will have a wide readership and circulation, and that it will be a seed for many more studies to come. I certainly stand better informed and inspired.

Prakash N. Desai, M.D.
Professor of Clinical Psychiatry
Univ. of Illinois, Chicago
And
Associate Medical Director
Medical Center
Univ. of Illinois, Chicago.

Annotated Bibliography

Compiled by
Purnima Khanna

This bibliography is a descriptive annotation of the body of literature on Aging, Gender and Mental Health available at the Women's Studies Research Centre, M. S. University Baroda. The key words for selection of materials for annotation were 'aging', 'mental health', and 'women'.

Over fifty relevant works were located. These included both primary and secondary research and reviews published as articles in reputed journals (Journal of Clinical Psychiatry, Indian Journal of Gerontology, American Journal of Psychiatry, Social Science and Medicine), as chapters of edited books, essays, seminar/symposium papers, and as Internet publication and news paper article. These works cover a wide range of topics – beginning with psycho-social, economic and adjustment problems of the elderly, geriatric depression, geriatric psychiatry, health concerns of elderly women, diet pattern and diseases of elderly, postmenopausal women, in gender differentials in the prevalence of mental disorders, issues in the classification of mental disorder, causative factors of mental disorders, to alternative treatment options that go beyond psychotherapy, and reviews of the mental health practices, policies and programs, and non-governmental interventions in the mental health sector. The bibliographic entries are in alphabetical order, according to the names of the authors.

This annotated bibliography is by no means an exhaustive one. It is however hoped that these annotations will provide readers a quick overview about the existing body of research on the situation of the elderly, women in particular, and their mental health problems.

1. **Balambal, V. (2005). Problems of aging in lower strata, with case study. In Indira Jai Prakash (Ed.), *Aging in India: Retrospect and Prospect* (pp. 187-194). Bangalore: Bangalore University.**

This paper is an analysis of a case study of a woman senior citizen in a slum in Chennai. Due to the decline of joint family system, the elders face problems of loneliness, dependency, poverty and lack of security. In rural areas and slums in the cities they have to work for their survival too as they do not have any savings or pension. The elders at the lower strata of society suffer due to inadequate finance, health and hygienic conditions. There are innumerable women in Chennai slums bearing witness to male exploitation, overwork, responsibility, humiliation, sacrifice and service to the family.

2. **Bali, A. P. (1997). Elderly females: An ignored silent majority. In Kalyan Bagchi (Ed.), *Elderly females in India: their status and suffering* (pp-23-38). New Delhi: Society for Gerontological Research and HelpAge India.**

This paper was presented at the National Seminar on 'The Need for Focusing Attention on the Plight of Elderly Females in India' in 1996, New Delhi. The well-being of elderly females is dependent on several factors, namely social, economic and psychological as also their health. The cumulative effect of social vulnerability that started earlier in life has an impact on a woman's well-being by the time she reaches the later years of her life. In the domain of the family, elderly women suffer loss in status, when parental care-giving gives way to parental dependency, thus making them vulnerable to marginalization and social isolation. Other common factors for distress among elderly females are the 'empty nest' syndrome, widowhood and economic dependency, which bring in several changes for the individual in terms of their role playing and adjustments to be made at various stages.

3. **Barkham, M., and Hardy, G. H. (2001). Counselling and interpersonal therapies for depression: Towards securing an evidence-base. *British Medical Bulletin, 57,* 115-132.**

Both generic counseling (delivered by BACP level counselors in primary care settings) and the interpersonal therapies place a central value on the role and function of relationships – both within and outside the practice setting – as a vehicle for understanding and treating people presenting with depression. Recent studies have compared generic counseling with antidepressant medication, usual General Practitioner (GP) care, cognitive-behavior therapy (CBT) and as an adjunct to GP care (i.e., in combination with GP care). Findings suggest either that there is no difference between generic counseling and other treatment conditions, or that there are small advantages to counseling over usual GP care but only in the short term with such differences disappearing at 1-year. Studies investigating the interpersonal therapies have established that the content of such therapies differ in their content from behavioral and cognition therapies despite the outcomes being broadly similar. Considerable research effort has focused on the process of change in IP therapies. Important factors include the level of prior commitment by the patients to psychological therapy and their confidence in the therapist. Patents with well assimilated problems tend to do better in CBT than psychodynamic-interpersonal therapy. Therapists need to be flexible and responsive to patients needs particularly concerning interpersonal and attachment issues. Future research in counseling needs to identify the effective components of generic counseling and relate these to a theoretical base. In the interpersonal therapies, there needs to be a greater focus on the change outside the therapy session and on the effectiveness of such therapies in non-research settings.

4. **Blazer, D. G. Geriatric psychiatry. Chapter 37. In Robert E. Hales and Stuart C. Yudofsky (Eds.), *The American Psychiatric Publishing Textbook of Clinical Psychiatry* (4th. Edition) (pp. 1535-1549). Arlington, VA: American Psychiatric Publishing Inc.**

The seven geriatric syndromes – Acute confusion, insomnia, suspiciousness, hypochondriasis, memory loss, anxiety and depression - discussed in this chapter account for most of the psychopathology that both psychiatrists and geriatricians encounter while working with older adults. The syndromal approach permits the clinician to focus on the functional impairment that results from psychopathology and on the day-to-day management of the older person in both the hospital and the out-patient clinic. A syndromal approach also provides a more realistic conceptualization of late life psychopathology which often is comorbid across psychiatric diagnoses and comorbid with physical illnesses.

5. **Cherian, J. (2003). Adjustment of the Elderly in relation to living arrangement, gender and family life satisfaction. *Indian Journal of Gerontology, 17*(1&2), 99-108.**

This research explored the impact of living arrangement, gender and family life satisfaction on adjustment of the elderly. The study used factorial design, which analyzed the data collected through an Adjustment Inventory and Family life satisfaction Inventory for the elderly from 300 subjects aged between 60-79 years from Kottayam and Kozhenchery Talukas in Kerala, India. The Adjustment inventory has six measures such as home, social emotional, self, health and general adjustment. An analysis of variance done on the data revealed that there is a significant effect of (a) Living arrangement on emotional adjustment (b) Gender on general adjustment and (c) Family life satisfaction on emotional and general adjustment. The findings, in general, underscore implications of organizing programs for the elderly focusing on strengthening the familial bond with a particular note on the widowed group.

6. **Cohen, L. (1999). *No Aging in India: Modernity, Senility and the Family*. New Delhi: Oxford University Press.**

This book is about age, and about its appearance and disappearance in the making of knowledge. It is a study that focuses on how people comprehend the body and its behavior in time. The focus is on loss and decay: decay of the body, its reason, and its voice, its ability to be heard as a speaking subject. In other words the focus is on senility. The author has answered the question – Is senility best understood in terms of neuropathology and genetics; normative understandings and expectations of old age, dependency and individualism; or the economics and politics of families, nations and the world system. Snowball sampling has been used but on a different scale continually adding different sites and methods of inquiry to the project. The voices of older people are full with unsolicited memories, opinions and stories. The author (in a span of a decade) interviewed people in each of the Varanasi neighborhoods and institutions, in institutions in several other cities and towns across India and institutions in Boston, Montreal and Miami.

7. **Davar, B. (1999). Prevalence of mental distress in Indian women. In B. Davar (Ed.), *Mental health of women – A Feminist Agenda* (pp. 37-43). New Delhi: Sage.**

This is a review of the available information on prevalence of mental disorders in Indian women. The review points out that most Indian epidemiological studies have been based on hospital samples and not community samples. This data cannot be treated as prevalence data because there is no gender parity of access to hospital services. Various reviews such as Guttentag et al. (1980), Dennerstein et al. (1993) for the WHO, Russo and Green (1993), ECA study by NIMH have been analyzed. All studies point towards a greater prevalence of major depression, simple phobias, schizophrenia and somatization disorder among women. Men suffer more from alcohol and drug related disorders. Studies by Dube (1970), Sethi et al (1972), Verghese et al (1973), Nanti et al.(1975), Carstairs and Paun (1976) and Chakraborty (1990) have all shown gender difference. Diagnostic tools for mental disorders have also been discussed here.

8. **Davar, B. (2003, June). Women and mental health: Some concerns. *Perspectives* (double issue), 24-26.**

This paper traces the contribution of the women's movement in the area of women's mental health. In the women's movement, there was earlier a reluctance to talk in terms of 'mental illnesses.

It was realized that while it was necessary to guard against pathologizing female ways of being and expression, the experiential realities of psychological distress could not be ignored. The women's movement itself is a positive mental health movement as it gave multitudes of women the psychological strength to grapple with the social and political realities of their lives. Two major moves have been made by women's groups towards a woman-friendly mental health discourse 1) critique of mainstream practices in mental health and 2) creating an alternative woman-centered thinking in mental health. The paper also raises concern about the reliability of diagnosis across clinics in India as also over-prescription of drugs, needless psycho-surgeries and the use of electroconvulsive therapy.

9. **De Sousa, A. (2005). Geriatric Depression: A clinical update. *Indian Journal of Gerontology, 19*(1), 23-36.**

This review aims to provide the basic clinical features, the etiology of geriatric depression and the various treatment modalities available to tackle the problem of elderly generation. In geriatric depression it is not enough to get well, but it is staying well that matters. Women outlive men and the former outnumber the latter for all the types of depression. Presence of hypogonadins and thyroid abnormalities in the elderly risk factors for geriatric depression is widely suspected, besides cerebrovascular and neuroanatomical pathways. Depression is more common in left hemisphere stokes and is more common when lesions are anterior than posterior. Unfortunately very few elders admit the presence of depression. Most of them present with somatic complaints, multiple aches and pains and a large amount of anxiety, fear and hypochondriacal symptoms. A sizable number of the depressed complain of recurrent pain not responding to any medication.

10. **Department of Health and Family Welfare, Government of Gujarat. (2003). *The Mission Report 2003: Priorities for Mental Health Sector Development in Gujarat.* Gandhinagar: Author, pp. 57-63.**

This report has been commissioned and published by the Government of Gujarat. The report acknowledges the importance given to mental disorders in the global public health agenda of the last decade. It recognizes that meeting the enormous mental health needs in developing countries is complex; it must take into account diverse influences such as limited availability and utilization of services, low awareness and the associated stigma of mental disorders. Policy formulation must be informed by local research, which reflects the diverse realities and influences on the mental health sector. In this report common mental disorders, substance abuse, and severe mental disorders have been discussed. Data on special populations like children and women have been reviewed. The needs of children and women are addressed and risk factors for mental disorders identified. Some interventions to prevent mental disability have been suggested.

11. **Dutta Ray, S. (1993). The field of mental health in India: A contemporary and futuristic viewpoint. In P. Mane and K. Y. Gandevia (Eds.), *Mental Health in India: Issues and concerns* (pp. 327-34). Bombay: Tata Institute of Social Sciences.**

In this paper grim socio-cultural realities such as increasing population, urbanization, growth of urban slums, poverty, unemployment, illiteracy, disabled population have been discussed. The paper warns that these ground realities are significant in etiological terms or in preventive terms. If these crucial factors are not tackled the prevalence of mental ill health is likely to worsen in the form of neuroses, psychosomatic disorders, interactional and personality adjustment problems including substance abuse. The paper stresses the need for primary preventive policies and programs.

12. **Goldberg, C. (2005, June 16, Thursday). Emotional health checked by wire. *Health Science. International Herald Tribune*, p. 10.**

This article reports on a groundbreaking experiment at the Massachusetts General Hospital (Boston), wherein a handful of patients battling depression had agreed to be wired for all day mobile monitoring of their palm sweat, heart rate, voice dynamics and movement (using a system called LIVE NET). The study seeks to prove that technology has reached the point where it can monitor a persons' basic emotional tenor through ordinary days. To that end researchers are developing an easy-to-wear system that continuously gathers masses of information, then quickly crunches and transmits it, providing objective data to help with diagnoses and provide early warning when crisis nears. This study by D. Carl Marci, the Massachusetts General psychiatrist was expected to last about a year and observe 20 patients. In another study at the University of California at San Diego, researchers used a "Life Shirt" (a monitoring system that combines a variety of sensors in a shirt that patients wear all day and night) to record the chaotic movements that patients with bipolar disorders make during a manic phase. The article concludes citing Lisa Feldman Barret, a Boston College professor who researchers emotion, that for all their computerized sophistication, systems such as LIVE NeT and Life Shirt are not mind readers, they cannot for example say definitively that a patient is feeling anger or happiness

13. **Harris, T. (2001). Recent developments in understanding the psychosocial aspects of depression. *British Medical Bulletin*, *57*, 17-32.**

This paper discusses the recent developments in understanding the psychosocial aspects of depression. According to the author, recent advances in the psychosocial understanding of depression have elaborated an already complex etiological model. Although recent stressors have for some time been recognized predictors of onset, new insights about the origins of these stressors have overlapped with other new work on depression and childhood adversity to identify a group who 'produce' their own severe life events in response to early negative experience. And recent studies have traced the well known gender differences in depressive prevalence to differences both in gender role involvement with the provoking life events and in styles of support seeking/support giving.

14. **Jai Prakash, I. (2004). Mental health of older people in India. In P. V. Ramamurti and D. Jamuna (Eds.), *Handbook of Indian Gerontology* (pp. 176-207). New Delhi: Serials Publications.**

India is in the middle of a demographic transition and will soon join the ranks of an ageing nation with an older population of more than 7.7 per cent. There are an estimated 4 million old people with serious mental disorders and another 25-30 million with minor disturbances. This paper examines the mental health needs of older people and the response of the concerned professions to such demands. The material focuses more on recent findings and research carried out in the 90s.

15. **Jai Prakash, I. (1997, October). Women and ageing. *Indian Journal of Medical Research 106*, 396-408.**

This paper highlights the particular vulnerability of elderly women in graying populations. Demographic changes have forced gerontologists to focus attention on the gender based character of population aging. Aging is likely to become a 'gender issue' with a large number of women surviving into very old age in almost all the countries of the world. Elderly women, especially in Third World countries like India face several jeopardies. They are likely to be illiterate or have low level of education, unlikely to be employed, most likely to be widowed and dependent on others and they suffer from malnutrition and debilitating symptoms as well as report higher psychological distress. The paper calls for better understanding of the vulnerability of the aging women, special types of problems they are likely to encounter over the life span, and factors that marginalize them. It also recommends that strategies to ensure health and well-being of older women be developed.

16. **Jai Prakash, I. (2004, October). Health concerns of older women in India. *Helpage India – Research and Development Journal, 10*(3), 7-10.**

Longevity poses several human problems – probability of chronic illness and disability with aging, chances of dementia, increased health costs and reduced savings and absence of family support. In women most dramatic change occurs around the age of 50 with menopause. According to the author, the problem with Indian women is that they are married early during adolescence when the body is still developing and multiple pregnancies deprive the body of its nutrients. Therefore in old age there is an accumulation of disadvantages that reduce quality of life. Early intervention, health education and improved nutrition are needed. Since health is not isolated from social status, power and prestige an egalitarian society is needed.

17. **Jamuna, D., Lalitha, K., and Ramamurti, P. V. (2004). Psycho-social contributants to self-esteem among older widows. *Indian Journal of Gerontology, 18*(2), 151-158.**

Widowhood, an inevitable life event for many older women has an impact on their psycho-social status. Consequent upon widowhood many older widows are vulnerable to the development of psychosocial problems and low self-esteem. This study is an attempt to investigate the psychosocial factors contributing to self-esteem of widows. The sample consists of 320 community-dwelling elderly widows from the age groups of 60-89 years living in rural and urban areas of Chittoor and Cuddapah Districts of Andhra Pradesh. The results indicate that the economic status, age and psychological health were the significant contributants to self-esteem of widows. Implications of the findings in the context of intervention for the better of older widows are indicated.

18. **Jaswal, S. K. P. (2001). Gynecological morbidity and common mental disorders in low income urban women in Mumbai. In Bhargavi V. Davar (Ed.), *Mental Health from a Gender Perspective*, 138-154, New Delhi: Sage.**

Urbanization has produced major transformations in Third World societies which have been particularly critical for women. Several studies in developing countries have also suggested associations between the mental ill health of poor women and factors such as migration, marital status and occupation. The main objective of this study was to understand women's experience of gynecological morbidity and its association with common mental disorders and social supports and networks. A total of 660 women were interviewed in three contiguous low-income communities. In this study 50.6% of the women reported gynecological morbidity. Further 27.5% of these women also reported common mental disorders. Most women were tired most of the time, had limited social activities and a poor self-image.

19. **Kendler, K. S. Thornton, L. M. and Gardner, C. O. (2001, April). Genetic risk, number of previous depressive episodes, and stressful live events in predicting onset of major depression. *American Journal of Psychiatry, 158*(4), 582-586.**

The association between stressful life events and the onset of major depression decreases as the number of previous depressive episodes increases. Using discrete – time survival analysis, the authors examined the interaction between genetic risk, number of previous depressive episodes and life event exposure in the prediction of episodes of major depression in (Caucasian) female-female twin pairs from a population based registry of Virginia. The twins were interviewed four times over a 9-year period, producing 92521 person-months of exposure. The result led to the conclusion that genetic risk factors for depression produce a 'prekindling' effect rather than increase the speed of kindling. The 'kindled' state, wherein depressive episodes occur with little provocation may be reached by two pathways: many previous depressive episodes, perhaps driven by multiple adversities, and high genetic risk.

20. **Khandelwal, S. (2000). Classification of mental disorders: Need for a common language. In R. Srinivasa Murthy (Ed.), *Mental health in India 1950-2000: Essays in honour of Prof. N. N. Wig* (pp. 60-73). Bangalore: People's Action for Mental Health (PAMII).**

The need for a classification of mental disorders has been felt throughout the history of medicine, though consensus has eluded the scientists about which disorders should be included and what should be the optimal method for their organization. The author has given a brief history of psychiatric classification (i.e. ICD (6-10) International Statistical Classification of Diseases, Injuries and Causes of Death and DSM – i.e., Diagnostic and Statistical Manual (I to IV). The Indian contributions to psychiatric classification and Indian Perspective have been discussed in this paper. The most recent revisions of classificatory systems, viz. ICD-10 and DSM – IV have come out with far greater clarity and applicability making their use almost universal all over the world.

21. **Khandelwal, S. K. (2003). Mental health of older people. In A. B. Dey (Ed.), *Aging in India: Situation analysis and planning for the future* (pp. 73-78). New Delhi: Rakmo Press Pvt. Ltd.**

This article deals with the issues that have a direct bearing on the physical and mental health of older people. It discusses the nature of mental morbidity in older people and examines issues relevant to its management. The principal mental disorders of late life are dementias and mood disorders. Others that are clinically important, but for which precise epidemiological data is not available, are personality disorders, drug and alcohol abuse, delirium and chronic psychoses.

22. **Lalitha, K. and Jamuna, D. (2004). Memory status in the elderly and its correlates: An intervention study. *Indian Journal of Gerontology, 18*(1), 34-57.**

Memory is the crux around which all the life gets organized. It is expected that with the increase of age there is a fading in memory. This piece of research aimed to assess the memory status in the elderly (memory performance) and study the contribution of a set of psychological factors. These were assessed by using standard tests. The sample consisted of 300 community-dwelling older men and women who were drawn by a multistage random sampling technique. Results showed that self rated memory, self esteem and locus of control were found to be significantly correlated with Memory performance. Implications of an intervention are also discussed by the authors.

23. **Manber, R., Allen, J. J. B., and Morris, M. M. (2002, July). Alternative treatments for depression: Empirical support and relevance to women. *Journal of Clinical Psychiatry 63*(7), 628-40.**

This article is a critical review of the efficacy of select alternative treatments for unipolar depression, including exercise, stress management techniques (meditation, relaxation, massage, acupuncture), herbal compounds: Hypoericum, St. John's Wort, Bright Light and sleep deprivation. Issues related to women across the life span, including pregnancy and lactation are highlighted. This review indicates that some unconventional treatments hold promise as alternative or complementary treatments for unipolar depression in women and have the potential to contribute to its long-term management.

24. **Mane, P. (1993). Mental health of Indian Women: Realities and Needed Response. In Purnima Mane and Katy Y. Gandevia (Eds.), *Mental health in India: Issues and concerns* (pp. 129-143). Bombay: Tata Institute of Social Sciences.**

In this article, the factors affecting the Indian women's mental health are examined from the socio-cultural perspective; the response from the mental health field is also briefly explored in the conclusion to identify areas for potential intervention. The duality and contradictions in the female image – the nurturant one and the destroyer (Wadley 1988; 24) and the nurturant and the helpless one (Taylor, 1990; 107) – can make for a schizophrenic existence and prove to be highly stressful. Socialization of women has always been oriented towards passivity, submission and a life of self-denial – the net result is a self image of being unwanted, inferior, a burden to one's family and deprived. Since marriage and motherhood are the primary status roles, their absence, suspension or disruption in any form may cause serious threats for a woman's mental health.

25. **Marcus, S. M., Flynn, H. A. Young, E. A., Ghaizuddin, N., and Mudd, S. (2001). Recurrent depression in women throughout the life span (Chapter 2). In John F. Greden (Ed.), *Treatment of Recurrent Depression* (pp. 19-50). Arlington, VA: American Psychiatric Publishing Inc.**

Depression impacts an astounding 20% to 23% of women at some point in their lives. This high prevalence in women is probably mulitfactorial, involving a complex interplay of genetic, neuro-endocrine, psychosocial and stress factors. In this chapter the impact of gender on recurrent major depressive disorder (MDD) is discussed, emphasizing the clinical features and treatment of the illness during three key periods of hormone transition – adolescence, pregnancy, and the post partum period and the menopausal period. Clinical features and sex differences are described first followed by a focus on recurrences and strategies for prevention.

26. **Mehta, P., and Laddu, K. (2002). A study on diet, nutritional status and disease profile of the elderly suffering from depression. Indian *Journal of Gerontology, 16*(3&4), 250-257.**

The present investigation was planned to see the effect of depression on food intake. Depression is known to affect the overall nutritional status of the individuals by lowering their food intake. Ninety subjects both men and women were selected from the free living population of Baroda and screened for depression using the Beck's Depression Inventory (BDI scale). The case group of depressed individuals included 15 men (above 60 yrs.) and 30 women (15 in age group of 45-60 and 15 over 60 yrs), while the control group also included the same number. Diet related information was collected using a 24-hour dietary recall and food frequency questionnaire. Nutritional status was assessed in terms of anthropometric measurements such as height, weight, MUAC, Body Mass Index and biochemical parameters such as hemoglobin and serum cholesterol. A gross inadequacy of nutrients was observed among the depressed individuals with respect to energy, vitamin-B6, vitamin-C and vitamin B12.

27. **Nambiar, V. S. and Seshadri, S. (2004). Dietary patterns and its relation to disease profile in postmenopausal women. *Indian Journal of Gerontology*, *18*(1), 59-72.**

Changes in dietary patterns, physical activity and lifestyle occurring during late middle age in women, may have an impact on the health of the individuals as they grow old. The objectives of this research were to study the dietary pattern, disease profile and anthropometric profile in relation to income of 150 women, aged 45-48 years belonging to affluent (Gp A; n=75) and middle income (Gp M; n=75) groups. A highly significant difference was seen in the intake of pulses, fruits, milk and milk products between the two groups – the total consumption for Group A being much higher than Group M subjects. The major confirmed chronic degenerative diseases reported were hypertensions (34%), osteoarthritis (27%), multiple disorder (CVD, diabetes and blood pressure, 7%), and 59 subjects (39.3%) complained of symptoms which were suggestive of disorders of one or more systems of the body. Of the 150, the percent of subjects who reported to be healthy having no symptoms of disorders or disease was 31.3%. Forty five per cent of the subjects from Gp A and 33% from Gp M had reached menopause. Another 15% of the women were suffering from irregular periods.

The mean age for menopause was 46 years. The complaints of these women were mental irregularities, gastric upsets, hot flushes, depression, diminished stamina, fluctuations in moods, irritability, stiffness and pain in joints, memory lapses and headaches. The results indicated that, as age advanced there was a tendency for the subjects to make changes in their dietary habits. Some of these changes occurred because of the presence of disease in the subject or in the family. Others were apparently mediated by an increased health consciousness and a desire to avoid excess gain in body weight.

28. **Patel, V. (2004, January). *Gaining ground on mental health*. Available at http://www.indiatogether.org/2004/jan/wom-mnthlt.htm**

Mental health issues of women are gaining ground in the women's studies discourse. The author reports on the current developments and advocates progressive directions. The women's movement has provided fresh inputs in terms of individual and group counseling, popularly know as 'consciousness raising' exercise, a form of mutual counseling that enables women as a group to share experiences, problems, feelings, dreams, utopia and plan for rebuilding shattered lives. It empowers women to come to a realization of their own potential, makes them autonomous, self-dependent in their decision making power and emotionally self-reliant. The author has discussed the various approaches to mental illness and the association of mental health with sexual violence, domestic violence, and reproductive rights. As compared to institutionalization based mainly on medical intervention, community or family-based rehabilitation of mentally ill women based on human touch is far more effective.

29. **Patel, V. and Thara, R. (2003). *Meeting the mental health needs of developing countries. NGO interventions in India*. New Delhi: Sage Publications.**

The health concerns of a population are multi-factorial in etiology, presentation, and their impact on people's lives. Therefore health issues require multiple and varied sources of concern and care. NGOs with their roots firmly entrenched in the community which is largely dependent on them for their resources and their activities, have played a lead role in the care and acceptance of the mentally ill and the distressed NGOs in India have evolved from being amorphous, unstructured organizations to well established and professionally managed institutions. The broad areas of work of the NGOs are covered in this book and a critical analysis of the strengths, innovations and limitations of these NGO programs is presented in the last chapter of the book.

30. **Purewal, J. (2003). Gender, violence, sexuality and health: Redefining the Matrix. In Vikram Patel and R. Thara (Eds.), *Meeting the mental health needs of developing countries: NGO Innovations in India* (pp. 229-244). New Delhi: Sage.**

Feminism has reworked its strategy to include participation of men in its efforts to effect changes in gender dynamics. The evolution of IFSHA (Interventions for Support, Healing and Awareness) a Delhi based NGO is an attempt at one such creative confluence – constructed around formulating spaces, strategies and perspectives on how to prevent violence and protect women and children. Research was carried BY IFSHA on 245 women – who were in-patients consulting psychiatric services. 64.1% reported gender violence as a primary life event prior to the onset of mental illness and symptoms. The research established the need for designing a matrix of therapy by combining mainstream practices with alternative and creative techniques for addressing trauma in men, women and children. A package of interventions which included counseling, legal support, healing processes, rehabilitation, advocacy and awareness were put together to stem the trend of violence and professionals from all spheres became part of IFSHA's awareness outreach. Between July 1998 and October 2001 eight sexuality workshops were conducted with 126 service providers in NGO and allied settings. These workshops have formed the basis of the development of research on sexuality as well as the construction of a clear mandate of sexual healing and therapy.

31. **Rider, E. A. (2000). *Over Voices: Psychology of Women. Chapter 14 – Mental Health* (pp. 516-551). Belmont, CA: Wadsworth/Thomson Learning.**

This paper emphasizes that women's mental health is influenced by gender in several ways. First cultural constructions of mental health often equate good mental health with masculine characteristics such as independence and assertiveness and poor mental health with feminine characteristics of dependence and nurturance. Further when men exhibit problems the problems are often assumed to originate externally, such as stress at work, whereas women's problems are often assumed to originate internally. These assumptions have led to different philosophies for men and women often aimed at changing women themselves rather than changing social conditions. Some mental disorders are more common among women than men. These include depression, anxiety and eating disorders. The greater incidence among women is because women live in poverty, have less power than men, experience violence and exploitation within their close relationships and are regularly exposed to media messages that promote the beauty of thinness and 'supermom'. Substance use and abuse are less common in women. Traditional, non-sexist and feminist therapies have been discussed. A major racial-ethnic concern regarding therapy is underutilization of services due to lack of a good fit between clients and therapists.

32. **Rikhi, M., and Chadha, N.K. (2004). The status of empirical research in issues related to the social support of the elderly. *Indian Journal of Gerontology, 18*(2), 237-264.**

This paper deals with the investigation carried out in India and abroad pertaining to the issues related to social support network of the elderly: giving an empirical account of the literature and also bring forth the related factors of the variables investigated. This review of literature was carried out from a number of journals and the recent books on the related topics conducted in India and abroad on the elderly population on the chosen variables, namely social support, subjective well being, life satisfaction, physical health and leisure activities.

33. **Rodrigues, M., Patel, V., Jaswal, S., and De Souza, N. (2003). Listening to mothers: Qualitative studies on motherhood and depression from Goa, India. *Social Science and Medicine, 57*, 1707-1806.**

The objective of the study in this paper was to use qualitative methods to investigate the cultural validity of the construct of postnatal depression and its local and cultural contexts. In-depth interviews were held with 39 mothers (19 of whom were found to be suffering from postnatal depression as defined by a cut-off score on the Edinburgh PND scale) and their husbands purposively recruited from the cohort. An illness narrative was conducted with mothers who were categorized as suffering from PND and their husbands to elicit their explanatory models. The two groups (PND and non-PND) of mothers were comparable in terms of socio-demographic characteristics. The study provides validity for the construct of PND in an Indian setting, but also shows that the emotional distress is interpreted from the context of social adversity, poor marital relationships and cultural attitudes towards gender rather than a biomedical psychiatric category. Contrary to the assumption that socio-cultural contexts associated with childbirth in non-Western societies protect mothers from depression, factors unique to the culture such as gender preference and the low involvement of the husbands in child care are major causes of stress to mothers.

34. Shah, A. (2001). Gender issues in mental health: A clinical psychology perspective. In Bhargavi Davar (Ed.), *Mental Health from a gender perspective* (pp. 61-81). New Delhi: Sage.

This is an overview of the theoretical developments and research-related issues over the last two decades. The psychological theories utilized in the clinical settings are psycho-dynamic theories, cognitive theories, behaviour theories, humanistic-existential theories and family systems theory. Women's mental health can be addressed through various perspectives. Mental health professionals are examining it through issues like physical and sexual violence, stress and coping patterns and reproductive functions. Other theoretical explanations offered are: restrictions placed on female sexual expression, power and personal freedom, conflict over the role of child-rearer and the need for self-development; women's concerns with relationships; learned helplessness and explanatory styles in women along with more helplessness training, received by them over a lifetime (Nolen-Hocksema 1987). Citing the works of

Brown and Harris (1978), Beach and O'Leary (1986) and Barnet and Gotlieb (1988) the author states that marital discord and depression are associated.

35. **Shah, G. Parker, S and Maheshwari, R. (1993). Suicide: A Mental Health Perspective. In P. Mane and K. Y. Gandevia (Eds.), *Mental Health in India: Issues and concerns* (pp. 182-211). Bombay: Tata Institute of Social Sciences.**

This paper examines the concept of suicide and reviews available empirical studies on it. The phenomenon is examined in relation to specific target groups, for example, women, the physically and mentally ill, and in terms of specific developmental life stages. Availability of statistics and research findings has been the main criterion for selecting the above target groups. The last section presents a rationale for prevention and the need to initiate and popularize mental health services and programs at the community level. Specific areas of intervention are proposed in the form of mental health services not merely for the population at risk but also for the population at large.

36. **Singh, R. (2002). Book review: Beyond Psychotherapy: Introduction to psychoenergetic Healing, by Martin E. Luthke and Linda Stein - Luthke, Expansion Publishing, Chagrin Fall, Ohio, USA 2001. *Indian Journal of Gerontology, 16*(1&2), 194-196.**

This book is on healing for the Body, Mind and Spirit, past life trauma, anxiety, anger, addictions, depression, pain and other physical complaints. Psychoenergetic Healing takes into account the fact that human beings are not only physical, emotional and mental beings, but also spiritual beings. Psychoenergetic Healing simply means to shift the balance of energies within an energy field towards harmony and higher vibration, or conversely, to reduce the prevalence of disharmony and lower vibrations. This book deals with healing by rays and concepts of 'chakras' and 'Kundalini'.

37. **Sloan, D. M. E., and Kornstein, S. G. (2003, September). Gender differences in depression and response to**

antidepressant treatment. *The Psychiatric Clinics of North America: Women's Mental Health, 26*(3), 581-594.

This is a review. Epidemiological studies have shown that the prevalence of major depressive disorder is about twice as high in women than in men, particularly during the child bearing years. There have also been differences reported between men and women in the nature of depressive symptoms, course of illness, and response to treatment. However, until recently women of childbearing age were not routinely included in clinical trials. As such, our understanding of gender differences in the phenomenology of depression and response to treatment has been limited. The inclusion of women in recent studies and a greater interest in examining the effect of gender on outcome in clinical trials have contributed to a growing body of literature in this area.

38. **Social Care: Call for Mental Health Rethink. *Public Agenda*, 14 June 2005, London, UK.**

A study by the Institute for Public Policy Research sets out a vision for mental health care and includes recommendations that it says could transform the way governments and the public approach mental health. It has recommended that 'access workers' in locations such as libraries and community health centers would reduce the burden on general practitioners and offer 'everything from a friendly ear to professional counseling.'

39. **Sonar, G. B. (2004). Old Age Pensioners: A Socio-psychological Study. *Indian Journal of Gerontology, 18*(2), 187-200.**

This study aimed to understand the socio-psychological and economic conditions and level of depression among old age pensioners. It was carried out in Shahbad town and few villages of Gulbarga district in Karnataka state, with a sample of 112 old age pensioners. The results showed that marital status, domicile, nature and composition of family, annual income, style of living, social contacts, having friends, involvement in decision making, adjustment with old age, feeling of isolation, time activities, recreation, sufficiency of food, satisfaction of needs, savings and feeling of insecurity had a bearing on geriatric depression. A non-significant association was observed between geriatric depression and age, education, gender, religion, nature of work, performance of rituals and intergenerational conflict.

40. **Srinivasa Murthy, R. (1993). Evolution of the concept of mental health – from mental illness to mental health. In P. Mane and K. Y. Gandevia (Eds.), *Mental Health in India: Issues and concerns* (pp. 17-42). Bombay: Tata Institute of Social Sciences.**

This paper traces the evolution of the concept of mental health. The evolution of the concept of mental health is linked to the larger developments in the understanding of human behavior. Starting from explanaticns of supernatural causation, we have arrived at understanding the states of mind and mental health from a holistic point of view. Rapid advances in the understanding of the human brain and individual and group behavior open up new possibilities for non-medical and wider psychosocial actions towards promotion of mental health. Indian mental health professionals now have the advantage of structuring mental health programs with these new understandings. Some important measures to prevent mental handicaps in the community have been suggested.

41. **Srinivasa Murthy, R. (2002). Community mental health in India. . In R. Srinivasa Murthy (Ed.), *Mental health in India 1950-2000: Essays in honor of Prof. N. N. Wig* (pp. 150-176). Bangalore: People's Action for Mental Health (PAMH).**

The scope and importance of mental health range from care of the ill to the promotion of mental health. This chapter reviews the community mental health programs in India in terms of (i) what has happened since Independence; (ii) evaluation of the developments and (iii) how future community mental health programs could be planned in the country.

42. **Srinivasa Murthy, R. and Bruno, Barbara. J. (Eds.) (1992). *Community Mental Health: Proceedings of the Indo-US Symposium*. Bangalore: NIMHANS.**

The Indo-US Symposium under NIMHANS-ADAM agreement was held in October 1987. The topic chosen was the development of community mental health in the two countries. Speakers from USA discussed the various aspects of community mental health, specifically issues of hospital care, community care, and involvement of families and role of para-professionals. Indian speakers had to speak on the same topics – though the differences with USA regarding community health movement, infrastructural facilities and trained mental health professionals are very large and striking. However against these contrasts, there are common needs across the two countries – the problems of the homeless mentally ill and the involvement of families. All these aspects were discussed in this Symposium.

43. **Srivastava, S. K. and Agrawal, Shweta. (2002). Effect of living arrangements and gender differences on emotional states and self-esteem of old aged women. *Indian Journal of Gerontology, 16*(3&4), 312-320.**

The purpose of the present investigation was to study the effect of living arrangement and gender differences on emotional states and self-esteem of old age people. Eight state questionnaire and self-esteem inventory were administered to 120 old people aged 65 years and above (60 aged living with their children and 60 living in institutions/ashrams). The results indicate that emotional states like anxiety, depression and guilt are more in old people living in institutions/ashrams. Living away from their children, family and relatives, economic insecurity, establishing living conditions or a sense of lost youth and approaching death are the major causes of emotional states in old institutionalized people. Gender differences were also found in this study. Old aged females suffer more from stress, depression, guilt and extraversion feelings. Findings also reveal that the living arrangement of the aged was significantly related with the self-esteem of these subjects.

44. **Stefanis, C. N., and Stefanis, N. C. (2002). Diagnosis of depressive disorders: A review. In Mario Maj and Norman Sartorius (Eds.), *Depressive Disorders* (2nd. edition). (pp. 1-42) Bangalore: Panther Publishers.**

Depression is a complex diagnostic construct applied to individuals with a particular set of symptoms among which the essential ingredients are a depressed mood and a loss of interest. The general issues surrounding the diagnosis of depression and the classification of Depressive Disorders are discussed in this chapter. Also discussed are its association with and differential diagnosis from normal sadness and other mental disorders and association with and differential diagnosis from medical illness. (the ultimate goal of the clinical investigator is to reach a diagnostic characterization that goes beyond the descriptive level and provides construct validity that will not only increase the diagnostic confidence but will also ensure an empirically-based explanatory scheme.

45. **Ushasree, S. and Basha, S. A. (2003). Religiosity as a contributor to meaning in life. *Indian Journal of Gerontology, 17*(1&2), 85-98.**

How satisfied are the aged persons living in ashrams, the religious retreats, devoting most of their time in religious practices? Do they cope better with their physical and psychosocial demands compared to their age mates living in out side the ashram? Are there differences in their motivational styles and meaning in life of these two groups? The present study attempts to seek answers to the above in a purposive sample of 80 (60-80 years old) male and female subjects residing in ashrams and outside the ashrams. Data were collected in-person interviews with the help of standardized questionnaires. Analyses of results showed no difference in the religiosity and meaning in life scores of the two groups. Women were found with better feeling of meaning in life. Majority of ashram residents used religious coping to familial problems and both the groups were found to use to some extent non-religious coping also to health problems. Subjects in depressive state were found more motivated and used more of religious coping.

46. **Varghese, M. (2005). Issues in old age: Psychiatry in India. In I. Jai Prakash (Ed.), *Aging in India: Retrospect and Prospect* (pp.15-19). Fifth Volume of the Aging and Development Project, Proceedings of the National Conferences on Aging and Development, August 2004. Bangalore: Bangalore University.**

This paper makes an attempt to look at studies of common psychiatric problems faced by older persons namely depression and dementia and the impact on the caregivers. Community studies report widely varying rates of psychiatric morbidity for the elderly ranging from 2.2% to 33.3%. Risk factors for mental disorders are poverty, lower levels of literacy, low social status and ill health. Biological factors play an important role in determining the risk to some mental disorders, in particular dementia. There is poor awareness about these disorders. Health education should aim to stress that depression and dementia are real disorders and not just the natural consequences of aging. Improvement in access to health care for the elderly with mental illness is required.

47. Venkoba Rao, A. (2004). Psychiatry of old age (Gero Psychiatry). In P. V. Ramamurti and D. Jamuna (Eds.), *Handbook of Indian Gerontology* (pp. 117-151). New Delhi: Serials Publications.

The elderly form a vulnerable group for multiple morbidities: physical, mental and social among others. Psychiatric illness is seldom an 'isolated' event in the elderly. The number of symptoms range from 6 to 12. These are associated with physical illness and/ or disabilities or handicaps. Psychiatric disorders sans physical illness either causal or co-existing accounts for less than 1 per cent of all illnesses. Co-morbidity marks geriatric medicine. The author has discussed depression, bipolar affective disorders, dysthymia, other psychoses and psycho-organic disorders. References to old age in Ancient Indian writings has also been discussed as these have a bearing on the development of modern geriatric medicine and its psychiatric component.

48. Venkoba Rao, A. (1997, October). Psychiatric morbidity in the aged. *Indian Journal of Medical Research, 106*, 361-369.

Mental morbidity in the elderly comprises mainly affective disorders (manic depressive psychosis) and psycho-organic syndrome, delirium and dementia. The prevalence rate is around 89/1000. The elderly form a high risk group for multiple morbidities; physical, mental and social. The overall prevalence rate of psychiatric morbidity rises for those over 60 to 124/1000 in their 70s to 155/1000 in those over 80. Psychiatric illness is seldom an isolated event. These are associated with physical illness and/or disabilities. In this paper quality ageing, dementia, depression, vascular depression, dysthymia, mania, suicidal behavior, depressive psuedodementia, anxiety disorders other psychoses (delusional disorder and late onset schizophrenia) and hallucinosis have all been studied on various people and the symptoms, co-morbidity and precipitating factors have been analyzed.

49. Venkoba Rao, A. (1992). Mental Health of the elderly in the community. In R. Srinivasa Murthy and Barbara J. Bruno (Eds.), *Community Mental Health: Proceedings of the Indo-US Symposium* (pp. 459-471). Bangalore: NIMHANS.

On the basis of hospital data, the author reports that those aged 60 or above formed 1.6 to 2.6% of the total outpatients attendances and 1.2% to 2.6% among the total inpatients in the department of psychiatry. The major psychiatric disorders in the elderly are: affective disorders, organic brain syndrome and late paraphernia. The prevalence of depression in the community varies from 60/100 to 241/1000. The primary health centre at the village Kallandhiri (16 km from Madurai) was chosen for research and a geriatric clinic was started within its premises in July 1984. Medical and paramedical personnel were roped into the program. Psychiatric illness alone was diagnosed in about half a dozen instances among the groups of 1910 elderly subjects. In associations with physical illness, they occurred in 155 individuals (8.1%). This fact justifies a total care for older patients besides social and other forms of support.

50. Vishnu Vandana, K., and Subramanyam, V. (2004). Counseling needs of the elderly. *Indian Journal of Gerontology, 18*(2), 219-226.

The present study was planned to examine the psychological and social counseling needs in a sample of community dwelling middle aged and older men and women. They were individually tested using a problem inventory. Analysis showed that with the increase of age, problems faced by them also increased. Based on the results, the counseling needs are discussed in different areas. The implications of the findings are discussed.

51. **Vishwanathan, N., and Wood Wetzel, J. (1993). Concepts and trends in mental health: A global overview. In P. Mane and K. Y. Gandevia (Eds.), *Mental Health in India: Issues and concerns* (pp. 43-69). Bombay: Tata Institute of Social Sciences.**

In this paper the author feels that both the prevention and treatment of mental illness and the promotion of mental health should be culture specific and not blindly based on Western forms of intervention. Mental health practice models such as psychoanalytic model, biochemical model, family treatment models, and education program models have been discussed. The contribution of media is needed for the increased emphasis being placed by medicine and other helping professions on prevention of mental illness through strengthening the social fabric and promoting attitudes conducive to improved quality of life, both globally and locally.

52. **World Health Organization (WHO). *World Health Report 2001. Mental Health: New understanding, new hope.* Geneva.**

This report presents information on the current understanding of mental and behavioral disorders, their magnitude and burden, effective treatment strategies, and strategies for enhancing mental health through policy and service development. The report recognizes mental health to be as important as physical health to the overall well-being of individuals, societies and countries. There are 450 million people in the world suffering from a mental or behavioral disorder, yet only a small minority of them is receiving treatment. In developing countries most individuals with severe mental disorders are left to cope as best they can with their private burdens such as depression, dementia, schizophrenia, and substance dependence. Globally many are victimized for their illness and become the targets of stigma and discrimination. More than 40% of countries have no mental health policy and over 30% have no mental health program. And so the suffering continues and the difficulties grow.

Index

F

G

H

I